VETERINARY MEDICAL TERMINOLOGY

Authored and Illustrated by

Dawn E. Christenson, L.V.T.

Instructor
College of Veterinary Medicine
Michigan State University
East Lansing, Michigan

W. B. SAUNDERS COMPANY
A Division of Harcourt Brace & Company
Philadelphia   London   Toronto   Montreal   Sydney   Tokyo

W.B. SAUNDERS COMPANY

A Division of Harcourt Brace & Company

The Curtis Center
Independence Square West
Philadelphia, Pennsylvania 19106

Library of Congress Cataloging-in-Publication Data

Christenson, Dawn E.
    Veterinary medical terminology / Dawn E. Christenson. — 1st ed.
        p.   cm.
    Includes bibliographical references and index.
    ISBN 0-7216-4859-2
        1. Veterinary medicine —Terminology.   I. Title.
    SF610.C48   1997
    636.089′2′0014—dc20   96-14266

VETERINARY MEDICAL TERMINOLOGY   ISBN 0-7216-4859-2

Last digit is the print number: 9   8   7   6   5   4   3   2

Preface

This text has been designed for veterinary technician students and veterinary students for use with a self-study format. Instructors may wish to assign chapters as "adjuvants" to related course materials. The text is intended to provide students with a basic foundation in the language of veterinary medicine—veterinary medical terminology. Additionally, the text is designed to familiarize students with introductory level anatomy, physiology, and selected disease topics. The anatomic, physiologic, and disease concepts reinforce the medical terms through immediate application in relevant contexts. The fundamental knowledge gained from this text provides a base from which instructors and their students may springboard to higher levels of understanding, hopefully engaging students in a lifelong quest for knowledge in veterinary medicine.

Whether used in a self-study situation or as part of a course, it is strongly recommended that students complete chapters 1–3, in succession, before proceeding to any subsequent chapters. The rest of the text has been organized by body-systems. Each chapter presents information about a given body-system. Therefore, most chapters, other than 1–3, may be completed in any sequence.

Use of an unabridged, medical dictionary (such as Dorland's Illustrated Medical Dictionary) in conjunction with this text is highly recommended. Note that all directional terminology used in this text adheres to the standardized nomenclature accepted by most veterinary anatomists and the American College of Veterinary Radiologists (ACVR).[1]

This book is dedicated to all students pursuing careers as veterinary technicians, veterinary technologists, and veterinarians. You are the future of veterinary medicine. It is the author's sincere hope that this text will provide you with a strong foundation on which to build your professional education and career.

---

[1]Smallwood, J.E., et al.: A Standardized Nomenclature for Radiographic Projections Used in Veterinary Medicine; *Veterinary Radiology,* Vol. 26, No. 1, 1985, pp. 2–9./Shively, M.J.: Synonym Equivalence Among Names Used for Oblique Radiographic Views of Distal Limbs, *Veterinary Radiology,* Vol. 29, No. 6, 1988, pp. 282–284.

Acknowledgements

This book is a culmination of innumerable hours of painstaking work at the computer and at the drafting table. Although I am recognized on the cover as the author and illustrator, I am indebted to many others for helping bring this text to fruition. It never would have come to pass if it weren't for the insight and vision of my editor, Selma Kaszczuk. Selma, you saw something in me which, frankly, I didn't think that I had. I sincerely appreciate the opportunity you have afforded me to mold the minds of future veterinary professionals.

I am very grateful to my sister, Sharon. Sis, I can't begin to tell you how much I appreciate your willingness to learn about a completely foreign subject, proofread the entire document (arrrgh!), and play the role of the student by completing all of the testing sections in each chapter. I can't tell you how refreshing it was for me to hear you get excited about learning this information. Your student perspective was a strong guiding force for me. Thanks!

I must express my appreciation to my colleagues in the MSU Veterinary Technology Program. Cindi, Donn, Helen, Jolynne and Mel, you guys are topnotch people. It truly is a privilege working with you. I can't thank you enough for supporting and encouraging me throughout this project. Thank you too for letting me bounce ideas off of you. Your insights have helped me focus many of the ideas in this text.

I cannot forget to thank two outstanding medical professionals, Dr. Tom Lindsey and Dr. Dorothy Mondejar, who restored my health so that I could complete this task. You two are a credit to physicians everywhere. Certainly, what you have done for me goes far beyond the scope of this book and I cannot thank you enough. In light of the book, Dr. Mondejar, I appreciate your tolerance of me as a patient. Without your help in keeping the discomfort in my drawing arm tolerable, the illustrations for this book could never have been completed. Now that it is finished, I shall follow through with your directives to rest it.

I am grateful to so many individuals that I could not begin to name them all. I must, however, express my appreciation to my family and friends. I am indebted to you for all of your support, love, encouragement, and belief in my abilities. You have always stood by me through thick and thin and have always seen past my shortcomings (no pun intended). I am also grateful to my students who, through the years, have taught me so much. I am thankful for Mongo, Sadie, and Porky who provided me with subjects to illustrate. More so than that, Mongo and Sadie, I appreciate all of the unconditional love that you bestowed upon me, even at times when I was less than receptive to you.

They say that one should always save the best for last, and so I have. Galen, you are by far the very best husband that any woman could ever wish for. I can't thank you enough for the years of love and companionship that you've given me. You truly are my best friend. They say that there are no heroes left in the world today, but they're wrong. You are, and always will be, my hero. Thank you so much for putting up with me during the long, arduous process of writing and illustrating this book. Honestly, you are the most tolerant person I know. Your love and support are appreciated beyond that which words can express.

Dear Student:

I remember, when I was a student, the way that I struggled with learning medical terminology. The intensity and complexity of my professional education were overwhelming at times. This "foreign language" just complicated matters. If that wasn't bad enough, the subject by itself was boring beyond belief. Medical terminology has at times confused me, frightened me, and put me to sleep.

Through my experiences as a student, as a practicing veterinary technician, and as a teacher, I have found that medical terminology does not have to be an ominous "monster". Learning medical terminology can actually be an adventure. Put yourself in the shoes of Sherlock Holmes. How would he solve the mystery hidden within each medical term? If you can pursue this subject in a curious, positive way you'll change it from a millstone into a fun experience.

I know that medical terminology "feels" awkward at first. You're probably wondering how you will ever remember all of the terms, what they mean, and (Oh, my!) how to spell them. Once you begin to use them on a regular basis, they will become a part of you. You'll take them for granted. Someday you'll be in a casual conversation with family or friends and someone will stop you. "What did you say? Why do you always have to use such big words?" You'll feel like you've really arrived when you're having a conversation with practitioners, who are experts in the field, and you understand everything that they're talking about. That is *so* gratifying. You'll get there. Just give it time. When will you "arrive"? No one knows. It sneaks up on you. Someday you'll simply recognize, "I'm there!" Being persistent and consistent with anything is the key to success. Someone once said that success is a journey, not a destination. Enjoy the journey. I hope that this book will help you on that journey and I hope that you'll have some fun along the way.

Sincerely,

ATTENTION!

Student, the following information is IMPORTANT to YOUR SUCCESS:

Many of the definitions given in the introductory sections of each chapter are literal translations from the Greek and Latin roots. These literal translations serve to simplify definitions and to reduce the volume of information to be absorbed initially. This approach eases the process of learning to recognize and rapidly interpret medical terms. It is important to read each chapter in its entirety to gain a greater understanding of the meanings and applications of these terms. As stated in the preface, it is strongly recommended that students complete chapters 1–3, in sequence, before proceeding to any subsequent chapters. Use of a medical dictionary (such as Dorland's Illustrated Medical Dictionary) in conjunction with this text is also highly recommended.

Contents

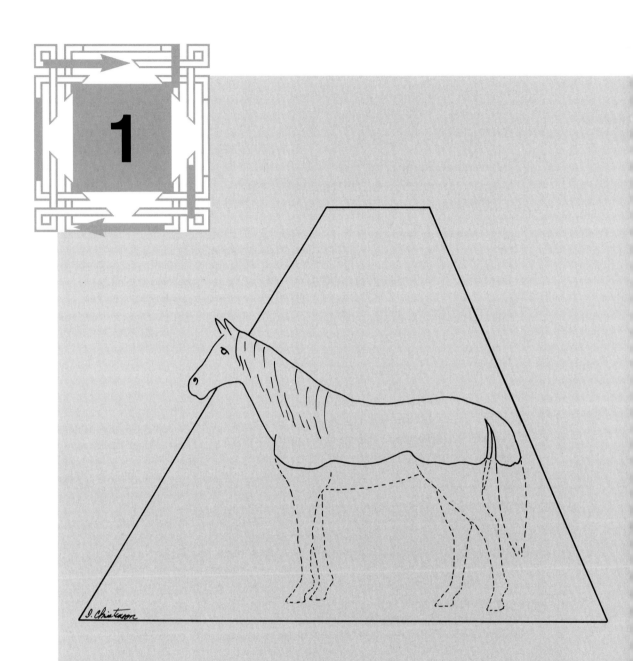

1

Introduction to Veterinary Medical Terminology

GOALS AND OBJECTIVES

By the conclusion of this chapter, the student will be able to:

1. Recognize common root words, prefixes, suffixes, and combining vowels.
2. Understand the function of root words, prefixes, suffixes, and combining vowels.
3. Divide simple and compound words into their respective parts.
4. Understand the function of combining forms.
5. Recognize, correctly pronounce, and appropriately use common directional terms.
6. Recognize the planes of the body.
7. Demonstrate a basic understanding of directional terminology as it relates to the body and to radiography.

1.1. Introduction to Word Structure

1.1.1. ROOT WORD

The root word is the **foundation of a word.** It is from the root that the majority of the meaning for a given word is derived. Words may contain one or more roots, as in football (root 1 = foot, root 2 = ball).

1.1.2. PREFIX

A prefix is a word part that **precedes the root, modifying the root's meaning.** Generally, prefixes may not stand alone as words. When written alone, prefixes are followed by a hyphen (e.g., *pre-*, a prefix meaning "before").

1.1.3. SUFFIX

A suffix is a word part that **follows the root word, modifying the root's meaning.** Generally, suffixes may not stand alone as words. When written alone, suffixes are preceded by a hyphen (e.g., *-ad*, a suffix meaning "toward"). When reading the meaning of a word containing a suffix, begin by reading the meaning of the suffix first. For example, in the word *craniad* (crani / ad), the root *crani(o)-* [head], when combined with the suffix *-ad*, is interpreted as meaning "toward the head."

1.1.4. COMPOUND WORD

A word constructed of **two or more roots** is a compound word. The roots may or may not be joined by a combining vowel. *"Mediolateral"* is a compound word. Given the following information, *medi(o)-* [middle] / *o* / *later(o)-* [side] / *al* [pertaining to], the correct interpretation of the word *mediolateral* would be "pertaining to the middle and the side."

1.1.5. COMBINING FORM

A combining form is an incomplete word constructed of **a root word, prefix, or suffix with a combining vowel.** In combining forms, the standard combining vowel (shown in parentheses) is "o." *Medi(o)-* is a combining form meaning "middle". *Later(o)-* is a combining form meaning "side." When joined in the compound word *mediolateral*, note that the combining vowel "o" is used between the two roots. However, the second combining vowel "o" is dropped before the suffix *-al*. In most cases, the combining vowel should be dropped when it precedes a suffix beginning with a vowel. The combining vowel "o," shown in most combining forms, may not be appropriate for use in the creation of some words. For example, with the adjective *posterior* (poster / i / or; "pertaining to the rear"), the combining form *poster(o)-* is joined to the suffix *-or* by the combining vowel "i."

Consult an unabridged medical dictionary to ensure correct spelling of any medical term.

1.1.6. GENERAL RULES

1. Read the meaning of medical terms beginning with the suffix, then proceed to the first part of the word and follow through.
2. Drop the combining vowel before a suffix beginning with a vowel.
3. Retain the combining vowel between two roots.

These rules hold true for most medical terms.

1.1.7. INTRODUCTION TO RELATED TERMS

Divide each of the following terms into its respective parts ("R" root, "P" prefix, "S" suffix, "CV" combining vowel).

1. **Anterior**   (R) _anter_   (CV) _i_   (S) _or_

   anterior (an-te're-or; pertaining to the front)

2. **Caudad**   (R) _caud_   (S) _ad_

   caudad (kaw'dad; toward the tail)

3. **Cranial**   (R) _crani_   (S) _al_

   cranial (kra'ne-al; pertaining to the head)

4. **Caudocranial**   (R) _caud_   (CV) _o_   (R) _crani_   (S) _al_

   caudocranial (kaw"do-kra'ne-al; pertaining to the tail and head; directionally pertaining to coursing from the tail to the head)

5. **Craniocaudal**   (R) _crani_   (CV) _o_   (R) _caud_   (S) _al_

   craniocaudal (kra'ne-o-kaw"-dal; pertaining to the head and tail; directionally pertaining to coursing from the head to the tail)

6. **Dorsal**   (R) _dors_   (S) _al_

   dorsal (dor'sal; pertaining to the back; clinically refers to the dorsum of the head, neck, trunk, and tail.)

7. **Palmar**   (R) _palm_   (S) _ar_

   palmar (pal'mar; pertaining to the palm; in veterinary medicine refers to the sole of the forefeet of domestic animals)

8. **Dorsopalmar**   (R) _dors_   (CV) _o_   (R) _palm_   (S) _ar_

   dorsopalmar (dor"so-pal'mar; pertaining to the dorsum and palm; directionally pertaining to coursing from the dorsum to the palm [forefoot])

9. **Plantar**   (R) _____ (S) _____

plantar (plan'tar; pertaining to the sole; in veterinary medicine refers to the sole of the hindfeet of domestic animals)

10. **Dorsoplantar**   (R) _____ (CV) ___ (R) _____ (S) _____

dorsoplantar (dor"so-plan'tar; pertaining to the dorsum and sole; directionally pertaining to coursing from the dorsum to the sole [hindfoot])

11. **Ventral**   (R) _____ (S) _____

ventral (ven'tral; pertaining to the belly; clinically refers to those surfaces of the head, neck, trunk, and tail oriented the same as the belly surface)

12. **Dorsoventral**   (R) _____ (CV) ___ (R) _____ (S) _____

dorsoventral (dor"so-ven'tral; pertaining to the back and the belly; directionally pertaining to coursing from the dorsum to the belly)

13. **Lateral**   (R) _____ (S) _____

lateral (lat'er-al; pertaining to the side)

14. **Medial**   (R) _____ (S) _____

medial (me'de-al; pertaining to the middle)

15. **Mediolateral**   (R) _____ (CV) ___ (R) _____ (S) _____

mediolateral (me"de-o-lat'er-al; pertaining to the middle and the side; directionally pertaining to coursing from the middle to the side)

16. **Palmarodorsal**   (R) _____ (CV) ___ (R) _____ (S) _____

palmarodorsal (pal'mar-o-dor"sal; pertaining to the palm and dorsum; directionally pertaining to coursing from the sole to the dorsum [forefoot])

17. **Plantarodorsal**   (R) _____ (CV) ___ (R) _____ (S) _____

plantarodorsal (plan'tar-o-dor"sal; pertaining to the sole and dorsum; directionally pertaining to coursing from the sole to the dorsum [hindfoot])

18. **Posterior**   (R) _____ (CV) ___ (S) _____

posterior (pos-ter'e-or; pertaining to the rear)

19. **Rostral**   (R) _____ (S) _____

rostral (ros'tral; pertaining to the nose)

1.2. Introduction to Body Planes

The body is divided by four basic planes. The **median plane** (*me′de-an*) divides the body into equal right and left halves (Fig. 1–1). **Sagittal planes** (*saj′ĭ-tal*) are any planes that lie parallel to the median plane (Fig. 1–2 on p. 6). Sagittal planes divide extremities longitudinally into medial and lateral aspects. The *midsagittal plane* and the *median plane* are synonymous. The **dorsal plane** divides the animal into dorsal and ventral portions (Fig. 1–3 on p. 7). Last, the **transverse plane** (*trans-vers′*) intersects the body perpendicular to the body's axis, dividing the trunk of the animal into cranial and caudal regions (Fig. 1–4 on p. 8). An extremity is also considered to have its own axis; therefore, a transverse plane of a limb divides the limb into *distal* (*dis′tal*; [distant]) and *proximal* (*prok′sĭ-mal*; [close]) portions.

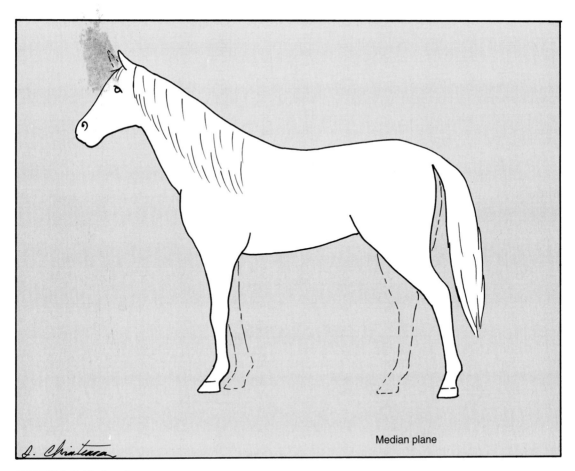

Median plane

FIGURE 1–1. Median plane.

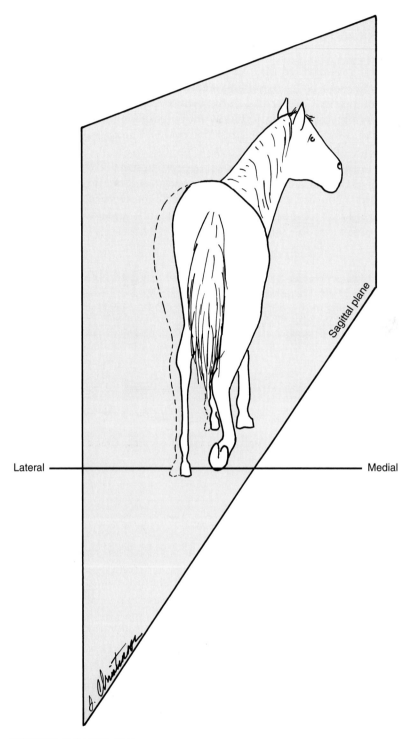

Lateral ———————————————— Medial

Sagittal plane

FIGURE 1–2. Sagittal plane.

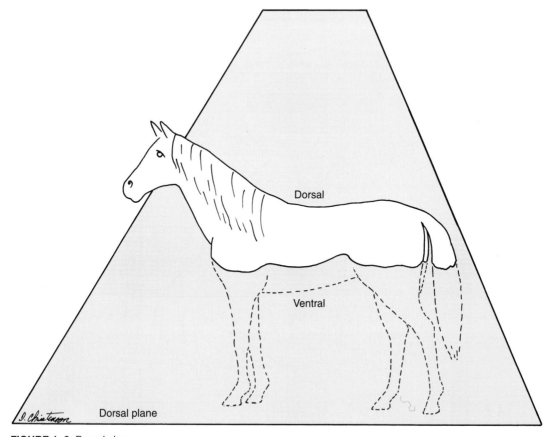

FIGURE 1–3. Dorsal plane.

1.3. Application of Directional Terms

Whether describing the location of a wound on an animal or producing radiographs (x-rays) of its body parts, directional terminology is critical. The key to using directional terminology appropriately is to use a suitable point of reference on the animal. For example, if one were to try to describe the location of the right elbow of a dog, it could be said that the right elbow lies at a midpoint *proximal* to the right front foot and *distal* to the right shoulder. Without the reference points, the terms "proximal" and "distal" would have no value in locating the right elbow. It is also important to remember that domestic animals walk on four limbs. Therefore, the basic structure and orientation of their bodies make reference to various aspects appropriate in some circumstances and inappropriate in others (Table 1–1 on p. 9). Along the head, neck, trunk, and tail, references are made to physical attributes, such as the back and belly, to describe *dorsal* ("upper") and *ventral* ("lower") surfaces. Because the neck, trunk, and proximal

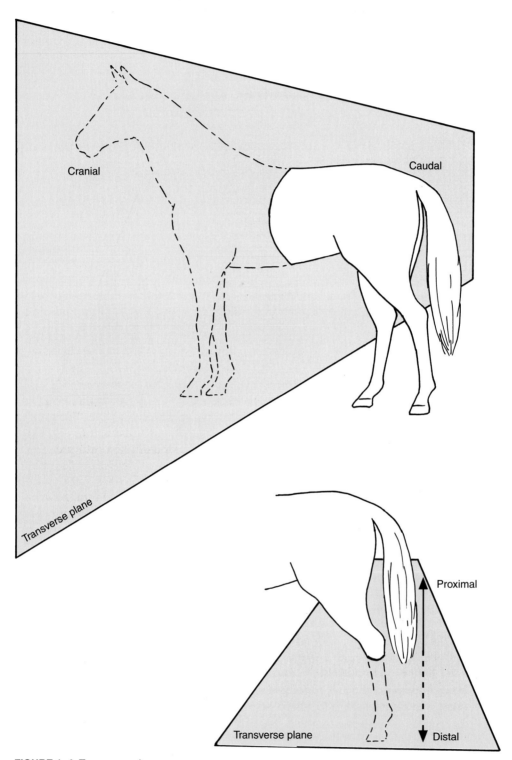

FIGURE 1–4. Transverse plane.

TABLE 1–1. Directional Terms Applicable to Radiographic Views of Body Parts			
HEAD	**NECK, TRUNK, AND TAIL**	**LIMBS***
Left	Left	Cranial (proximal limb only)
Right	Right	Caudal (proximal limb only)
Rostral	Cranial	Dorsal (distal limb only)
Caudal	Caudal	Palmar (distal forelimb only)
Dorsal	Dorsal	Plantar (distal hindlimb only)
Ventral	Ventral	Proximal
		Distal
		Medial
		Lateral

*Radiographs of extremities must always be marked with regard to right versus left limbs.

limbs (i.e., proximal to the carpus and tarsus[1]) are physically connected between the head and the tail, it is appropriate to use the terms *cranial* and *caudal* to describe *anterior* and *posterior* locations, respectively, on those body parts. "Distal" and "proximal" are inappropriate for use directionally along the trunk, because the trunk serves as the reference point for attributes of the extremities. Each limb has a *lateral* surface and a *medial* surface (i.e., nearest the median plane). Regarding anterior and posterior aspects, the extremities are subdivided into proximal and distal parts. As stated earlier, on the proximal portions of the limbs, "cranial" is used to refer to the anterior surfaces and "caudal" is used to refer to the posterior surfaces. Distal to the carpus and tarsus, "dorsal" is used to refer to the anterior aspects of the limbs and feet. The posterior aspect of the distal forelimb and the sole of the forefoot are referred to as the *palmar* surfaces. The posterior aspect of the distal hindlimb and the sole of the hindfoot are referred to as the *plantar* surfaces. Finally, because the most anterior structure on the head of any domestic animal is the nose, it is used as a common point of reference on the head. Therefore, rather than referring to anterior locations on the head, *rostral* is used. For visualization of appropriate directional terms as they relate to the body, refer to Figures 1–5 and 1–6 (on pp. 10 and 11).

We begin to combine many of the directional terms for the production of radiographs. The combination of terms is based on the direction of passage of the beam of radiation through the body part. If it is difficult to visualize a beam of radiation penetrating the body, the analogy of the penetration of a bullet may help. The directional terms are combined in the order of passage of the "bullet" (beam)

---

[1]If necessary, see Figure 6–8 in this text for an illustration of canine joints.

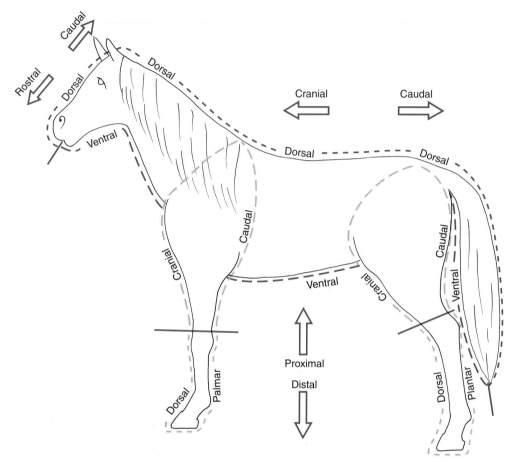

FIGURE 1–5. Directional terms related to body surfaces of large animals.

sequentially through each body surface (i.e., entry and exit points). For example, if a bullet were fired straight through the left thigh of an animal with the entry wound on the lateral aspect of the thigh and the exit wound on the medial thigh, the directional term used to describe the path of the bullet would be *lateromedial* (LM). A radiograph taken of an animal's chest, such that the beam of radiation penetrates from his back to the underside of his chest, before reaching the x-ray film, describes a *dorsoventral* (DV) radiographic view of the chest. A radiograph taken of the proximal limb of an animal, such that the beam of radiation passes through the limb from front to rear, describes a *craniocaudal* (CrCd) view. A similar view of the distal forelimb is called a *dorsopalmar* (DPa) view, whereas a similar view of the distal hindlimb is called a *dorsoplantar* (DPl) view. Note that these types of radiographic views orient the beam of radiation parallel or perpendicular to the various planes of the body. In special circumstances, to help visualize particular aspects of a body part, the beam may be angled so that it is neither parallel nor perpendicular to any body plane (i.e., tangent). Any radiographic view

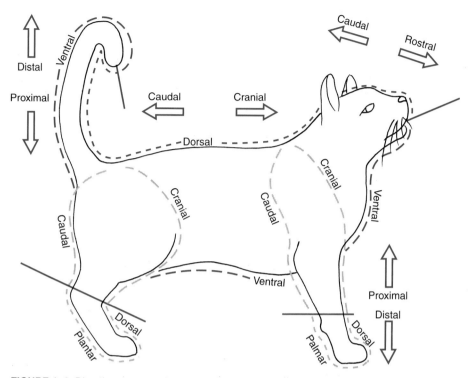

FIGURE 1–6. Directional terms related to body surfaces of companion animals.

that is neither parallel nor perpendicular to any body plane is said to be *oblique* (o-blĭk, o-blēk). In such a view, the term "oblique" usually follows the directional terms used to describe the overall beam penetration. For instance, if the overall penetration of the beam through a limb was in a dorsomedial direction (i.e., with the beam angled such that it was tangent to the limb, entering on the dorsal aspect and exiting on the medial aspect), the radiographic view would be labeled as a *dorsomedial oblique* (DMO) of that body part. Because the directional terminology in radiography can become lengthy at times, Table 1–2 provides standard-

TABLE 1–2. Directional Terms and Abbreviations

DIRECTIONAL TERM	ABBREVIATION	DIRECTIONAL TERM	ABBREVIATION
Left	Lt	Medial	M
Right	Rt	Lateral	L
Dorsal	D	Proximal	Pr
Ventral	V	Distal	Di
Cranial	Cr	Palmar	Pa
Caudal	Cd	Plantar	Pl
Rostral	R	Oblique	O

TABLE 1–3. Comparison of Standardized Radiographic Nomenclature and Obsolete Terminology	
OFFICIAL/STANDARDIZED TERMINOLOGY	**OBSOLETE TERMINOLOGY**
Craniocaudal (CrCd)	Anteroposterior (AP)
Caudocranial (CdCr)	Posteroanterior (PA)
Dorsopalmar (DPa)	Anteroposterior (AP)
Dorsoplantar (DPl)	Anteroposterior (AP)
Palmarodorsal (PaD)	Posteroanterior (PA)
Plantarodorsal (PlD)	Posteroanterior (PA)

ized abbreviations for the terms. Standardized nomenclature is still being adopted by some veterinary practitioners and technicians; therefore, Table 1–3 provides comparisons between some standardized and obsolete terminology.

1.4. Self-Test

Using the previous information in this chapter, respond to each of the following questions using the most appropriate term. Do not use abbreviations.

1. The word part that is considered to be the foundation of a word is the
   root.

2. A single-letter word part that is used to join other word parts is a(n)
   combining vowel.

3. A word part that follows a root word modifying its meaning is a(n)
   suffix.

4. An incomplete word that is formed by the joining of a root word followed by a vowel, like the letter "o," is called a(n) _combining form_.

5. A word part that precedes a root word modifying its meaning is a(n)
   prefix.

6. A flea was found crawling from the brow of a cat toward his nose. What simple directional term would best describe the direction of travel for the flea?
   rostral

7. A radiograph of a dog's abdomen was taken to visualize the stomach. The animal was positioned on the x-ray table on his back so that the beam of radiation had to penetrate his belly first, before reaching the x-ray film in the cassette beneath the table top. What compound directional term would best describe this radiographic view?
   ventrodorsal

8. A vertical body plane that runs in a craniocaudal direction, dividing the body into unequal right and left portions is a(n) _____Sagittal plane_____ plane.

9. A body plane that divides a limb into proximal and distal portions is a(n) _____transverse_____ plane.

10. A radiographic view taken of a distal forelimb, such that the beam penetrates straight through the front of the limb first before reaching the x-ray film in the cassette, which lies behind the limb, is best termed a(n) _____ view.

11. When describing the relationship between the chest and the abdomen to the head of an animal, the animal's chest would be described as lying _____cranl_____ to the abdomen.

12. When describing the relationship between the chest and abdomen to the tail of an animal, the animal's abdomen would be described as lying _____caudal_____ to the chest.

13. The horizontal body plane that runs in a craniocaudal direction, dividing the body into dorsal and ventral portions, is the _____dorsal_____ plane.

14. The surface of a limb that lies nearest to the median plane of the body is the limb's _____medial_____ surface.

15. The side of a limb that lies parallel to the median plane but is furthest from that plane is the limb's _____lateral_____ surface.

16. A vertical body plane that crosses the body laterally, dividing it into cranial and caudal portions, is a(n) _____transverse_____ plane.

17. When describing the relationship of a front limb to the trunk of the body, the foot would be described as the most _____distal_____ portion of the extremity.

18. When describing the relationship of a rear limb to the trunk of the body, the hip would be described as the most _____proximal_____ point of the extremity.

19. A radiograph is required of the right front foot of a dog. The patient will be positioned in right lateral recumbency with the film and cassette directly beneath the foot. The radiographic beam will be set at an angle tangent to the foot, penetrating first on the dorsomedial aspect and exiting on the palmarolateral aspect. This radiographic view would be most appropriately called a dorsomedial-palmarolateral _____ view.

20. The vertical body plane that divides the body into equal right and left halves is the _____median_____ plane.

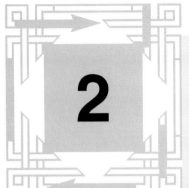
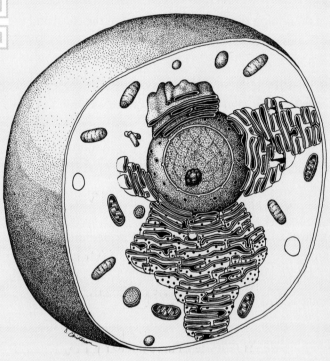

The Cell

GOALS AND OBJECTIVES

By the conclusion of this chapter, the student will be able to:

1. Recognize common root words, prefixes, and suffixes related to cells.
2. Divide simple and compound words into their respective parts.
3. Recognize, correctly pronounce, and appropriately use common medical terms related to cells.
4. Recognize anatomic components of animal cells.
5. Demonstrate a basic understanding of animal cell physiology.

2.1. Introduction to Related Terms

Divide each of the following terms into its respective parts ("R" root, "P" prefix, "S" suffix, "CV" combining vowel).

1. **Microscopic**   (P) _____   (CV) ___ (R) _____   (S) _____

   microscopic (mi"kro-skop'ik; pertaining to a small view; clinically refers to something that requires visualization by use of a microscope)

2. **Cytology[1]**   (R) _Cyt_ (CV) _O_ (S) _logy_

   cytology (si-tol'o-je; the study of cells)

3. **Lysosomal**   (R) _lys_ (CV) _O_ (R) _som_ (S) _al_

   lysosomal (li"so-so'mal; pertaining to a dissolving/destructive body)

4. **Intracellular**   (P) _intra_ (R) _cellul_ (S) _ularar_

   intracellular (in"trah-sel'u-lar; pertaining to within cells)

5. **Extracellular**   (P) _extra_ (R) _cellul_ (S) _ar_

   extracellular (eks"trah-sel'u-lar; pertaining to outside of cells)

6. **Nuclear**   (R) _nucle_ (S) _ar_

   nuclear (nu'kle-ar; pertaining to a nucleus)

7. **Chromosome[2]**   (R) _chrom_ (CV) _O_ (S) _some_

   chromosome (kro'mo-sōm; a colored body)

8. **Nucleolus**   (R) _nucle_ (S) _olus_

   nucleolus (nu-kle'o-lus; a small nucleus)

9. **Endoplasmic**   (P) _endo_ (R) _plasm_ (S) _ic_

   endoplasmic (en"do-plaz'mik; pertaining to within matter)

---

[1]Cytology: Note that the true suffix for the word is technically the letter "y." The interpretive meaning of "y" as a suffix is "the process of." It implies action. Therefore, any word ending in the letter "y" will have action implicated in it and should be used accordingly. For the purpose of simplifying medical terms in this text, the letter "y" will be shown collectively with the adjacent word part as a suffix. In the case of *cytology*, the adjacent word part is -*log*-. The collective meaning of the "suffix" -*logy* is "the study of." Hence, the meaning of *cytology* is interpreted as "the study of cells."

[2]Chromosome: Note that the true suffix for the word is technically the letter "e." The interpretive meaning of "e" as a suffix is "the presence of." As a suffix, "e" creates nouns (i.e., persons, places, or things). For the purpose of simplifying medical terms in this text, the letter "e" will be shown collectively with the adjacent word part as a suffix. In the case of *chromosome*, the adjacent word part is the root -*som*-. The collective meaning of the "suffix" -*some* is "a body." Hence, the meaning of *chromosome* is interpreted as "a colored body."

10. **Centriole**   (R) _Centri_ (CV) _o_ (S) _le_

centriole (sen'trĭ-ōl; a small center)

11. **Cytoplasmic**   (R) _Cyt_ (CV) _o_ (R) _plasm_ (S) _ic_

cytoplasmic (si"to-plaz'mik; pertaining to cell matter [cytoplasm])

12. **Vacuole**   (R) _vacu_ (S) _ole_

vacuole (vak'u-ōl; a small emptiness)

13. **Chromatic**   (R) _Chromat_ (S) _ic_

chromatic (kro-mat'ik; pertaining to color)

14. **Phagocytosis[3]**
    (R) _phag_ (CV) _o_ (R) _cyt_ (CV) _o_ (S) _sis_

phagocytosis (fag"o-si-to'sis; process of eating [by] cells)

15. **Pinocytosis**
    (R) _pin_ (CV) _o_ (R) _cyt_ (CV) _o_ (S) _sis_

pinocytosis (pi"no-si-to'sis; process of drinking [by] cells)

16. **Exocytosis**   (P) _ex_ (CV) _o_ (R) _cyt_ (CV) _o_ (S) _sis_

exocytosis (eks"o-si-to'sis; processing out of a cell)

17. **Mitosis**   (R) _mit_ (CV) _o_ (S) _sis_

mitosis (mi-to'sis; a condition of "thread"; clinically refers to cellular reproduction)

18. **Nuclei[4]**   (R) _nucle_ (S) _i_

nuclei (nu'kle-i; plural of nucleus)

19. **Intercellular**   (P) _inter_ (R) _cellul_ (S) _ar_

intercellular (in"ter-sel'u-lar; pertaining to between cells)

20. **Organelle**   (R) _organ_ (S) _elle_

organelle (or"gan-el'; a tiny organ)

21. **Physiology**   (R) _physi_ (CV) _o_ (S) _logy_

physiology (fiz"e-ol'o-je; the study of function)

---

[3]Phagocytosis: Note that the suffix -sis may appear alone or with a number of combining vowels (e.g., -osis, -asis, -esis, -iasis). The interpretive meaning of the suffix -sis is usually "the process of" or "a condition of."

[4]Nuclei: As a general rule, many medical terms ending in "i" or "a" indicate the plural form of the word.

22. **Reticular**   (R) _____   (S) _____

    reticular (rĕ-tik'u-lar; pertaining to a net)

23. **Ribosomal**   (R) _____ (CV) ___ (R) _____   (S) _____

    ribosomal (ri'bo-so-mal; pertaining to an RNA body)

24. **Centromere**   (P) _____ (CV) ___ (S) _____

    centromere (sen'tro-mēr; a central part)

2.2. Cellular Anatomy and Physiology

Cells are the smallest functional units of the body. They are so small that they cannot be studied without the aid of a microscope. In fact, many of the *intracellular organelles* are so small that an electron microscope must be used to visualize them. There are a plethora of cell types within the body of any animal, each uniquely different both anatomically (structurally) and physiologically. For the purpose of this discussion, an average, basic cell is presented. The reader should recognize that the intracellular organelles and details of cellular physiology may appear in varying degrees in other cells of the body.

2.2.1. CELLULAR ANATOMY

A basic animal cell is depicted in Fig. 2–1. A portion of the cell has been removed for easy visualization of its anatomic features.

1. **Cellular membrane.** The cellular membrane is the outermost structure of a cell that forms an envelope around all of the intracellular components. It is composed of lipids[5] and proteins.
2. **Cytoplasm.** The cytoplasm is a colorless fluid that gives the cell mass and suspends all of the intracellular organelles.
3. **Smooth endoplasmic reticulum.** The smooth endoplasmic reticulum is a complex network of canals and flattened sacs throughout the cytoplasm of the cell. It is devoid of ribosomes.
4. **Rough endoplasmic reticulum.** The rough endoplasmic reticulum is also a network of canals and flattened sacs throughout the cytoplasm of the cell. It appears rough microscopically because of the many ribosomes attached to it.
5. **Ribosomes.** The ribosomes are tiny, spherical organelles attached to the membrane of the rough endoplasmic reticulum.
6. **Mitochondrion** (mitochondria, plural; *mi"to-kon'dre-on, mi"to-kon'dre-ah*). The mitochondria, under the electron microscope, appear as tiny, elongated gran-

---

[5]Lipid is derived from [Gr. *lipos* fat]; *lip(o)-* is a combining form meaning "fat."

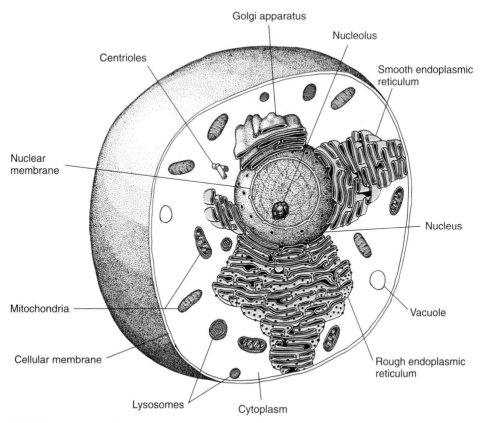

FIGURE 2–1. Animal cell.

ules with thread-like ridges over their surfaces. The texture is created by the intricate maze of partitions within the mitochondrial interior.

7. **Lysosome.** The lysosomes are small, enzyme-filled sacs. The enzymes within them literally dissolve particles with which they come in contact.

8. **Vacuole.** Vacuoles often appear microscopically as small, empty, cytoplasmic spaces, much like the appearance of holes in Swiss cheese. Actually, vacuoles are vesicles[6] that often contain either food for the cell or waste products to be removed from the cell.

9. **Golgi apparatus.**[7] The Golgi apparatus is a specialized series of flattened sacs and vesicles near the nucleus.

10. **Nucleus.** The nucleus is a large, intracellular organelle formed of loosely woven chromatin. The chromatin, when the cell is stained in the laboratory,

---

[6]*Vesicle* is derived from [L. *vesicula*], meaning "tiny bladder." A vesicle is a small sac-like structure.

[7]The Golgi (*gol'je*) apparatus is named after Comillo Golgi, an Italian scientist who was the co-winner of the Nobel Prize for medicine and physiology in 1906.

readily accepts the stain, giving it a colorful appearance microscopically. The chromatin is actually made up of loosely woven DNA, which when undergoing mitosis will become organized into the rod-like chromosomes that contain the blueprints of the cell.

11. **Nuclear membrane.** The nuclear membrane forms a porous envelope around the nucleus.

12. **Nucleolus.** Nucleoli are small, dense structures within the nucleus that are composed mainly of RNA and protein. They usually are visible only in very active cells.

13. **Centriole.** The centrioles are two cylindrical structures found near the nucleus and the Golgi apparatus. The centrioles lie perpendicular to one another and are of importance during mitosis.

2.2.2. CELLULAR PHYSIOLOGY

It was stated previously that cells are separate, functional compartments that make up the tissues of the body. A strong understanding of cellular anatomy and physiology is essential to gaining an understanding of individual body systems and the body as a whole. Unfortunately, many students have found cellular physiology difficult to comprehend. Actually, the structure and function of cells are quite basic, comparable to those of a large corporation.

The basic structure of both the cell and the corporation are based on very detailed blueprints. The design of each structure and the materials used to build it may differ in various respects, but the overall organization of the cell and the corporation are much the same. Each has a protective outer construction (i.e., the *cellular membrane* and the corporation's foundation, roof, and walls). The cement, mortar, and brick used to fabricate the outer building of the corporation are replaced by strong, water-impervious lipids and proteins in the cellular membrane. Whereas the corporation uses vents and windows to provide ventilation for the interior, the *semipermeable*[8] cellular membrane provides for easy passage of lipid-soluble molecules such as oxygen and carbon dioxide. Thus, by *simple diffusion*[9] cellular respiration is accomplished; that is to say, oxygen and carbon dioxide diffuse freely to and fro across the cellular membrane between the *intracellular* and the *extracellular* fluids.

Just as the corporation has doors and service doors to allow entry of people, supplies, and products, the cellular membrane provides for passage of liquids and large molecules. Rather than having actual doors that open and close, however, the cellular membrane indents and forms a *vesicle* around the substance to be taken into the cell. The vesicle, when completely formed, breaks free from the

---

[8]Semipermeable: [*semi-* partial + *permeable* to pass through] a semipermeable membrane permits passage of some things but not others.

[9]Diffusion is the *movement of particles* (molecules) across a semipermeable membrane from an area of high concentration to an area of low concentration (cf. *osmosis* Chap. 5, p. 71).

cellular membrane and can then be transported to an area of need intracellularly. *Pinocytosis* is the name given to the intake of liquids by a cell through such a process. Small, water soluble molecules, like glucose, are taken into the cell through a mechanism called *active transport* (facilitated diffusion). For active transport to take place, the extracellular glucose molecule is temporarily attached to a protein molecule on the surface of the cellular membrane. This protein molecule actively transports the glucose molecule through the cellular membrane, much like a mechanical arm or a conveyor belt would carry small packages through a service port into the corporation.

    Phagocytosis (Fig. 2–2) is a process whereby a cell takes in large objects, such as large protein particles or organisms like bacteria. The process begins much like pinocytosis, with the formation of a vesicle around the object. The object itself is like the raw ore and other crude materials taken into the corporation; it must be refined before it can be used. Therefore, the "food" vesicle of the cell will be joined with a *lysosome*. Just as a foundry would melt down the ore, the lysosomal enzymes digest the object into usable components. Some of the refined byproducts may provide fuel for the cell, whereas others provide building blocks (amino acids) for other production purposes within the cell. Waste products are expelled

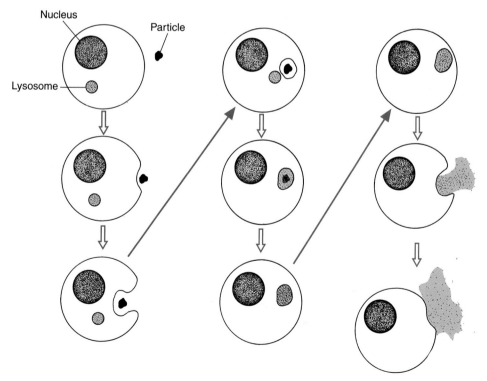

FIGURE 2–2. Phagocytosis.

from the cell using a reverse process called *exocytosis*. Similar to corporate dumping of wastes into rivers and streams, cells send waste vesicles to the surface of the cell where the cellular membrane opens, exposing and expelling the contents of the vesicles into the *intercellular fluid* of the body (cf. *interstitial* Chap. 5, p. 66).

All energy for cellular function is provided through the *mitochondria*, just as the internal physical plant and generators provide needed electricity for the corporation. Glucose, rather than coal or petroleum products, provides the fuel for these little powerhouses. Without the energy generated by the mitochondria, other cellular organelles could not carry out their functions.

The smooth and rough endoplasmic reticula provide mechanisms for transporting fuel, products, and byproducts throughout the cell, much like hallways and elevators provide for transport of products and the like throughout the corporation. The *rough endoplasmic reticulum* is of particular importance because of its close association with the *ribosomes*. The ribosomes are small production units. Whereas one production unit within the corporation may be responsible for making oblong widgets, another unit may be responsible for producing round gadgets. The principal ribosomal products are proteins of all shapes and sizes. Some of the products may be used for internal needs, such as repairs and general maintenance. Any of the products intended for export and global distribution must be packaged. Only one packaging department exists within the cell, the *Golgi apparatus*. All products and byproducts are sent, by way of the endoplasmic reticula, to the Golgi apparatus, where they are packaged into small vesicles. Again using the endoplasmic reticula, the packaged proteins, like mucus from a secretory cell, can be transported to the cellular membrane for exocytosis. Other proteins, like lysosomal enzymes, are packaged and distributed as lysosomes throughout the cytoplasm of the cell for later use.

The core of any corporate operation is the executive offices. All detailed information about corporate structure, products, production rates, profits, and losses is stored in the executive offices. The *nucleus* of a cell is much like the executive offices of the corporation. The nucleus is not enclosed in lavish oak and mahogany woodwork with bright brass fixtures; rather, it is enclosed in a porous *nuclear membrane*. All of the critical information (DNA [deoxyribonucleic acid]) about the cell and its functions are stored within the chromatin of the nucleus, as opposed to filing cabinets. The *nucleolus*, like any good executive secretary, is responsible for communicating with the other intracellular organelles. For example, work orders and blueprints are sent to the ribosomes in the form of RNA (ribonucleic acid) messages and information. Each ribosome receives from the nucleolus an RNA "photocopy" of an original DNA template for a protein to be produced, along with the work order for the quantity needed. Thereby, the nucleolus controls protein production. The nucleolus even has the authority and ability to form new ribosomes, if the need exists for additional production units. If the communication needs of a corporation exceed the capabilities of one executive secretary, temporary help may be hired. Temporary employees in the case of a cell come in the form of additional *nucleoli*. Whenever multiple nucleoli are visible in a nucleus, the cell is assumed to be very active.

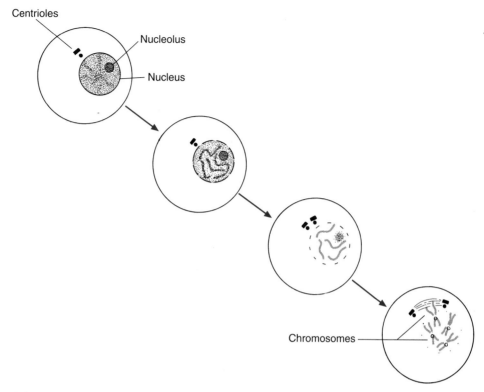

FIGURE 2–3. Mitosis: Prophase.

A peak time of activity for a cell is before *mitosis* or cellular reproduction. During this process, every aspect of the cell must be reproduced in fine detail. This situation could be likened to a corporation developing a daughter plant out of state or perhaps out of the country. To be as successful as the original, the plant must be duplicated in every detail. Likewise, the cell must duplicate its every detail. The actual phases of mitosis are explained in the following paragraphs.

During the *prophase*[10] (Fig. 2–3), the nuclear membrane is temporarily disassembled. The nuclear chromatin begins to reorganize and become tightly coiled into *chromosomes*. The DNA chains have been duplicated so that each chromosome is actually formed of two *chromatids* (the original and a duplicate), joined by a temporary attachment called a *centromere*. This gives the chromosomes the appearance of an "X" shape. At this time, too, the *centrioles* are duplicated. The two pairs of centrioles begin to move to opposite sides of the cell, while forming thin, spindle-like fibers between them.

---

[10]*pro-*, a prefix meaning *"before."*

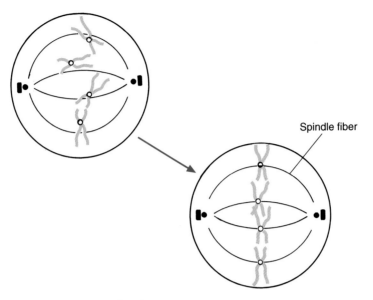

Spindle fiber

FIGURE 2–4. Mitosis: Metaphase.

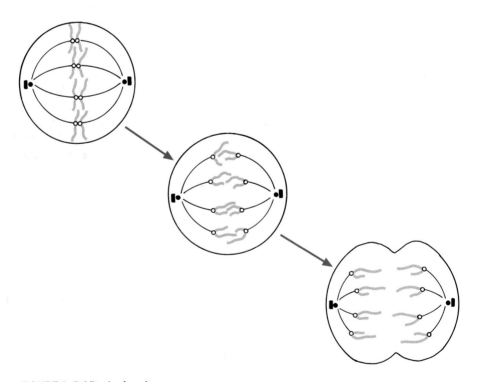

FIGURE 2–5. Mitosis: Anaphase.

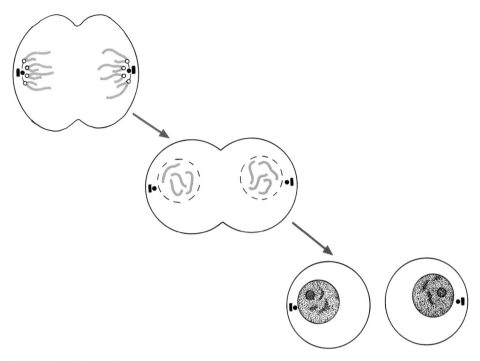

FIGURE 2–6. Mitosis: Telophase.

During the *metaphase*[11] (Fig. 2–4), the chromosomes line up midway between the centrioles. The centromere of each chromosome is attached to a *spindle fiber.*

During the *anaphase*[12] (Fig. 2–5), the chromatids separate and each (the original and the duplicate) is drawn in opposite directions by the attached spindle fibers, toward the associated centrioles. Microscopically, the spindle fibers and chromatids have a thread-like appearance, hence the term "mitosis." The other cellular organelles and the cytoplasm are also equally divided between the two sides. The cellular membrane begins to constrict, outlining the two daughter cells.

During the *telophase*[13] (Fig. 2–6), migration of the chromosomes to the centrioles is completed. Soon, the cytoplasmic and cellular membrane divisions will also be completed. Within each new daughter cell, the chromosomes unwind into loosely woven chromatin, while new nuclear membranes envelope the new nuclei. The new daughter cells are identical, yet separate, fully functional entities. Each is smaller than the parent cell. Heavy protein production within each new cell is required for further cellular development, such that the reproductive cycle may be repeated.

---

[11]*meta-*, a prefix meaning *"after"* or *"beyond."*

[12]*ana-*, a prefix meaning *"backward."*

[13]*telo-*, a prefix meaning *"end."*

2.3. Self-Test

Using the previous information in this chapter, respond to each of the following questions using the most appropriate medical term(s).

1. The study of cells is medically termed _____.

2. The "powerhouses" of the cell that provide energy for all cellular functions are the ___mitochondria___.

3. Anything contained within a cell is referred to as a(n) ___intra-cellular___ structure.

4. The fluid between cells is called ___interacellular___ fluid.

5. ___phagocytosis___ is a process by which cells consume large particles and organisms.

6. The colorless fluid that suspends all of the organelles within a cell is called ___cytoplasm___.

7. The cellular organelle responsible for packaging secretory products is the ___Golgi apparatus___.

8. The cellular process by which waste products are expelled from the cell is termed _____.

9. The ___ribosomes___ is the cellular organelle that produces proteins.

10. A cytoplasmic inclusion that appears microscopically as a hole is medically termed a(n) ___vacuole___.

11. The ___nucleus___ is the control center of the cell, containing all of its necessary DNA information.

12. In a cell not in the process of reproducing itself, DNA is stored in the form of loosely woven _____.

13. Anything outside of a cell is termed _____.

14. A cytoplasmic vesicle containing "digestive" enzymes for the cell is a(n) ___lysomes___.

15. The cellular organelle that is composed of highly organized networks of tubes for the transport of proteins produced by its attached ribosomes is the ___rough endoplasmatic reticulum___.

16. Cellular reproduction is medically termed ___mitosis___.

17. _____ are tightly coiled, connected strands of original and duplicate DNA that are visible only during cellular reproduction.

18. The process by which a carrier protein on the surface of the cell carries a molecule through the cellular membrane into the cell is called _____.

19. The _nucleolus_ is the cellular organelle composed of RNA and protein that is responsible for interorganelle communication.

20. Movement of molecules, such as oxygen, across the semipermeable cellular membrane from an area of high oxygen concentration to an area of low oxygen concentration is termed _____.

21. Cellular _anatomy_ is another way of saying cell "structure."

22. To learn about cellular _physiology_ is another way of saying that one is studying the function of cells.

23. The paired, cylindrical organelles that are responsible for chromatid migration during cellular reproduction are called _centrioles_.

24. _pinocytosis_ is the process by which cells "drink" fluids.

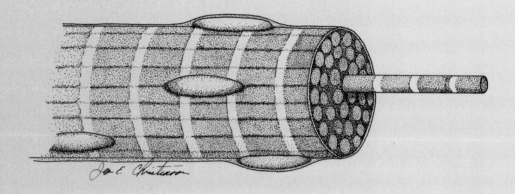

Body Structure and Organization

GOALS AND OBJECTIVES

By the conclusion of this chapter, the student will be able to:

1. Recognize common root words, prefixes, and suffixes related to the body and biology.
2. Divide simple and compound words into their respective parts.
3. Recognize, correctly pronounce, and appropriately use common medical terms related to the body and animal physiology.
4. Demonstrate an understanding of basic chemistry, including atomic structure and molecular bonds.
5. Demonstrate an understanding of general body structure and organization.
6. Demonstrate an understanding of the functional relationships of body tissues and organs.

3.1. Introduction to Related Terms

Divide each of the following terms into its respective parts ("R" root, "P" prefix, "S" suffix, "CV" combining vowel).

1. **Hematopoietic**   (R) hemat (CV) o (R) poiet (S) c

   hematopoietic (hem"ah-to-poi-et'ik; pertaining to blood production)

2. **Lymphatic**   (R) lymph (CV) a (S) tic

   lymphatic (lim-fat'ik; pertaining to lymph [L. "water"])

3. **Musculoskeletal**   (R) muscul (CV) o (R) skelat (S) al

   musculoskeletal (mus"ku-lo-skel'ĕ-tal; pertaining to the muscles and skeleton)

4. **Cardiovascular**   (R) cardi (CV) o (R) vascul (S) ar

   cardiovascular (kar"de-o-vas'ku-lar; pertaining to the heart and vessels)

5. **Respiratory**   (P) re (R) spirat (S) ory

   respiratory (rĕ-spi'rah-to"re; pertaining to again breathing)

6. **Neurological**   (R) neur (CV) o (R) log (CV) i (S) cal

   neurological (nu-ro-loj'ik-al; pertaining to nerve study)

7. **Alimentary**   (R) aliment (S) ary

   alimentary (al"ĕ-men'tar-e; pertaining to food)

8. **Urinary**   (R) urin (S) ary

   urinary (u'rĭ-ner"e; pertaining to urine)

9. **Reproductive**   (P) re (R) product (S) ive

   reproductive (re"pro-duk'tiv; pertaining to again producing [i.e., offspring])

10. **Endocrine**   (P) endo (R) crine

    endocrine (en'do-krin; to secrete inside)

11. **Integumentary**   (R) integument (S) ary

    integumentary (in-teg-u-men'tar-e; pertaining to covering over)

12. **Visceral**   (R) viscer (S) al

    visceral (vis'er-al; pertaining to the viscera [organs])

13. **Cranium**   (R) crani (S) um

    cranium (kra'ne-um; the head)

14. **Thoracic**   (R) _____   (S) _____

thoracic (tho-ras'ik; pertaining to the thorax [chest])

15. **Abdominal**   (R) _____   (S) _____

abdominal (ab-dom'ĭ-nal; pertaining to the abdomen [belly])

16. **Epithelial**   (R) _epithel_   (S) _al_

epithelial (ep"ĭ-the'le-al; pertaining to epithelium[1])

17. **Endothelial**   (R) _endothel_   (S) _al_

endothelial (en"do-the'le-al; pertaining to endothelium[2])

18. **Cuboidal**   (R) _cuboid_   (S) _al_

cuboidal (ku-boi'dal; pertaining to resembling a cube)

19. **Squamous**   (R) _squam_   (S) _ous_

squamous (skwa'mus; pertaining to scales)

20. **Columnar**   (R) _colum_   (S) _ar_

columnar (ko-lum'nar; pertaining to columns [pillars])

21. **Myocyte**   (R) _my_   (CV) _o_   (S) _cyte_

myocyte (mi'o-sīt; a muscle cell)

22. **Homeostasis**   (R) _home_ (CV) _o_   (S) _stasis_

homeostasis (ho"me-o-sta'sis; standing unchanged; clinically refers to that state of balance or equilibrium, albeit normal function within the body)

23. **Pathology**   (R) _____ (CV) ___ (S) _____

pathology (pah-thol'o-je; the study of disease)

24. **Synergism**   (P) _syn_   (R) _erg_   (S) _ism_

synergism (sin'er-jizm; the state of working together; syn- [together], erg(o)- [work])

25. **Symbiosis**   (P) _sym_   (R) _bios_   (S) _is_

symbiosis (sim"bi-o'sis; the state of living together; sym- [together], bio- [life])

---

[1]Epithelium: derived from the prefix *epi-* [upon] and [L. *thele*, nipple] epithelium is a superficial tissue found on any exposed surface of the body.

[2]Endothelium: derived from the prefix *endo-* and [L. *thele*] endothelium is a type of epithelium found lining the interior surfaces of vessels and the like.

26. **Biology**   (R) _____   (S) _____

   biology (bi-ol'o-je; the study of life)

27. **Atomic**   (R) _____   (S) _____

   atomic (ă-tom'ik; pertaining to an atom)

28. **Molecular**   (R) _____   (S) _____

   molecular (mo-lek'u-lar; pertaining to a little mass [molecule])

3.2. Anatomy and Physiology

3.2.1. BASIC STRUCTURE OF MATTER

Every domestic animal is composed of billions of *organic* (containing carbon) and *inorganic* (noncarbon containing) compounds. All matter is composed of tiny, invisible particles called *atoms*. Each different element has a unique atomic structure consisting of a minute, central, positively charged mass (*nucleus*) and "orbiting," negatively charged particles (*electrons*). The nuclear mass of the atom determines the *atomic weight* of the element (Fig. 3–1). The *atomic number* for the element is determined by the number of *protons* (positively charged particles) within the nucleus[3] of an atom. A hydrogen atom contains a single proton; therefore, the atomic number of hydrogen is 1. A carbon atom contains six protons and so has the atomic number 6. The number and the arrangement of the electrons that encircle the nucleus determine all other properties of the element. Depending on the element, the electrons of an atom are arranged in one or more "shells" around the nucleus. For example, an atom of hydrogen appears as a nucleus circled by a single electron, whereas an atom of oxygen appears as a nucleus encircled by eight electrons (Fig. 3–2). The number of electrons of an atom equals the number of protons in the nucleus, rendering the atom neutral.

The *atomic weight* of an element is approximately equal to the number of protons and *neutrons* in the nucleus. For example, a hydrogen atom contains only one proton and no neutrons. Therefore, its atomic weight is 1.00. In comparison, a carbon atom contains six protons and six neutrons, giving it an atomic weight of approximately 12.0.

As stated earlier, the number of electrons is equal to the number of protons in an atom, rendering it neutral. Being electrically neutral does not mean that a given atom is "stable." The stability of an atom is determined by the number of electrons filling its outermost shell. For elements with atomic numbers 1 through

---

[3]The nucleus of most atoms is composed of both protons and neutrons. Each proton carries a single positive charge, whereas each neutron, being about equal in weight to a proton, carries no electrical charge.

Legend:
- 1 ← atomic number
- H ← element symbol
- 1.008 ← atomic weight

Ia	IIa	IIIb	IVb	Vb	VIb	VIIb		VIIIb		IB	IIB	IIIa	IVa	Va	VIa	VIIa	O
1 H 1.008																	2 He 4.00
3 Li 6.94	4 Be 9.01											5 B 10.81	6 C 12.01	7 N 14.00	8 O 15.99	9 F 18.99	10 Ne 20.18
11 Na 22.99	12 Mg 24.31											13 Al 26.98	14 Si 28.09	15 P 30.97	16 S 32.06	17 Cl 35.45	18 Ar 39.95
19 K 39.10	20 Ca 40.08	21 Sc 44.96	22 Ti 47.90	23 V 50.94	24 Cr 51.99	25 Mn 54.94	26 Fe 55.85	27 Co 58.93	28 Ni 58.71	29 Cu 63.54	30 Zn 65.37	31 Ga 69.72	32 Ge 72.59	33 As 74.92	34 Se 78.96	35 Br 79.91	36 Kr 83.8
37 Rb 85.47	38 Sr 87.62	39 Y 88.91	40 Zr 91.22	41 Nb 92.91	42 Mo 95.94	43 Tc (99)	44 Ru 101.97	45 Rh 102.91	46 Pd 106.40	47 Ag 107.87	48 Cd 112.40	49 In 114.82	50 Sn 118.69	51 Sb 121.75	52 Te 127.60	53 I 126.90	54 Xe 131.30
55 Cs 132.91	56 Ba 137.34	57-71 see below	72 Hf 178.49	73 Ta 180.95	74 W 183.85	75 Re 186.20	76 Os 190.20	77 Ir 192.20	78 Pt 195.09	79 Au 196.97	80 Hg 200.59	81 Tl 204.37	82 Pb 207.19	83 Bi 208.98	84 Po (210)	85 At (210)	86 Rn (222)
87 Fr (223)	88 Ra (226)	89-103 see below	104 Rf (261)	105 Ha (260)	106* 263												

* newly produced

Lanthanide series	57 La 138.91	58 Ce 140.12	59 Pr 140.91	60 Nd 144.24	61 Pm (147)	62 Sm 150.35	63 Eu 151.96	64 Gd 157.25	65 Tb 158.92	66 Dy 162.50	67 Ho 164.93	68 Er 167.26	69 Tm 168.93	70 Yb 173.04	71 Lu 174.97

Actinide series	89 Ac (227)	90 Th 232.04	91 Pa (231)	92 U 238.03	93 Np (237)	94 Pu (242)	95 Am (243)	96 Cm (247)	97 Bk (247)	98 Cf (251)	99 Es (254)	100 Fm (253)	101 Md (256)	102 No (254)	103 Lr (257)

Please note: Values in parentheses are approximate.

FIGURE 3–1. Periodic table of elements.

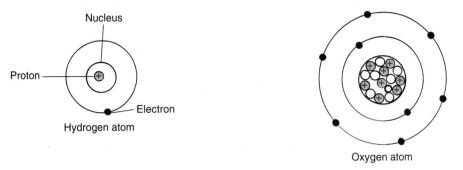

FIGURE 3–2. Atomic structure.

20, the maximum numbers of electrons that may be held by each shell are as follows:

First shell (closest to the nucleus)	2 electrons
Second shell	8 electrons
Third shell	8 electrons

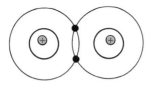

FIGURE 3–3. Hydrogen molecule.

Elements, like helium, whose outermost shell is filled to capacity are considered stable or *inert*. In comparison, an element like hydrogen is lacking an electron in its outer shell. Therefore, hydrogen atoms are unstable; they will try to bond with other atoms, either gaining or sharing electrons to achieve a stable state. Whenever two or more atoms bond together, they form a new larger particle called a *molecule*. A molecule of hydrogen (H_2) is stable, due to the sharing of each atom's single electron. The shared arrangement, in essence, fills the first (outer) shell of each atom (Fig. 3–3). Such a union between atoms is referred to as a *covalent*[4] bond. The most common molecule formed with hydrogen is water. Water is composed of two hydrogen atoms plus a single oxygen atom (H_2O). This stable molecule, like hydrogen gas (H_2), also forms by virtue of electron sharing (Fig. 3–4). Water is the most abundant, inorganic compound found in the body, comprising approximately two thirds of the total body mass.

Other molecules are formed through the giving up or taking on of electrons. Sodium chloride is an example of such a molecule. As separate atoms, the sodium atom has one electron in its outer shell, whereas the chlorine atom has seven electrons in its outer shell. To achieve a stable state, the sodium atom tends to give up the single electron from its outer shell. The chlorine atom, on the other hand, must gain an electron to become stable. When these atoms react, the sodium atom gives up the electron to the chlorine atom. The electron-proton ratio in each atom is no longer equal (i.e., 1:1). The sodium atom has one more proton than electrons and the chlorine atom has one more electron than protons. This imparts a net positive charge to the sodium atom and a net negative charge to the chlorine atom. As opposite, electrically charged particles, the two atoms are attracted to one another and are united in an *electrovalent bond* (Fig. 3–5).

Electrolytes are salts, acids, or bases that dissociate into *ions*[5] in body fluids. Sodium chloride is an example of a salt. When NaCl is dissolved in water, it releases sodium ions (Na^+) and chlorine ions (Cl^-). Bases are compounds that combine with hydrogen ions (H^+) in solution. Acids are compounds that release hydrogen ions in solution. Electrolytes affect many body functions. Salts, like

---

[4]Covalent (*ko-va'lent*): derived from the prefix *co-* [together/jointly] + [L. *valere*, to be strong].

[5]Ions are electrically charged atoms or molecules in solution. These atoms have become electrically charged by either gaining or losing electrons. Ions with a positive charge are referred to as *cations* and ions with a negative charge are referred to as *anions*.

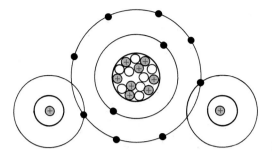

FIGURE 3–4. Water molecule

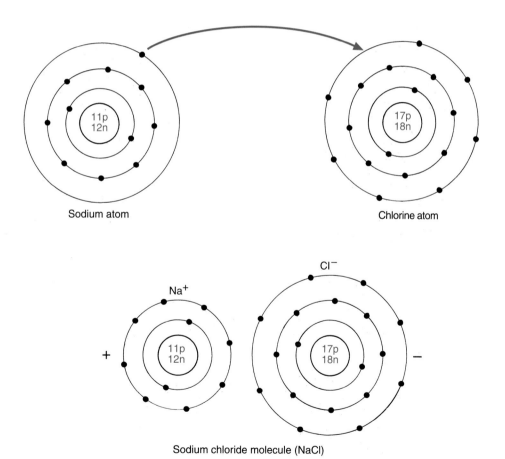

Sodium atom

Chlorine atom

Na⁺

Cl⁻

11p
12n

17p
18n

+

−

Sodium chloride molecule (NaCl)

FIGURE 3–5. Sodium chloride molecule.

NaCl, tend to attract water, which has an impact on the hydration[6] of the body. Neural impulses occur because of the net exchange of intracellular and extracellular ions. The acid–base balance (pH) of the body is determined by the numbers of hydrogen ions (H^+) versus bicarbonate ions (HCO_3^-). For every action, there is an equal and opposite reaction. Consequently, changes in the body, even at the atomic or molecular level, have an effect on the function and well-being of that animal.

Various molecules combine to form a diverse array of compounds in the body. *Amino acids* are a type of compound that are the "building blocks" for *proteins*. These amino acids are nothing more than large molecules composed of carbon, hydrogen, oxygen, and nitrogen atoms. As various amino acids join together in chains, they form proteins. Most cellular structure is formed from various proteins. The most fundamental molecular compounds for cells are the *nucleic acids*, which contain phosphorus in addition to C, H, O, and N. The two major types of nucleic acids are *ribonucleic acid* (RNA) and *deoxyribonucleic acid* (DNA). DNA molecules store cellular information in a kind of molecular code, unique to the given cell. For more information regarding cellular anatomy and physiology, refer to Chapter 2. As stated in Chapter 2, cells comprise the smallest functional units of the body. *En masse*, cells make up the tissues of the body.

3.2.2. BODY TISSUES

Body tissues are formed by numerous cells. Each of the major tissue types serves a particular function for the organ with which it is associated. The following are major tissue types found in domestic animals.

3.2.2.1. Epithelial Tissue

In general, *epithelial tissue* covers all body surfaces, inside and out. It covers all organs, forms the inner lining of body cavities, and lines hollow organs. Epithelial tissue is anchored to underlying connective tissue by a thin *basement membrane*. The tightly packed structure of epithelium provides an excellent protective barrier for underlying structures. If epithelial tissue is damaged, it has the capacity to regenerate rapidly to repair the wound. Surprisingly, most epithelial tissues do not have a direct blood supply. They receive nourishment by means of nutrients that diffuse from underlying connective tissues.

Epithelial tissues are classified according to the various shapes, arrangements, and functions of their cells. For example, those epithelial tissues composed of single layers of cells are called *simple*; those arranged in layers are called *stratified*; those that appear to be arranged in layers but actually are not are called *pseudostratified*[7]; those composed of thin, flattened cells are called *squamous*; those

---

[6]*Hydr(o)-* is a combining form meaning "water."

[7]The prefix *pseudo- (su'do)* means "false."

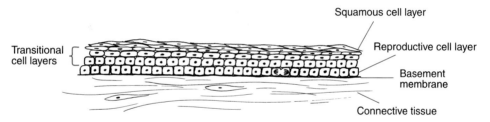

FIGURE 3–6. Stratified squamous epithelium.

composed of cube-like cells are called *cuboidal*; and those which are composed of tall, elongated cells are called *columnar*. Each type of epithelium is suited to a particular purpose.

Stratified squamous epithelium is made up of many layers, making it relatively thick (Fig. 3–6). The cells near the surface are flattened. Deeper into the tissue layers (i.e., near the basement membrane), the cells are usually cuboidal or columnar in shape. It is in these deeper layers that mitosis takes place. As the new cells grow and reproduce, they push the older cells toward the surface. The transitional cells tend to flatten out as they progress toward the surface. When they finally reach the surface, they are true squamous epithelium. Stratified squamous epithelium provides an excellent barrier against *pathogenic*[8] organisms. Areas that contain abundant stratified squamous epithelium include the skin and the urinary bladder.

Simple squamous epithelium is a thin layer of flattened cells that are interlocked, much like floor tiles (Fig. 3–7). It is designed to permit diffusion of some substances. For instance, simple squamous epithelium forms the walls of air sacs in the lungs and the walls of capillaries. Both of these structures must permit diffusion of O_2 and CO_2. Simple squamous epithelium may also be found lining body cavities and vessels. The term *"endothelium"* is usually used when referring to simple squamous epithelium that lines the interior of blood vessels and lymphatic vessels. Because it is so thin and delicate, simple squamous epithelium is easily damaged.

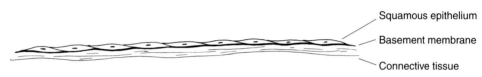

FIGURE 3–7. Simple squamous epithelium.

---

[8]Pathogenic is derived from *path(o)-* [disease] + *gen(o)-* [producing] + *-ic* [pertaining to].

Simple cuboidal epithelium consists of a single layer of cube-shaped cells (Fig. 3–8). This type of tissue is frequently found in glands and lining the tubules of such organs as the kidneys and the liver. Cuboidal cells generally aid with functions of absorption or secretion. For instance, in glands, these cells are concerned with secretion of glandular products. Along areas of the kidney tubules, cuboidal cells are concerned with absorption of compounds such as water.

Simple columnar epithelium consists of a single layer of cells that are taller than they are wide (Fig. 3–9). It is found in various regions of the body, such as the stomach and intestines. It serves functions similar to those of the cuboidal epithelium. For instance, some columnar epithelial cells of the intestines are very active in the absorption of nutrients, whereas others may be responsible for secreting substances such as mucus.

Pseudostratified columnar epithelium may appear to be layered, but is not. It appears to be layered because the nuclei of the cells are located at various levels throughout the tissue (Fig. 3–10). Pseudostratified columnar epithelium is commonly found lining certain areas of the body, such as the respiratory tract. Many of these columnar cells are *ciliated*.[9] In the respiratory tract, the cilia help move mucus up and out of the airways.

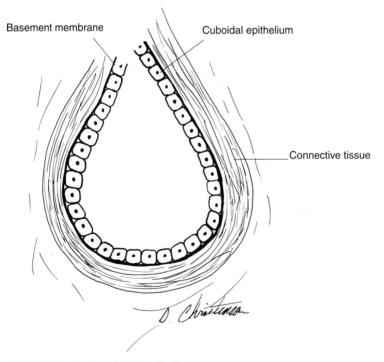

FIGURE 3–8. Simple cuboidal epithelium.

---

[9]Cilia are hair-like projections from the free (exposed) cell wall. They usually provide motion.

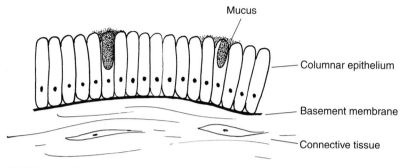

FIGURE 3–9. Simple columnar epithelium.

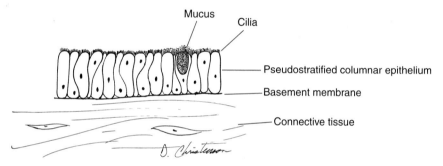

FIGURE 3–10. Pseudostratified columnar epithelium.

3.2.2.2. Connective Tissue

Connective tissue is found throughout the body. It connects structures together, providing support and protection. Unlike epithelial cells, connective tissue cells are further apart from one another. Between them lies an abundant matrix of fibers or other such substances. In addition, connective tissues usually have an abundant blood supply. Types of connective tissue are classified according to their basic structural characteristics. Some of the major types of connective tissue are discussed in the following.

Fibrous connective tissue is a very dense tissue composed of many tightly packed, thick collagen fibers and fine elastic fibers. The collagen fibers are very tough and can withstand extreme forces of pulling. That is why this tissue is crucial in holding bones together and providing attachments of muscles to bones. It is also found in the deeper layers of the skin (beneath the epithelium).

Elastic connective tissue is composed primarily of elastic tissue fibers, in addition to some collagenous fibers. As its name implies, it provides elasticity to the structures it forms. It is found predominantly in hollow internal organs and in vessel walls.

Loose connective tissue is a more delicate type of connective tissue. It generally forms thin membranes throughout the body, like the basement membrane that anchors epithelium to underlying tissues. Loose connective tissue provides a loose, flexible attachment of the skin to underlying tissues and organs. It is also found between muscles and in other spaces between organs. A specialized form of loose connective tissue is *adipose tissue,* commonly referred to as fat. Specialized cells that make up adipose tissue store fat droplets in their cytoplasm.

Cartilage is a more rigid form of connective tissue. Unlike other types of connective tissue, cartilage does not have a direct blood supply. It receives nutrients from other surrounding connective tissues that do have abundant blood supplies. Cartilage is found in abundance in joints formed between bones. In such areas, the cartilage provides a smooth joint surface, protecting the underlying bone.

Bone is the most dense, rigid type of connective tissue. The hardness of bone results from the presence of minerals and mineral salts in its matrix. Bones provide support for muscles and other body tissues and organs. They provide protection for viscera—for example, the rib cage with regard to the thoracic viscera and the skull with regard to the brain.

3.2.2.3. Muscle Tissue

Muscle tissue is divided into three different types: *smooth muscle, cardiac muscle,* and *skeletal muscle.* Unlike other types of tissue, muscle tissue has the capacity to contract and relax, thereby changing the given muscle's overall length. A description of each type of muscle tissue follows.

Smooth muscle (Fig. 3–11) is typically associated with unconscious, involuntary, muscular activity, like the diaphragm's activity with breathing. It is found predominantly in the walls of hollow organs, such as the stomach, intestines,

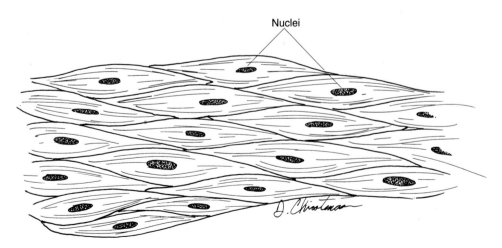

Nuclei

FIGURE 3–11. Smooth muscle tissue.

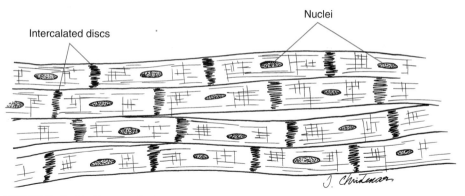

FIGURE 3–12. Cardiac muscle tissue.

blood vessels, and the urinary bladder. It is called smooth muscle because its cells lack *striations* (stripes).

   Cardiac muscle (Fig. 3–12), like smooth muscle, is also under unconscious, involuntary control. Cardiac muscle is found only in the heart. Its cells are striated and uniquely joined together end to end. These specialized intercellular junctions (*intercalated* discs; *in"ter-ka'la-ted*) are found only in cardiac muscle, and give this muscle extraordinary strength and contractile ability.

   Skeletal muscle (Fig. 3–13) is composed of billions of *myocytes* (also called muscle fibers). Each myocyte (Fig. 3–14) has a long, thin, cylindrical shape with rounded ends and numerous nuclei along its length. The rounded ends of the myocytes are attached to fibrous connective tissue. Inside each myocyte are long, thin, thread-like structures called *myofibrils* (*mi"o-fi'brilz*). These myofibrils are

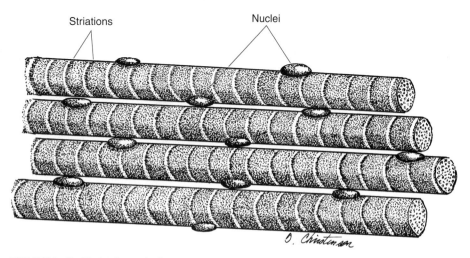

FIGURE 3–13. Skeletal muscle tissue.

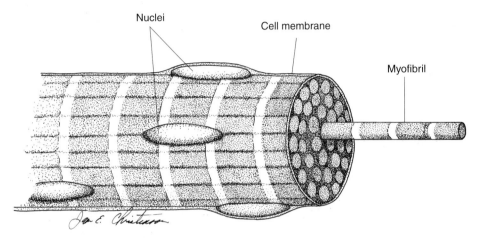

FIGURE 3–14. Myocyte.

tightly packed and lie parallel to one another, much like the wires within an electrical cord. Unlike wire, however, the myofibrils are very elastic and have tremendous contractile ability. When a myocyte is stimulated by a nerve, the myofibrils inside synchronously contract. When the nervous stimulation is removed, the myofibrils relax. Numerous muscle fibers are bundled together with fibrous connective tissue. An actual muscle is made up of innumerable bundles of muscle fibers. Muscles are separated from one another by sheets of fibrous connective tissue called *fascia* (*fash'e-ah*). The fascia surrounding a muscle extends beyond the ends of the muscle to form the cord-like attachments to the bones (i.e., *tendons*).

3.2.2.4. Neural Tissue

Neural tissue is found in the brain, spinal cord, and peripheral nerves. It is composed of nerve cells or *neurons*, which are highly specialized cells responsible for transmitting neuroelectrical impulses. Neurons are supported by other specialized cells and connective tissues, which are discussed in more detail in Chapter 9. Nerves are a culmination of bundles of neurons. They transmit impulses to all areas of the body, eliciting various responses from the target organs (e.g., muscle contraction).

3.2.3. BODY CAVITIES

Domestic animals have three principal body cavities. The *cranial vault*, formed by the bones of the cranium, houses the brain. The *thoracic cavity* contains visceral components such as the heart and the lungs. *Abdominal viscera* include such organs as the liver, stomach, intestines, and urinary bladder. The thoracic and abdominal cavities are separated by a large muscle called the *diaphragm*. Only a small region of the diaphragm permits passage of major blood vessels and other such structures. That region is called the *hiatus* (hi-a'tus).

3.2.4. ORGANS AND ORGAN SYSTEMS

The body is organized into larger functional culminations of tissues and organs. Although each organ system is discussed in detail as a separate entity in subsequent chapters, one should remember that all organ systems function interdependently. They each have principal tasks they must carry out, but they must do so without disturbing the normal function of other organ systems. Complete discussions of each system's anatomy and physiology are detailed in subsequent chapters. The specific organ systems and their principal functions are summarized in the following list.

1. The *hematopoietic system* is comprised of the blood and blood-forming tissues.
2. The *lymphatic system* is composed of a network of vessels and glands that are largely responsible for immunity within the body.
3. The *musculoskeletal system*, formed of bones, muscles, and connective tissues, provides for the overall structure and movement of the body.
4. The *cardiovascular system*, comprised of the heart and blood vessels, provides continual circulation of the blood.
5. The *respiratory system*, consisting of airways running from the nose to the lungs, provides for the needed exchange of gases like O_2 and CO_2.
6. The *neurologic system*, made up of the brain, spinal cord, and peripheral nerves, controls many of the other organ systems with neuroelectrical input.
7. The *alimentary system*, or digestive system, provides for the intake of nutrients for the body and disposal of some wastes.
8. The *urinary system*, composed of the kidneys and urinary bladder, is also critical for the removal of toxic wastes from the body as well as the maintenance of water and electrolyte balance.
9. The *reproductive system* provides the means for animals to propagate their species.
10. The *endocrine system*, comprising various glands, provides chemical (hormonal) control over many body functions.
11. The *integumentary system* comprises the largest organ of the body, the skin, and its associated structures.

3.2.5. HOMEOSTASIS

Each of the body's organs/organ systems must carry out specific functions. However, they must function in such a way so as not to disturb *homeostasis*. All of the organ systems must function *synergistically* to maintain a balanced, normal state for the body. Whenever a portion of the body deviates from the homeostatic state, disease will result. As stated earlier, the various body systems each are discussed in detail later in this text. Although diseases may be discussed in relation to a given body system, one must remember that disease in any body system will, to one degree or another, have an impact on the rest of the body. Fortunately, the body has built-in mechanisms that attempt to correct abnormalities, to bring the whole body back into a state of homeostasis. At times, these mechanisms may be efficient enough to provide for the *symbiotic* relationship between domestic animals and other organisms. For example, in the digestive tract of an animal are many *commensal* (kŏ-men'sal, cf. symbiotic) microorganisms, such as bacteria. The digestive tract provides an environment suitable to support life for the bacteria, whereas the bacteria aid in the digestion of food for the animal without causing disease. If these same bacteria were somehow to gain entry to areas of the body other than the digestive tract, disease would likely ensue. Veterinary professionals must acquire knowledge of normal *physiology*, as well as *pathophysiology*. The understanding of how domestic animals function in health and disease will guide the medical decisions and therapies rendered to veterinary patients. Our ultimate goals are to restore and maintain homeostasis in our patients.

3.3. Self-Test

Using the previous information in this chapter, respond to each of the following questions using the most appropriate medical term(s).

1. Two or more atoms bonded together are called a(n) _____.

2. _____ is the state of working together, as in various organ systems working together for the well-being of the body.

3. A small, almost weightless, negatively charged particle that is in constant motion around the nucleus of an atom is a(n) _____.

4. In the periodic table of elements, each element has a specific atomic number. This number is derived from the number of _____ in the nucleus of an atom.

5. A(n) ___Symbiotic___ relationship is one in which two organisms live together, providing for the mutual benefit of one another.

6. The ___thoracic___ cavity is another name for the chest cavity.

7. The body system which is composed of blood and blood-forming tissues is the ___hematopoietic___ system.

8. ___homeostasis___ is the balanced, stable state of the body.

9. All free or exposed body surfaces are covered by ___epithelial___ tissue.

10. _____ are complex molecules of carbon, oxygen, hydrogen, and nitrogen, and are referred to as the "building blocks" of proteins.

11. ____pathology____ is literally the study of disease.

12. The ____integumentary____ system is composed of the largest organ in the body, the skin.

13. A(n) _____ bond is a type of molecular bond in which two atoms share an electron.

14. _____ is the most abundant inorganic compound found in the body, comprising approximately two thirds of the total body mass.

15. _____ is literally the study of life.

16. Elements, like helium, whose outermost shell is filled to capacity with electrons, are considered stable or _____.

17. _____ are compounds, such as salts, that dissociate into ions in body fluids.

18. The ____endocrine____ system is comprised of various glands that exert hormonal control over other organs and body tissues.

19. ____pseudostratified____ columnar epithelium gives the false impression of being layered, but it is not.

20. ____adipose____ tissue is a specialized type of loose connective tissue, composed of cells that store fat in their cytoplasm.

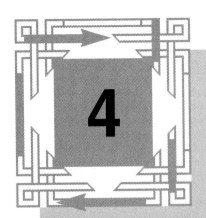

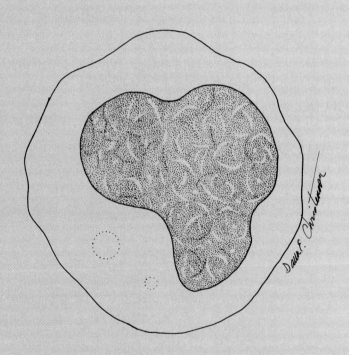

The Hematopoietic System

GOALS AND OBJECTIVES

By the conclusion of this chapter, the student will be able to:

1. Recognize common root words, prefixes, and suffixes related to blood.
2. Divide simple and compound words into their respective parts.
3. Recognize, correctly pronounce, and appropriately use common medical terms related to blood.
4. Demonstrate an understanding of the composition of blood.
5. Recognize basic morphologic characteristics of normal blood cells.
6. Demonstrate an understanding of the basic physiology of hematopoiesis and the function of each major constituent of the blood, including specific cell types.
7. Demonstrate a basic understanding of hematology, including the clinical determination of the packed cell volume (PCV), total protein (TP), and morphologic evaluation of blood smears.

4.1. Introduction to Related Terms

Divide each of the following terms into its respective parts ("R" root, "P" prefix, "S" suffix, "CV" combining vowel).

1. **Hematology**   (R) _____ (CV) ___ (S) _____

   hematology (hēm"ah-tol'o-je; the study of blood)

2. **Morphology**   (R) _____ (CV) ___ (S) _____

   morphology (mor-fol'o-je; the study of form)

3. **Erythrocyte**   (P) _____ (CV) ___ (S) _____

   erythrocyte (e-rith'ro-sīt; a red cell; clinically refers to red blood cells)

4. **Reticulocyte**   (R) _____ (CV) ___ (S) _____

   reticulocyte (re-tik'u-lo-sīt"; a "net" cell; clinically refers to a young red blood cell containing remnant ribosomes and endoplasmic reticulum)

5. **Polychromasia**   (P) _____ (R) _____ (S) _____

   polychromasia (pol"e-kro-ma'ze-ah; a condition of many colors; clinically refers to erythrocytes with varied staining qualities)

6. **Anisocytosis**   (P) _____ (CV) ___ (R) _____ (CV) ___ (S) _____

   anisocytosis (an-e"so-si-to'sis; a condition of unequal cells; clinically refers to size variations of red blood cells)

7. **Polycythemia**   (P) _____ (R) _____ (R) _____ (S) _____

   polycythemia (pol"e-si-the'me-ah; a condition of many cells; clinically refers to excess numbers of erythrocytes)

8. **Anemia**   (P) _____ (R) _____ (S) _____

   anemia (ah-ne'me-ah; a condition without blood; clinically refers to a deficiency of erythrocytes)

9. **Pancytopenia**   (P) _____ (R) _____ (CV) ___ (S) _____

   pancytopenia (pan"si-to-pe'ne-ah; a deficiency of all cells; clinically refers to a deficiency of all blood cells)

10. **Leukocyte**   (P) _____ (CV) ___ (S) _____

    leukocyte (lu'ko-sīt; a white cell; clinically refers to white blood cells)

11. **Leukopenia**   (P) _____ (CV) ___ (S) _____

    leukopenia (lu"ko-pe'ne-ah; a deficiency of white; clinically refers to a deficiency of white blood cells)

12. Leukocytosis   (P) _____   (CV) ___   (R) _____   (CV) ___   (S) _____

leukocytosis (lu"ko-si-to'sis; a condition of white cells; clinically refers to increased numbers of white blood cells)

13. Neutropenia   (P) _____   (CV) ___   (S) _____

neutropenia (nu"tro-pe'ne-ah; a deficiency of neutrophils; clinically refers to decreased numbers of neutrophilic leukocytes in the blood)

14. Basophilic   (P) _____   (CV) ___   (R) _____   (S) _____

basophilic (ba-so-fil'ik: pertaining to blue affinity; clinically refers to things that stain readily with basic or blue dyes)

15. Eosinophilia   (P) _____   (CV) ___   (R) _____   (S) _____

eosinophilia (e"o-sin"o-fil'e-ah; a condition of red affinity; clinically refers to increased numbers of eosinophilic leukocytes in the blood)

16. Lymphocytosis   (R) _____   (CV) ___   (R) _____   (CV) ___   (S) _____

lymphocytosis (lim"fo-si-to'sis; a condition of lymph cells; clinically refers to increased numbers of lymphocytic leukocytes in the blood)

17. Monocytosis   (P) _____   (R) _____   (CV) ___   (S) _____

monocytosis (mon"o-si-to'sis; a condition of one cell; clinically refers to increased numbers of monocytic leukocytes in the blood)

18. Polymorphonuclear   (P) _____   (R) _____   (CV) ___   (R) _____   (S) _____

polymorphonuclear (pol"e-mor"fo-nu'kle-ar; pertaining to a multishaped nucleus)

19. Thrombocyte   (R) _____   (CV) ___   (S) _____

thrombocyte (throm'bo-sīt; a clot cell; clinically refers to blood platelets)

20. Hemostasis   (R) _____   (CV) ___   (S) _____

hemostasis (he"mo-sta'sis; the process of blood stoppage [i.e., the process of clotting])

21. Thrombus   (R) _____   (S) _____

thrombus (throm'bus; a clot)

22. Phagocyte   (R) _____   (CV) ___   (S) _____

phagocyte (fag'o-sīt; an eating cell; clinically refers to leukocytes that ingest foreign organisms and particles)

23. Macrophage   (P) _____   (CV) ___   (S) _____

macrophage (mak'ro-faj; a large eater; clinically refers to phagocytic leukocytes found wandering outside the bloodstream, in the tissues of the body)

24. **Anticoagulant**   (P) _____   (R) _____   (S) _____

anticoagulant (an"ti-ko-ag'u-lant; one that is against clotting; clinically refers to any chemical agent that prevents coagulation of blood)

25. **Hemolysis**   (R) _____   (CV) ___   (S) _____

hemolysis (he-mol'ĭ-sis; the process of destroying blood; clinically refers to lysis or breakage of erythrocytes)

26. **Hemorrhage**   (R) _____   (CV) ___   (S) _____

hemorrhage (hem'or-ij; escape of blood; i.e., bleeding)

27. **Hematoma**[1]   (R) _____   (S) _____

hematoma (he"mah-to'mah; a blood swelling; clinically refers to a localized accumulation of blood between tissues or tissue layers, due to a break in a blood vessel)

28. **Hematocrit**   (R) _____   (CV) ___   (S) _____

hematocrit (he-mat'o-krit; to separate blood)

29. **Megakaryocyte**   (P) _____   (R) _____   (CV) ___   (S) _____

megakaryocyte (meg"ah-kar'e-o-sīt; a large nucleated cell; clinically refers to a cell found in the bone marrow that contains a very large nucleus and from which platelets are formed)

30. **Poikilocytosis**   (R) _____   (CV) ___   (R) _____   (CV) ___   (S) _____

poikilocytosis (poi"kĭ-lo-si-to'sis; a condition of varied/irregular cells; clinically refers to varied shapes of erythrocytes)

4.2. Hematopoietic Anatomy and Physiology

4.2.1. WHOLE BLOOD

Blood is composed of a liquid component (*plasma*) and a cellular component. If whole blood, mixed with an *anticoagulant,* were left to stand in a tube over a period of time, these two major components would separate (Fig. 4–1). The heavier cellular component containing *erythrocytes, leukocytes,* and *thrombocytes* would settle in the tube. The transparent *plasma* would be left at the top of the tube. The erythrocytes, being the heaviest of the cells, would settle to the bottom, while the

---

[1]Note that the suffix *-oma* usually denotes the presence of a tumor. The suffix *-oma* is thought to have been originally adapted from the Greek word *onkoma,* meaning "a swelling." In the case of the word *hematoma,* the suffix meaning is derived from this early interpretation.

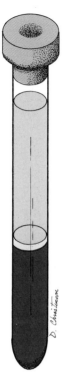

FIGURE 4–1. Whole blood components.

leukocytes and thrombocytes would form a thin layer between the erythrocytes and the plasma. This thin layer of leukocytes and thrombocytes is often referred to as the *"buffy coat."* In clinical practice, the settling of cells is hastened by the use of a centrifuge (*sen-trĭ-fūj'*). Whole blood is placed in a *hematocrit tube*; a clay plug in one end of the tube prevents the blood from escaping. The hematocrit tube is then placed into a centrifuge and spun at a very high rate of speed. The centrifugal force quickly forces the cells to the bottom (plugged end) of the hematocrit tube. The spun sample is removed from the centrifuge and measured. The measurement from the bottom to the top of the column of erythrocytes is called the *packed cell volume* (PCV; Fig. 4–2). The PCV, recorded as a percentage, is the percentage of erythrocytes compared to the total sample volume in the hematocrit tube (Fig. 4–3). Whole blood specimens must be carefully handled during and after collection to prevent *hemolysis. Hemolyzed* specimens render much of the laboratory testing invalid. Hemolyzed specimens may be quickly recognized because of the variable red discoloration of the plasma. The degree of discoloration depends on the amount of *hemoglobin (he-mo-glo'bin)* that is released into the plasma from destroyed erythrocytes.

Plasma is predominantly composed of water. Dissolved and suspended in that water are many proteins, lipids, sugars, and electrolytes. The concentration of these dissolved particles may be determined in many ways. One of the most

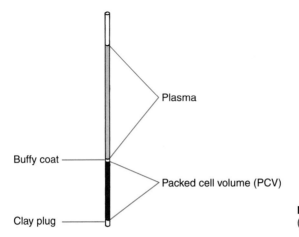

Plasma

Buffy coat

Packed cell volume (PCV)

Clay plug

FIGURE 4–2. Packed cell volume (PCV).

frequently used tests is for the determination of *total protein* (TP). Because proteins are building blocks for cells, the concentration of blood proteins reflects the general well-being of the body. Evaluation of the TP is simple. The column of plasma contained in a spun hematocrit tube is used for this determination. The plasma is placed on an instrument called a *refractometer (re"frak-tom'et-er;* so called because it uses the refraction of light through the sample to determine the concentration of particles in a solution). The greater the concentration of particles,

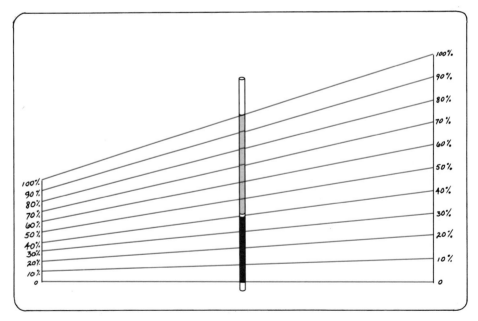

FIGURE 4–3. Spun hematocrit reading.

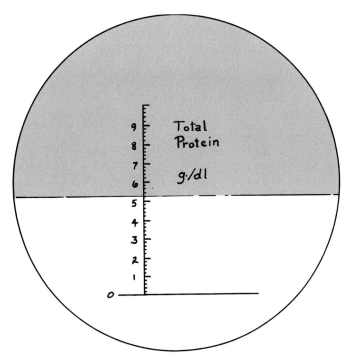

FIGURE 4–4. Total protein (TP) determination with a refractometer.

the more the light will be refracted or bent. The TP is read where the light intersects a calibrated scale within the instrument (Fig. 4–4). Both the TP and the PCV are valuable pieces of laboratory data for determining the health or disease state of veterinary patients. Quantitation of erythrocyte, leukocyte, and thrombocyte numbers, as well as evaluation of their *morphology*, are also of great diagnostic value.

4.2.2. BLOOD CELLS

Most of the blood cells are formed in the bone marrow by a process known as *hematopoiesis.* In general, only the more mature cells are found in the circulating blood. It is those mature cells in normal domestic animals that are discussed in this chapter.

Erythrocytes originate in the bone marrow. The kidney produces a hormone called *erythropoietin* that stimulates the bone marrow to produce erythrocytes. While in the bone marrow, the developing red blood cells are nuclear. Just prior to being released from the bone marrow, the erythrocytes discard their nuclei. Therefore, erythrocytes in the circulating blood of most domestic animals are

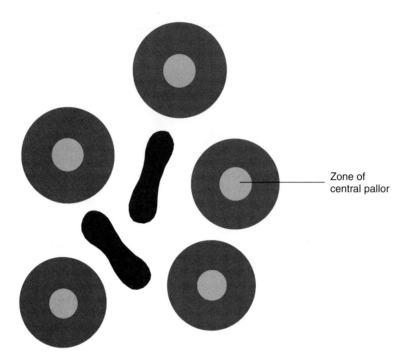

Zone of central pallor

FIGURE 4–5. Erythrocytes in circulating blood.

anuclear, biconcave, disc-shaped cells (Fig. 4–5). Erythrocytes contain a protein compound called *hemoglobin* that is essential for the transport of oxygen and carbon dioxide. The primary role of erythrocytes is to transport oxygen to the tissues of the body and carbon dioxide away from those tissues. It is the hemoglobin, when bound with oxygen, that gives the cells their red coloration. Hemoglobin when bound to carbon dioxide exhibits a darker bluish coloration, which may be seen grossly through the skin of animals. Laboratory *morphologic* evaluation of blood cells is important in determining the overall health status of the body. This morphologic evaluation is achieved through making a smear of the patient's blood on a glass microscopic slide. *Eosinophilic* and *basophilic* stains are then applied to the dried blood smear to enhance morphologic characteristics of the cells. Mature erythrocytes accept the eosinophilic stains and, therefore, appear red on a blood smear. Less mature, newly released erythrocytes are somewhat larger (*macrocytic*) than fully mature erythrocytes, and may stain with a slightly basophilic hue in addition to the red. This staining characteristic is reported clinically as *polychromasia. Anisocytosis* would also be noted in such a patient, as a result of the size variation between mature and immature erythrocytes (Fig. 4–6). Some of the *polychromatophilic* erythrocytes may still contain ribosomes and portions of the endoplasmic reticulum. Such red blood cells are called *reticulocytes*. Special staining procedures may be used to make the ribosomes and endoplasmic

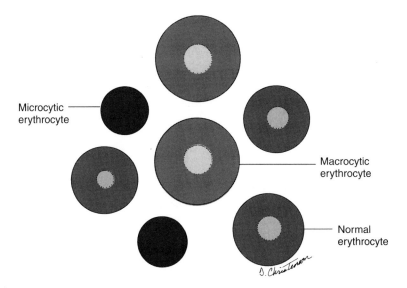

Microcytic
erythrocyte

Macrocytic
erythrocyte

Normal
erythrocyte

D. Christenson

FIGURE 4–6. Anisocytosis.

reticulum of the reticulocytes visible microscopically, allowing for quantitation of these cells (Fig. 4–7). Reticulocyte counts are valuable for determining the bone marrow's ability to respond in *anemic* states. When studying the blood smear of an anemic patient, identification of reticulocytes and polychromasia are considered positive signs for the patient because they show that the bone marrow is trying to respond to the loss of mature erythrocytes.

Many different types of leukocytes are produced by the bone marrow. All are larger than erythrocytes. The three *granulocytes* are the *neutrophil,* the *basophil,* and the *eosinophil.* They are referred to as "granulocytes" because they each contain many cytoplasmic granules. Each specific name is indicative of the staining characteristics of the cytoplasmic granules of the cell type. The neutrophil is so named because its granules do not readily accept stain, rendering a neutral coloration to them. Basophils contain basophilic cytoplasmic granules. Last, eosinophils contain many eosinophilic cytoplasmic granules. In most domestic animals, the neutrophils comprise the largest portion of the circulating leukocytes. *Agranular*[2] leukocytes are the *monocyte* and the *lymphocyte.* Each of these different leukocytes plays a somewhat different role in the fighting of disease.

Morphologically, **neutrophils** are *polymorphonuclear* (Fig. 4–8). That is to say, the nucleus of the neutrophil tends to take many shapes, but is usually very linear, curved, and somewhat lobulated. The nuclear chromatin of a mature neutrophil is very condensed, rendering a characteristic dark purple staining. The

---

[2]Agranular: A- (without) + granul(o) + -ar; pertaining to without granules.

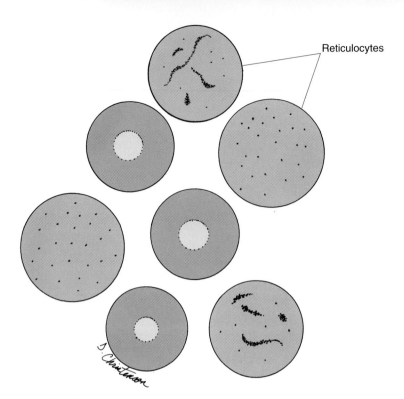

Reticulocytes

FIGURE 4–7. Reticulocytes.

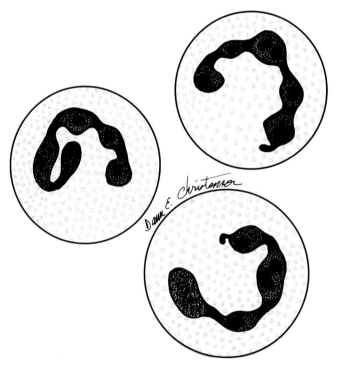

FIGURE 4–8. Neutrophils.

cytoplasm and granules are colorless to a very slight pink hue. This makes it difficult to visualize clearly distinct granules in the neutrophil, especially if the microscope is improperly illuminated. Neutrophils are important in ridding the body of foreign invaders. Their cytoplasmic granules contain potent enzymes, thus giving the neutrophil powerful phagocytic capabilities.

The other important phagocyte is the **monocyte**. The monocyte is the largest of the leukocytes (Fig. 4–9). The nucleus tends to be large and potentially multilobed, with a very loose, lightly basophilic staining chromatin pattern. The abundant cytoplasm of the monocyte is a homogenous, light gray color. Although monocytes may contain vacuoles, this is a very unreliable criterion for cell identification. Functionally, both monocytes and neutrophils can slip through blood vessel walls to provide phagocytic services out in the tissues of the body. Once these cells have left the circulating blood, they are referred to as *macrophages*.

Eosinophils have only marginal phagocytic abilities. Like the neutrophils, they are polymorphonuclear. However, the eosinophil's nucleus characteristically stains lighter than that of the neutrophil. The eosinophilic staining granules are important in allergic-type reactions (Fig. 4–10 on p. 58). **Basophils** are morphologically similar to neutrophils and eosinophils. The basophilic staining gran-

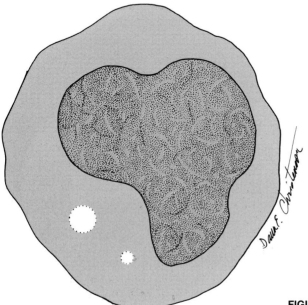

FIGURE 4–9. Monocyte.

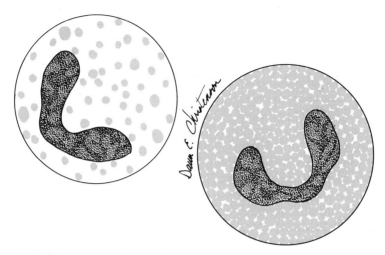

FIGURE 4–10. Eosinophils.

ules of basophils are also important in allergic-type reactions (Fig. 4–11). Generally, basophils have fewer cytoplasmic granules than the other granulocytes, and their cytoplasm stains lightly basophilic.

Lymphocytes, depending on their age, may range in size from just smaller than a monocyte to just larger than an erythrocyte (Fig. 4–12). The younger the lymphocyte, the larger it is, and the older the lymphocyte, the smaller it is, with very little cytoplasm. The nuclear morphology tends to be round to ovoid, with varying degrees of chromatin density. The condensation and dark, basophilic staining qualities of the nucleus increase with the age of the lymphocyte. The cy-

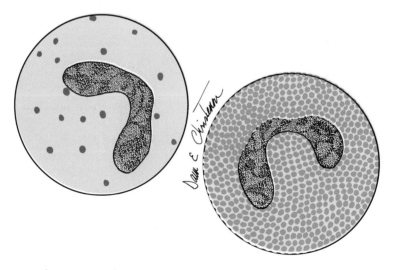

FIGURE 4–11. Basophils.

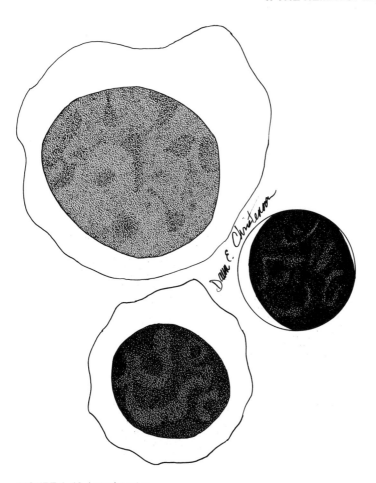

FIGURE 4–12. Lymphocytes.

toplasm is usually colorless, but may have a thin basophilic rim around its outer edges. Lymphocytes are important for body immunity and the production of *antibodies*. Antibodies are specialized proteins that when attached to foreign invaders, help the body recognize and rid itself of the invaders.

Thrombocytes, or *platelets*, are actually nuclear fragments of large, specialized cells (*megakaryocytes*) that are found in the bone marrow. These fragments, in the peripheral blood, generally appear as anuclear, mottled, lavender-staining objects (Fig. 4–13 on p. 60). They are much smaller than erythrocytes. As their name implies, thrombocytes are important for clot formation.

4.2.3. HEMOSTASIS

Hemostasis is the process by which *hemorrhage* is stopped. This happens in several stages. First, immediately after a blood vessel is injured, the smooth muscle in

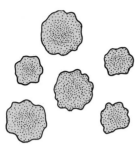

FIGURE 4–13. Thrombocytes.

that vessel constricts. This constriction makes the lumen of the vessel much smaller, thereby slowing the flow of blood from the wound. The thrombocytes tend to stick to exposed connective tissues surrounding the vessel. Soon, many platelets find themselves stuck to the edges of the wound and to each other, forming what is called a *platelet plug*. Until the platelet plug is formed, blood from a superficial vessel may ooze out under the skin, creating a *hematoma*. Once the platelet plug is formed, hemorrhage at the site ceases. The plug, however, is somewhat fragile and be dislodged easily. Therefore, many of the plasma proteins, specifically designed for coagulation, begin to coalesce and form a strong matrix of fibers that secure the platelet plug at the wound site. The ultimate *thrombus* that is formed contracts with the healing wound and is dissolved over time.

These same clotting mechanisms can be used to our advantage in the laboratory. Many blood chemistry tests cannot be run on plasma or whole blood. For such tests, the whole blood specimen is placed into a plain (i.e., not containing anticoagulant) blood tube. The sample is left undisturbed for a period of time, permitting it to clot. The plasma proteins coalesce, forming a strong matrix of fibers that entraps most of the cells in the sample. The final clot can be easily removed from the sample. Any remaining cells can be centrifuged out, leaving the transparent liquid called *serum*. This serum may now be used for numerous serum chemistry tests. If one were to compare the TP of serum to that of plasma, serum would contain far less protein than the plasma. This makes sense, because many of the proteins have been removed from the serum as a result of the clot formation.

4.2.4. DISEASE

Various diseases have different effects on the whole body, including the hematopoietic system. In general, one would expect the body to respond to the presence of pathogenic organisms by producing sufficient numbers of leukocytes to fight the invaders. Therefore, in many instances overwhelming numbers of white blood cells are released from the bone marrow, creating a *leukocytosis*. Once the pathogenic organisms are removed from the body, leukocyte numbers in the circulating blood return to normal. Some diseases, such as *Feline Panleukopenia,* render the body incapable of producing sufficient numbers of leukocytes to defend against the pathogenic organism. Cats with this disease cannot defend against the panleukopenia virus, and, because of the insufficient numbers of leukocytes, they cannot defend against secondary invading organisms such as bacteria. Other disease entities may affect only one specific cell type. For this reason, *differential counts* of the various cell types are important diagnostic tools. Concurrent changes in the numbers of the different leukocyte types may be indicative of specific disease conditions. For instance, although a *neutropenia* with an accompanying *lymphocytosis* may be indicative of one disease, an *eosinophilia* and an accompanying *monocytosis* may be indicative of another. Erythrocytes are also important indicators of disease conditions within veterinary patients. One would expect to see decreased numbers of erythrocytes on a blood smear from a patient with a *hemolytic anemia* or a patient with *hemorrhagic anemia.* Morphologically, the erythrocytes seen in the two types of anemia are quite different. Polychromasia and anisocytosis may be present in both types of anemia. However, the *poikilocytosis* present in the hemolytic anemia distinguishes it from a hemorrhagic anemia. Fragmentation of erythrocytes is often a characteristic of hemolytic anemias. Recognizing these differences is important not only for determining a specific diagnosis but for determining appropriate medical management of the patients as well. The medical management of these anemic patients is markedly different. Certainly, patients at the opposite end of the spectrum with *polycythemia* will present their own diagnostic and medical management challenges. It is through *hematology* that many diseases are identified, with painstaking acquisition of minute clues that may be found only in the blood.

4.3. Self-Test

Using the previous information in this chapter, respond to each of the following questions using the most appropriate medical term(s). Do not use abbreviations.

1. _____ are anuclear, biconcave, discoid blood cells whose primary function is the transport of oxygen to the tissues of the body.

2. _____ are granulocytes whose cytoplasmic granules do not readily accept stains and whose primary function is phagocytosis of foreign invaders of the body.

3. The largest of the white blood cells that is agranular and has phagocytic capabilities is the _____.

4. A(n) _____ is a swelling beneath the skin caused by a localized accumulation of blood.

5. The fluid component of the blood that suspends all of the cellular constituents and is rich in electrolytes and proteins is the _____.

6. Rough and improper handling of whole blood specimens has a destructive effect on the cells, which is clinically referred to as _____.

7. The blood cells that are collectively responsible for fighting disease in the body are the

_____.

8. The _____ is a specific granulocyte that contains red-staining cytoplasmic granules and is often involved in allergic responses.

9. Platelets or _____ are small, anuclear cell fragments involved in blood clotting.

10. _____ is the process by which hemorrhage is stopped.

11. The _____ is a type of white blood cell responsible for immunity and antibody production. It has a round to ovoid nucleus, and the generally colorless cytoplasm often stains with a thin basophilic rim at the periphery of the cell.

12. Clinically, numbers of white blood cells in excess of the normal range would be referred to as a(n) _____.

13. Diseases that impair the bone marrow's ability to produce white blood cells of all types would result in markedly reduced numbers of those cells in circulation. The resulting cellular deficiency would be medically termed a(n) _____.

14. Excessive numbers of the granulocyte with blue-staining granules would be clinically referred to as a(n) _____.

15. _____ is the intracellular protein compound of red blood cells that combines with oxygen, facilitating its transport throughout the body.

16. _____ are the cells that comprise the largest cellular portion of a spun hematocrit or packed cell volume.

17. A(n) _____ is any chemical agent that, when combined with whole blood, prevents clotting.

18. _____ are young red blood cells that still contain remnants of their ribosomes and endoplasmic reticulum.

19. Deficient numbers of platelets in the circulating blood is clinically referred to as a(n)

_____.

20. The morphologic term that refers to the variation in size of the red blood cells is

_____.

21. In a blood specimen, if the sample is permitted to clot, using up many of the proteins/clotting factors, the transparent fluid that is left is called _____.

22. A bone marrow disorder that impairs the marrow's ability to produce all blood cell types results in a(n) _____.

23. A patient's condition in which the individual has inadequate numbers of red blood cells due to hemorrhage is medically termed _____.

24. The packed cell volume (PCV) is the measure of the column of red blood cells compared to total sample volume in the _____ tube. The PCV is recorded as a percentage.

25. Abnormal shape changes due to fragmentation of red blood cells is medically termed

_____.

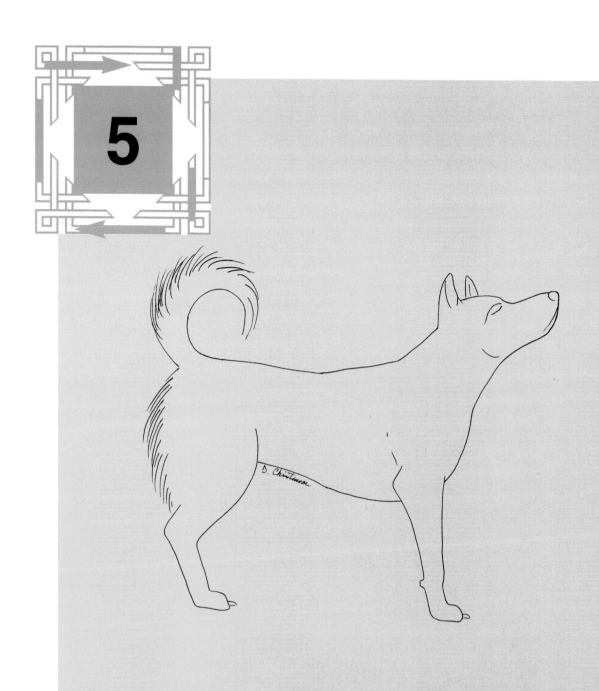

The Lymphatic System

GOALS AND OBJECTIVES

By the conclusion of this chapter, the student will be able to:

1. Recognize common root words, prefixes, and suffixes related to the lymphatic system.
2. Divide simple and compound words into their respective parts.
3. Recognize, correctly pronounce, and appropriately use common medical terms related to the lymphatic system.
4. Demonstrate an understanding of the basic anatomy and physiology of the lymphatic system.
5. Demonstrate an understanding of the lymphatic system as it relates to edema formation.
6. Demonstrate an understanding of the basic role of the lymphatic system in immunity.

5.1. Introduction to Related Terms

Divide each of the following terms into its respective parts ("R" root, "P" prefix, "S" suffix, "CV" combining vowel).

1. **Lymphadenopathy** (R) _lymph_ (R) _aden_ (CV) _o_ (S) _pathy_

   lymphadenopathy (lim-fad"ĕ-nop'ah-the; disease of the lymph glands; clinically refers to enlarged lymph nodes)

2. **Splenic**   (R) _splen_ (S) _ic_

   splenic (splen'ik; pertaining to the spleen)

3. **Lymphangitis**   (R) _lymph_ (R) _ang_ (S) _itis_

   lymphangitis (lim"fan-ji'tis; inflammation of lymph vessels)

4. **Lymphocyte**   (R) _lymph_ (CV) _o_ (S) _cyte_

   lymphocyte (lim'fo-sīt; a lymph cell)

5. **Splenomegaly**   (R) _splen_ (CV) _o_ (S) _megaly_

   splenomegaly (splĕ"no-meg'ah-le; a condition of splenic enlargement)

6. **Interstitial**   (P) _inter_ (R) _stiti_ (S) _al_

   interstitial (in"ter-stish'al; pertaining to between tissues)

7. **Macrophage**   (P) _macr_ (CV) _o_ (S) _phage_

   macrophage (mak'ro-faj; a large eater; clinically refers to large phagocytic cells)

8. **Phagocytosis**   (R) _phag_ (CV) _o_ (R) _cyt_ (S) _osis_

   phagocytosis (fag"o-si-to'sis; the process of cellular eating)

9. **Pathogenic**   (R) _path_ (CV) _o_ (R) _gen_ (S) _ic_

   pathogenic (path-o-jen'ik; pertaining to disease production)

10. **Tonsillectomy**   (R) _tonsill_ (S) _ectomy_

    tonsillectomy (ton"sĭ-lek'to-me; cutting out the tonsils; clinically interpreted as surgical excision of the tonsils)

11. **Tonsillitis**   (R) _tonsill_ (S) _itis_

    tonsillitis (ton"sĭ-li'tis; inflammation of the tonsils)

12. **Lymphoid**   (R) _lymph_ (S) _oid_

    lymphoid (lim'foid; resembling lymph)

5.2. Lymphatic Anatomy and Physiology

5.2.1. GENERAL

The lymphatic system is composed of the *tonsils, spleen, thymus (thi'mus)*, numerous glands, vessels, and cells that provide the body with *immunity* (resistance to disease) and destroy *pathogens*. The lymphatic system is also important for the constant transport of fluid (lymph) from the *interstitial* spaces to the general circulating blood.

5.2.2. TONSILS

The tonsils are made up of *lymphoid* tissue but they are not referred to as lymph nodes. Anatomically, the two tonsils are located in the throat (one tonsil on each side, near the base of the tongue; Fig. 5–1). Unless a disease process is present to create *tonsillitis*, they are usually contained (hidden) within the *tonsillar crypts* in the throat. Therefore, during physical examination of a normal patient, the tonsils

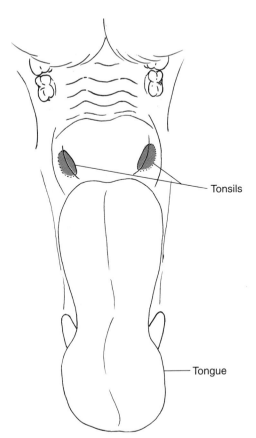

Tonsils

Tongue

FIGURE 5–1. Tonsils.

may not be visible. For those animals with persistent tonsillitis, such that it interferes with swallowing or breathing, a *tonsillectomy* may be performed.

5.2.3. SPLEEN

The spleen is a large, tongue-shaped organ located in the left craniodorsal abdominal cavity, closely associated with the stomach and protected by the caudal rib cage (Fig. 5–2). On routine physical examination, the spleen is not palpable in the abdomen unless *splenomegaly* exists. The spleen is highly vascular and contains many *macrophages*. The *splenic* macrophages are very important for repairing or removing damaged red blood cells from circulation. The splenic macrophages are also very important for *phagocytosis* of *pathogenic* organisms found in the blood. Last, the spleen serves as a storage area for red blood cells.

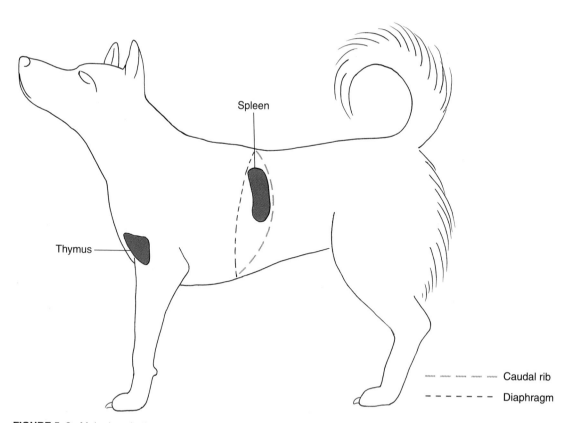

FIGURE 5–2. Major lymphatic organs.

5.2.4. THYMUS

The thymus is a glandular lymphoid organ located midline in the cranioventral thoracic cavity (see Fig. 5–2). The thymus is extremely important for the maturation of specialized *lymphocytes*. The lymphocytes that mature in the thymus are critical for the production of *antibodies*. Antibodies are specialized proteins that help the body recognize pathogenic organisms, so that macrophages can destroy the pathogens. Therefore, the thymus plays an integral role in the maintenance of immunity for the body. Interestingly, the thymus is quite large in young, developing animals. As animals age, the size and function of the thymus diminish. Consequently, the immune capabilities of very young and of geriatric animals is compromised. The very young have not yet produced sufficient amounts of antibodies, and geriatric animals no longer have the capacity to maintain sufficient antibody levels. This leaves these patients very susceptible to disease.

5.2.5. LYMPH NODES AND VESSELS

Lymph glands (also called *lymph nodes*) are located throughout the body. Many of them are named by virtue of the region of the body in which they are located. For example, lymph nodes located in the axillary region are called *axillary lymph nodes*.[1] Those peripheral lymph nodes that are clinically important for physical examinations in small animal medicine are the axillary lymph nodes, the *mandibular lymph nodes*,[2] the *prescapular lymph nodes*,[3] the *popliteal lymph nodes*,[4] and the *superficial inguinal lymph nodes*[5] (Fig. 5–3). The mandibular, prescapular, and popliteal lymph nodes should always be palpated during a physical examination of a small animal patient. Although palpation of the axillary, superficial

---

[1]Axillary *(ak'sĭ-lar"e; pertaining to the axilla)*; the axilla, also referred to as the "armpit" in humans, is that ventral region where the forelimb adjoins the thoracic wall; axillary lymph nodes are those lymph glands located deep in the tissues of the axilla.

[2]Mandibular *(man-dib'u-lar; pertaining to the mandible)*; the mandible is the lower jaw bone; mandibular lymph nodes are located caudoventral to the mandible.

[3]Prescapular *(pre-skap'u-lar; pertaining to before the scapula)*; prescapular lymph nodes are located craniomedial to the shoulder joint. For more information regarding the scapula and the shoulder joint, see Chapter 6 ("The Musculoskeletal System").

[4]Popliteal *(pop-lit'e-al, pop"lĭ-te'-al; pertaining to the "ham"* ["ham" is acquired from the semimembranosus/semitendinosus muscles of the caudal thigh]); popliteal lymph nodes are located caudal to the stifle (femorotibial) joint. For more information regarding the stifle joint, see Chapter 6 ("The Musculoskeletal System").

[5]Inguinal *(ing'gwĭ-nal; pertaining to the inguen [groin])*; the inguen is that ventral region where the hindlimb adjoins the abdominal wall; superficial inguinal lymph nodes are located deep in the tissues of the inguen.

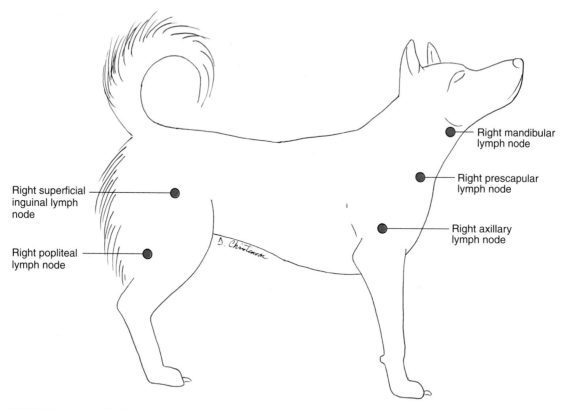

FIGURE 5–3. Superficial lymph nodes.

inguinal, and *mesenteric lymph nodes*[6] should be attempted, they may be felt only if lymphadenopathy is present. Many other lymph nodes are present throughout the thoracic cavity (*mediastinal lymph nodes*[7]). Obviously, the rib cage prohibits palpation of these latter glands. *Lymphadenopathy* of mediastinal nodes may be detected radiographically if significant enlargement is present.

---

[6]Mesenteric *(mes"en-ter'ik; pertaining to the mesentery)*; the mesentery is a tissue found in the abdominal cavity that provides support and attachments for the abdominal viscera; mesenteric lymph nodes are located in multiple sites throughout the mesentery. For more information regarding the mesentery, see Chapter 12 ("The Alimentary System").

[7]Mediastinal *(me"de-as-ti'nal; pertaining to the mediastinum)*; the mediastinum is a tissue found in the thoracic cavity that divides that cavity into right and left halves; mediastinal lymph nodes are located in multiple sites throughout the mediastinum. For more information regarding the mediastinum, see Chapter 8 ("The Respiratory System").

Lymph nodes are small, glandular structures that are partly responsible for the production of lymphocytes. Connected by an intricate network of lymphatic vessels, the lymph nodes are responsible for filtration of lymphatic fluid. Macrophages located in the lymph nodes phagocytize pathogenic organisms from the lymphatic fluid. It should be noted that, unlike blood, lymphatic fluid does not flow in response to pressure within the lymphatic system. Lymphatic fluid is passively absorbed from the *interstitium* into the lymphatic vessels. Gravity and movement of the muscles and other tissues that closely approximate the lymphatic vessels force the fluid to flow passively. Unidirectional (one-way) valves within the vessels keeps the fluid flowing in one direction. Ultimately, lymphatic fluid flows until it finds its way to the general circulating blood.

5.2.6. EDEMA

All of the tissues of the body are bathed in *interstitial fluid*. This fluid is constantly percolating through the tissues. It originates predominantly from capillaries (*cap-ĭ-lar-ēz*). Capillaries are the smallest blood vessels of the body, made up of simple squamous endothelium. The capillary structure facilitates diffusion of some molecules (O_2 and CO_2) and minor, normal "leakage" of fluid from the bloodstream. The constant replenishment of interstitial fluid ensures cellular respiration and nutritional support for even the most remote tissues of the body.

Excessive accumulation of interstitial fluid is clinically referred to as *edema* (*ĕ-de'mah;* swelling). If the lymphatic system is diseased in some way (e.g., *lymphadenopathy* or *lymphangitis*), it may not be able to accommodate the routine production and flow of the interstitial fluid. Absorption of the fluid into the lymphatic vessels may be impaired, or flow of lymphatic fluid within those vessels may be significantly impaired due to obstruction. In either case, interstitial fluid builds up and is clinically recognized as edema. One should realize that many other mechanisms may contribute to edema formation. Some of those mechanisms include lymphatic disease, changes in osmotic[8] pressures (e.g., hypoproteinemia—a condition of low protein in the blood), changes in hydrostatic pressures (e.g., pulmonary [lung] edema due to congestive heart failure), and inflammation due to tissue trauma. Often, edema results from a combination of causative factors. Knowledge of the lymphatic system's function may be very useful clinically for the prevention of or reduction of edema.

---

[8]Osmosis is the movement of water across a semipermeable membrane, from an area of low particle numbers to an area of high particle numbers. In essence, water moves to dilute an area of high particle concentration.

5.3. Self-Test

Using the previous information in this chapter, respond to each of the following questions using the most appropriate medical term(s).

1. The _____ lymph nodes are located caudal to the stifle joint.

2. __leukocytes antibodies__ are specialized proteins produced by lymphocytes that help the body recognize disease producing organisms.

3. Excessive accumulation of interstitial fluid is clinically referred to as ___edema___.

4. Splenic ___macrophage___ are large, phagocytic cells responsible for repairing or removing damaged red blood cells from circulation as well as removing disease-producing organisms from the blood.

5. Disease-producing organisms are medically referred to as ___pathogens___.

6. The ___thymadnus___, located in the cranioventral chest cavity, is responsible for the maturation of specialized lymphocytes and maintenance of immunity.

7. The _____ lymph nodes are located craniomedial to the shoulder joint.

8. _____, or an inflammation of the lymphatic vessels, could contribute to the formation of excess interstitial fluid.

9. Splenic enlargement is medically termed _____.

10. Inflammation of the tonsils is medically termed ___tonsillitis___.

11. A(n) ___tonsilectomy___ is a surgical procedure involving the removal of the tonsils.

12. The ___Spleen___ is a large, tongue-shaped lymphatic organ located in the left craniodorsal abdominal cavity that serves as a storage area for red blood cells.

13. Enlargement of the lymph glands is clinically referred to as _____.

14. The _____ lymph nodes are located in the "armpit" region of animals, and are not usually palpable unless enlarged.

15. The _____ lymph nodes are located in the "groin" region of animals, and are not usually palpable unless enlarged.

16. A(n) _____ is a surgical procedure involving excision of the spleen.

17. __Osmosis_____ is the movement of water across a semipermeable membrane from an area of low particle concentration to an area of high particle concentration.

18. __Capillaries_____ are the smallest blood vessels of the body and are composed of simple squamous endothelium.

19. __interstitial_____ fluid is found percolating through all tissues of the body in the intercellular spaces.

20. Resistance to disease is referred to as __immunity_____. This quality is provided through the lymphatic system.

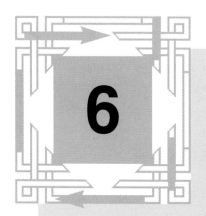

6

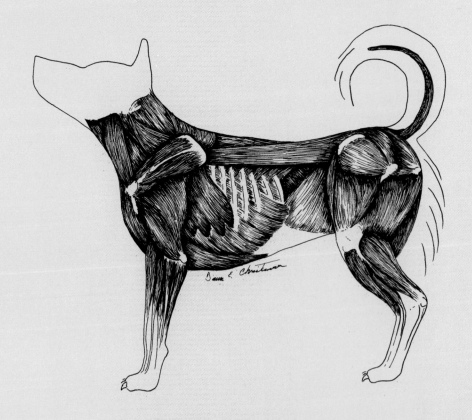

The Musculoskeletal System

GOALS AND OBJECTIVES

By the conclusion of this chapter, the student will be able to:

1. Recognize common root words, prefixes, and suffixes related to the musculoskeletal system.

2. Divide simple and compound words into their respective parts.

3. Recognize, correctly pronounce, and appropriately use common medical terms related to the musculoskeletal system.

4. Recognize major bones and joints of domestic animals.

5. Translate/compare musculoskeletal anatomy of the dog to that of a horse.

6. Recognize the parts of a bone.

7. Demonstrate a basic understanding of bone growth and repair.

8. Demonstrate an understanding of joint anatomy and function.

9. Recognize major muscle groups and common intramuscular injection sites of domestic animals.

10. Recognize common types of traumatic fractures.

6.1. Introduction to Related Terms

6.1.1. LIMB ANATOMY

The musculoskeletal system is composed of numerous muscles and bones. The bones provide support for muscles and other tissues of the body. They also provide protection for vital organs, such as the brain and thoracic viscera. Many joints of the body are named using the names of the bones that form the joint (*articulate*). Figure 6–1 identifies many of the bones of the canine limbs. Review the illustration and the descriptions that follow to familiarize yourself with canine limb anatomy before completing part 6.1.2. of this introductory section.

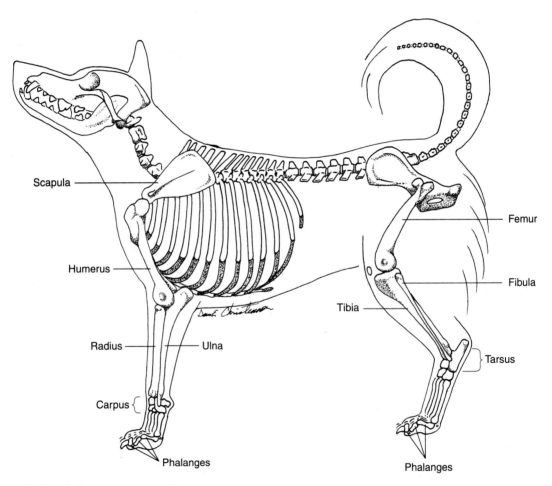

FIGURE 6–1. Bones of the canine limb.

1. Scapula (*skap'u-lah*)

   The *scapula* is a flat bone that is the most proximal bone of the forelimb. The thin, bony ridge found on its lateral surface is referred to as the *spine of the scapula*. The distal end of the scapula articulates with the humerus to form the shoulder joint.

2. Humerus (*hu'mer-us*)

   The *humerus* is a long bone of the proximal forelimb (i.e., *brachium*[1]). The proximal end of the humerus articulates with the scapula to form the shoulder joint. The distal end of the humerus articulates with the radius and ulna bones to form the elbow joint.

3. Radius (*ra'de-us*)

   The *radius* is a long bone of the forelimb (i.e., *antebrachium*[2]). The radius lies on the cranial aspect of the antebrachium. The proximal end of the radius articulates with the humerus to form, in part, the elbow joint. The distal end of the radius articulates with the bones of the carpus.

4. Ulna (*ul'nah*)

   The *ulna* is a long bone of the antebrachium. The ulna lies on the caudal aspect of the antebrachium. The proximal end of the ulna articulates with the humerus to form, in part, the elbow joint. On the caudal aspect of its proximal end, the ulna has a large, bony protuberance or process, the *olecranon* (*o-lek'rah-non*) which forms the *point of the elbow*. The distal end of the ulna articulates with the bones of the carpus.

5. Carpus (*kar'pus*)

   The *carpus* is a joint of the distal forelimb. It is composed of numerous small, short bones. The proximal border of the carpus articulates with the radius and ulna.

6. Phalanx (*fa'lanks*)

   A *phalanx* is a small bone of the foot. Each *digit* (*dij'it;* toe) is composed of three *phalanges* (*fah-lan'jēz*).

7. Femur (*fe'mur*)

   The *femur* is a long bone of the proximal hindlimb (i.e., thigh). The proximal end of the femur articulates with the pelvis to form the hip. On the lateral aspect of the proximal femur is a large, bony protuberance called the *greater trochanter* (*tro-kan'ter*). The distal end of the femur articulates with the tibia to form the stifle (*sti'ful*) joint.

8. Tibia (*tib'e-ah*)

   The *tibia* is a long bone of the hindlimb (i.e., *crus*[3]). The proximal end of the tibia articulates with the femur to form the stifle joint. The distal end of the tibia articulates with the tarsus.

---

[1]Brachium (*bra'ke-um;* [L. *brachium,* "arm"]); the proximal portion of the forelimb between the shoulder and elbow joints.

[2]Antebrachium (*an"te-bra'ke-um;* [*ante-* "before" + *brachium*]); the portion of the forelimb between the elbow and carpal joints.

[3]Crus (*krus;* [L. *crus,* "leg"]); the portion of the hindlimb between the stifle and tarsal joints.

9. Fibula (*fib'u-lah*)

The *fibula* is a thin, long bone of the crus. It lies lateral to the tibia. The proximal end of the fibula, in most domestic animals, falls just short of the stifle joint. The distal end of the fibula articulates with the tarsus.

10. Tarsus (*tahr'sus*)

The *tarsus* is a joint of the distal hindlimb. It is composed of numerous, small, short bones. The proximal border of the tarsus articulates with the tibia and fibula.

6.1.2. WORD EXERCISES

Divide each of the following terms into its respective parts ("R" root, "P" prefix, "S" suffix, "CV" combining vowel).

1. **Scapulohumeral**   (R) scapul   (CV) o (R) humer (S) al

scapulohumeral (*skap"u-lo-hu'mer-al; pertaining to the scapula and humerus; anatomically refers to the shoulder joint*)

2. **Humeroradioulnar**

(R) humer (CV) o (R) radi (CV) o (R) uln (S) ar

humeroradioulnar (*hu"mer-o-ra"de-o-ul'nar; pertaining to the humerus, radius, and ulna; anatomically refers to the elbow joint*)

3. **Carpal**   (R) carp (S) al

carpal (*kar'pal; pertaining to the carpus*)

4. **Metacarpal**   (P) meta (R) carp (S) al

metacarpal (*met"ah-kar'pal; pertaining to beyond/after the carpus; anatomically refers to the portion of the distal forelimb that lies between the carpus and the phalanges*)

5. **Metacarpophalangeal**

(P) meta (R) carp (CV) o (R) phang (CV) e (S) al

metacarpophalangeal (*met"ah-kar"po-fah-lan'je-al; pertaining to the metacarpus and phalanges; anatomically refers to any joint formed by a metacarpal bone and a phalanx*)

6. **Interphalangeal**   (P) inter (R) phalang (CV) e (S) al

interphalangeal (*in"ter-fah-lan'je-al; pertaining to between the phalanges; anatomically refers to those joints formed by phalanges*)

7. **Coxofemoral**   (R) cox (CV) o (R) femor (S) al

coxofemoral (*kok"so-fem'o-ral; pertaining to the hip and femur; anatomically refers to the hip joint*)

8. **Femorotibial**   (R) <u>femor</u> (CV) <u>o</u>   (R) <u>tibi</u>   (S) <u>al</u>

femorotibial (fem"o-ro-tib'e-al; pertaining to the femur and tibia; anatomically refers to the stifle joint)

9. **Tarsal**   (R) <u>tars</u>   (S) <u>al</u>

tarsal (tahr'sal; pertaining to the tarsus)

10. **Metatarsal**   (P) <u>meta</u>   (R) <u>tars</u>   (S) <u>al</u>

metatarsal (met"ah-tar'sal; pertaining to beyond/after the tarsus; anatomically refers to that portion of the distal hindlimb that lies between the tarsus and the phalanges)

11. **Metatarsophalangeal**

(P) <u>meta</u>   (R) <u>tars</u>   (CV) <u>o</u>   (R) <u>phalang</u>   (CV) <u>e</u>   (S) <u>al</u>

metatarsophalangeal (met"ah-tar"so-fah-lan'je-al; pertaining to the metatarsus and phalanges; anatomically refers to any joint formed by a metatarsal bone and a phalanx)

12. **Cervical**   (R) <u>cervic</u>   (S) <u>al</u>

cervical (ser'vǐ-kal; pertaining to the neck)

13. **Intervertebral**   (P) <u>inter</u>   (R) <u>vertebr</u> (S) <u>al</u>

intervertebral (in"ter-ver'tě-bral, in"ter-ver-te'bral; pertaining to between vertebrae;[4] anatomically refers to the joints formed between the bones of the spinal column)

14. **Lumbosacral**   (R) <u>lumb</u>   (CV) <u>o</u>   (R) <u>sacr</u>   (S) <u>al</u>

lumbosacral (lum"bo-sa'kral; pertaining to the lumbus and sacrum; anatomically refers to the joint formed by the last lumbar vertebra and the sacrum)

15. **Coccygeal**   (R) <u>coccyg</u>   (CV) <u>e</u>   (S) <u>al</u>

coccygeal (kok-sij'e-al; pertaining to the coccyx; anatomically refers to the tail)

16. **Epaxial**   (P) <u>ep</u>   (R) <u>axi</u>   (S) <u>al</u>

epaxial (ep-ak'se-al; pertaining to upon the axis; anatomically refers to the region along the dorsal vertebral column)

17. **Intercostal**   (P) <u>inter</u>   (R) <u>cost</u>   (S) <u>al</u>

intercostal (in"ter-kos'tal; pertaining to between ribs; anatomically refers to the spaces found between ribs)

---

[4]Vertebra (ver'tě-brah), singular; vertebrae (ver'tě-bre), plural.

18. **Costochondral**   (R) _Cost_   (CV) _O_   (R) _chond_   (S) _al_

costochondral (kos"to-kon'dral; pertaining to rib cartilage; anatomically refers to the cartilage which connects the bony ribs to the sternum)

19. **Sternal**   (R) _stern_   (S) _al_

sternal (ster'nal; pertaining to the sternum)

20. **Epiphysis[5]**   (P) _epiphy_   (R) _physis_

epiphysis (e-pif'ĭ-sis; to grow upon; anatomically refers to the end of a long bone, usually covered with cartilage)

21. **Metaphysis[6]**   (P) _meta_   (R) _physis_

metaphysis (me-taf'ĭ-sis; to grow beyond; anatomically refers to the wider portion of the shaft of a long bone that is found at each end and is adjacent to the epiphysis)

22. **Diaphysis**   (P) _dia_   (R) _physis_

diaphysis (di-af'ĭ-sis; to grow between; anatomically refers to the shaft of a long bone)

23. **Periosteal**   (P) _peri_   (R) _oste_   (S) _al_

periosteal (per"e-os'te-al; pertaining to around bone; anatomically refers to the periosteum, a specialized connective tissue that covers the outer surfaces of all bones)

24. **Endosteum**   (P) _endo_   (R) _oste_   (S) _um_

endosteum (en-dos'te-um; within bone; anatomically it is the specialized tissue membrane that covers the interior surfaces of all bones)

25. **Synovial**   (P) _syn_   (R) _ovi_   (S) _al_

synovial (sĭ-no've-al; pertaining to with egg; anatomically refers to the synovia, a thick, transparent fluid that is found in joints and resembles egg whites)

26. **Arthritis**   (R) _arthr_   (S) _itis_

arthritis (ar-thri'tis; inflammation of a joint)

27. **Myositis[7]**   (R) _myos_   (S) _itis_

myositis (mi"o-si'tis; inflammation of muscle)

---

[5]Epiphysis, singular; epiphyses (e-pif'ĭ-sēz), plural.

[6]Metaphysis, singular; metaphyses (me-taf'ĭ-sēz), plural.

[7]Myositis: note that the root myos- is derived from [Gr. myos muscle]. In general, the combining form used to indicate muscle is my(o)-.

28. **Orthopedic** (R) _Orth_ (CV) _O_ (R) _ped_ (S) _ic_

    orthopedic (or"tho-pe'dik; pertaining to straightening a child; clinically refers to the correction of deformities of the musculoskeletal system)

29. **Flexion** (R) _flex_ (S) _ion_

    flexion (flek'shun; the act of bending)

30. **Extension** (P) _ex_ (R) _ten_ (S) _sion_

    extension (ek-sten'shun; the act of out-stretching)

31. **Abduction** (P) _ab_ (R) _duc_ (S) _tion_

    abduction (ab-duk'shun; the act of abducting; to draw away; ab- = away)

32. **Adduction** (P) _ad_ (R) _duc_ (S) _tion_

    adduction (ah-duk'shun; the act of adducting; to draw toward; ad- = toward)

33. **Circumduction** (P) _circum_ (R) _duc_ (S) _tion_

    circumduction (ser"kum-duk'shun; the act of circumducting; to draw around)

34. **Intramuscular** (P) _intra_ (R) _muscul_ (S) _ar_

    intramuscular (in"trah-mus'ku-lar; pertaining to within muscle; clinically refers to a route of medication administration in which medication is injected into a muscle mass)

6.2. Musculoskeletal Anatomy and Physiology

6.2.1. BONE ANATOMY

Bones come in many different shapes and sizes: long, short, flat, sesamoid, and irregular. *Long bones* are generally found in extremities. *Short bones* are found in joints, like the carpus and tarsus. *Flat bones* are found in the skull, pelvis, scapula, and ribs. Vertebrae would be classified as irregular bones. Sesamoid bones are so called because they resemble sesame seeds. Sesamoid bones are found associated near joints, like the *patella* (*pah-tel'ah*; "knee cap"), which is associated with the stifle. For this discussion, a long bone is used because it is easier to demonstrate specific anatomic structures in a long bone.

    Long bones are divided into three major regions: the *epiphysis*, the *metaphysis*, and the *diaphysis* (Fig. 6–2). The epiphyses are found at the very ends of a long bone. The epiphysis is usually the portion of the bone that is covered with *articular* (joint) *cartilage*. The diaphysis is the shaft of a long bone. The metaphysis closely approximates the epiphysis, and is that portion of the long bone found between the epiphysis and the diaphysis that provides a gradual, broadening transition between the two.

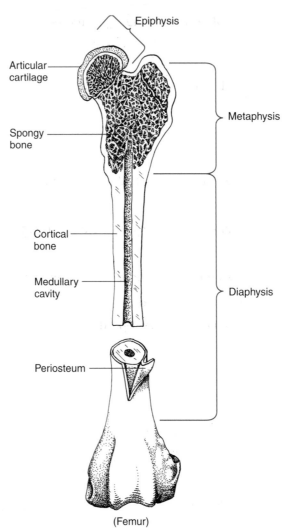

Epiphysis

Articular cartilage

Metaphysis

Spongy bone

Cortical bone

Medullary cavity

Diaphysis

Periosteum

(Femur)

FIGURE 6–2. Bone anatomy.

The wall of the diaphysis is composed of tightly *compact* (cortical) *bone. Cortical bone* is extremely dense and strong, to withstand forces of bending. The cortical bone of the diaphysis forms a central canal called the *medullary cavity*, which contains the *bone marrow*. The metaphyses and epiphyses are covered by a thin layer of cortical bone. Under the cortical bone of the metaphyses and epiphyses, however, is a network of numerous, thin, irregular, branching, bony (*osseous*) plates and interconnecting spaces. Because it looks like a sponge, it has been called *spongy bone*. Unlike a sponge, however, spongy bone is very strong and designed to withstand natural compression forces. The spaces found in spongy bone help to reduce the overall weight of the bone and, in the metaphyses, provide space for additional marrow. The medullary cavity and the spaces of the spongy bone are lined with a connective tissue membrane called the *endosteum*. Covering the entire bone, except for the articular cartilage on the epiphyses, is a tough connective tissue membrane called the *periosteum*.

6.2.2. BONE GROWTH

Bones in a developing fetus start off being made up of layers of fibrous connective tissue and cartilage. Eventually, much of the connective tissue and cartilage is replaced with hard, calcified bone. After birth, the bones continue to grow until the animal reaches maturity.

In a young, growing animal, the epiphyses are demarcated from the metaphyses by growth plates (*epiphyseal plates*; Fig. 6–3). The epiphyseal plate is made up of cartilage and bone-forming cells. During the growth process, bone-forming cells of the epiphyseal plates deposit calcified bone, causing the bone to grow in length. Bone-forming cells of the periosteum deposit calcified bone, causing the bone to grow in width. On reaching maturity, the epiphyseal plate is incorporated into the spongy bone of the epiphyses and metaphyses.

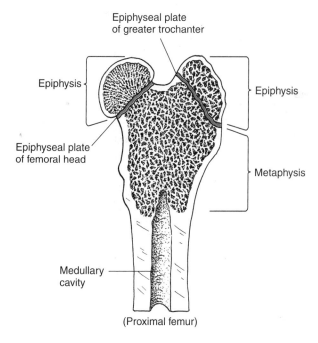

Epiphyseal plate
of greater trochanter

Epiphysis

Epiphysis

Epiphyseal plate
of femoral head

Metaphysis

Medullary
cavity

(Proximal femur)

FIGURE 6–3. Epiphyseal plates.

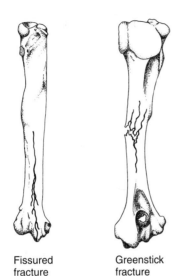
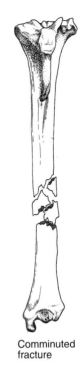
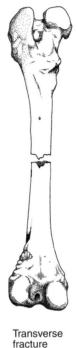
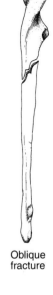

Fissured
fracture

Greenstick
fracture

Oblique
fracture

Transverse
fracture

Comminuted
fracture

FIGURE 6–4. Common traumatic fractures.

6.2.3. FRACTURES AND FRACTURE REPAIR

A *fracture* (*frak'tūr*) is the breakage of a bone. Many different types of fractures may occur for many different reasons. Trauma is the most frequent cause of fractures. Any fracture falls into one of two major categories: 1) *simple fracture*, one that is contained within the skin and soft tissues, or 2) *compound fracture*, one that is open to the environment through a penetrating soft tissue wound. Within these two categories, fractures are specifically named by the nature of the bone breakage. Figure 6–4 illustrates five of the common types of fractures in domestic animals:

1. *Fissured fracture:* an incomplete break, parallel to the longitudinal (length) axis of the bone.
2. *Greenstick fracture:* an incomplete break, involving predominantly one side of the bone, created by a bending force. It was so named because of the way it resembles the breakage of a young, supple, green twig.
3. *Transverse fracture:* a complete break that occurs perpendicular (at right angles) to the longitudinal axis of the bone.

4. *Comminuted fracture:* a complete break that results in numerous bony fragments.
5. *Oblique fracture:* a complete break that occurs at an angle oblique to the longitudinal axis of the bone.

Within days of a fracture occurring, cells that produce *fibrocartilage* (*fi"bro-kar'tĭ-lij*, a specialized type of cartilage) and bone infiltrate the area (Fig. 6–5). Most of these cells originate from the periosteum and the endosteum. Fibrocartilage and bone deposited at the fracture site provide the initial, but unstable union between the broken ends of the bone. The fibrocartilage matrix eventually is replaced by calcified bone. Orthopedic support devices are often warranted to stabilize the fracture site during these early stages of repair. Bone-forming cells continue to deposit spongy bone until all of the fibrocartilage is replaced. Once the fibrocartilage has been replaced by bone, it is referred to as a bony *callus*. Bone continues to be deposited and reorganized until the fracture site is fully

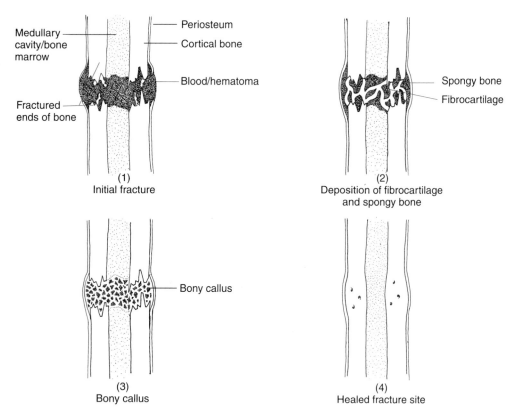

FIGURE 6–5. Fracture repair.

healed. Excess bone and fragments are removed from the site by specialized phagocytic cells.

6.2.4. JOINTS

A joint is formed wherever two or more bones meet. Joints differ structurally and functionally. Some joints are completely immobile and intended purely to hold opposing bones together, like those of the skull. Intervertebral joints are designed to allow minimal flexibility of the spinal column. In addition, the *intervertebral discs* act as small shock absorbers along the spinal column. The important type of joint found in the limbs of domestic animals is a *synovial joint* (Fig. 6–6).

The epiphyses of the bones in a synovial joint are covered with a layer of cartilage, called *articular cartilage*. It is designed to resist wear and produce minimal friction when the joint is moved. The joint is fully enclosed by a tubular *joint capsule*. Made of very tough, fibrous connective tissue, the joint capsule not only en-

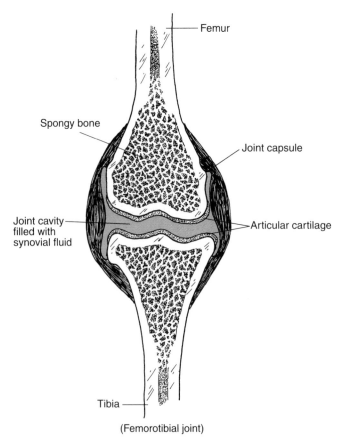

FIGURE 6–6. Synovial joint.

closes the joint cavity, it also helps prevent the articular surfaces of the bones from being pulled apart. *Ligaments* also play a major role in holding the bones together and minimizing movement. They are composed of bundles of fibrous connective tissue. Filling the joint cavity is a transparent, viscous fluid called *synovial fluid*. The synovial fluid acts as a lubricant for the articular surfaces.

Action or movement within a synovial joint depends on the bones that form it. For *hinged joints*, like the elbow, only *flexion* and *extension* are possible. *Rotation* (twisting around an axis) is made possible by *pivot joints* like those found between the head and neck, as well as the *lumbosacral joint*. For a *ball and socket joint* like the hip, multiple movements are possible, including *adduction, abduction* and *circumduction*. If joint range of motion (ROM) is requested for diagnostic or therapeutic reasons, the anatomic structure and natural movements of each joint involved must be considered to carry out the medical order fully.

6.2.5. COMPARATIVE SKELETAL ANATOMY

Horses differ from dogs and cats not just because they are much larger. The skeletal structure of the horse has evolved quite differently, particularly in the limbs, to support its massive weight. Refer to Figures 6–7 through 6–10 (pp. 88–91) for a comparative look at both species.

In comparing the forelimb of the horse to that of a dog, beginning proximally, the scapula and humerus appear quite similar. It is not until a point distal to the *humeroradioulnar joint* is reached that the anatomy begins to differ. In the dog, the radius and ulna are separate bones, the radius being the most cranial of the two. In the horse, the radius and ulna are fused. The carpus of the two animals is very similar, with numerous carpal bones, including an *accessory carpal bone* on the palmar aspect of the joint. Distal to the carpus, the most significant differences are observed. A normal dog stands on four of five digits. Digits are numbered in the dog from medial (#1) to lateral (#5). The first digit is *vestigial*,[8] on the medial aspect of the *metacarpus*, and is not used to bear weight. Each of the weight-bearing digits has associated with it three phalanges and a metacarpal bone. The horse, on the other hand, stands on only one digit! If compared to the dog, the horse is actually standing on the third digit. The *third metacarpal bone* of the horse has become massive to support weight. The vestigial second and fourth metacarpal bones are fused to the third metacarpal bone on the palmaromedial and palmarolateral aspects of the bone. The *proximal sesamoid bones* of the horse are apparent near the palmar aspect of the *metacarpophalangeal joint*. They help to support the large ligaments and tendons of the distal limb, as does the *distal sesamoid bone* (found cradled behind the *distal phalanx*). The distal phalanx of the horse cannot be seen, except radiographically, because it is found in the hoof. Even the *distal interphalangeal joint* is difficult to visualize in a horse because of the hoof. The

---

[8]Vestigial (*ves-tij'e-al; pertaining to a vestige*); rudimentary.

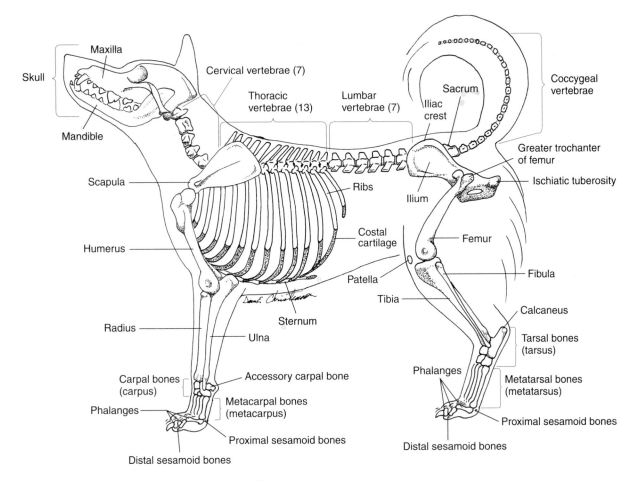

FIGURE 6–7. Comparative skeletal anatomy: Canine bones.

proximal interphalangeal joint, on the other hand, is quite easy to see and to palpate.

The next skeletal area in which major differences are found between the horse and the dog is in the rear. The pelvic structural differences are discussed first here. In the dog, the *ilium* is a wing-like portion of the pelvis that is oriented in a sagittal plane. The horse has an ilium, too; however, in the horse, it is as though the ventral border of the ilium has been twisted laterally and dorsally. That is why the most prominent osseous protuberance on the horse ilium is not the *iliac crest,* like in the dog. The most prominent osseous protuberance of the horse ilium is the *tuber coxae.*[9] The proximal hindlimb of the dog and the horse are similar. They both have a femur, and a patella that is associated with the

---

[9]Tuber coxae (*tu-ber koks'a*), derived from [L. *tuber,* a swelling or protuberance] and [L. *coxa,* "hip"].

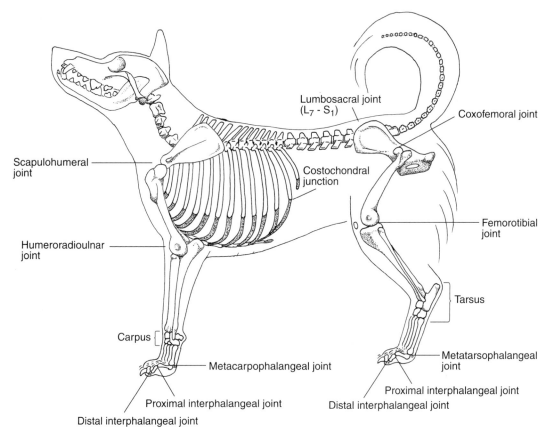

Lumbosacral joint
(L_7 - S_1)

Coxofemoral joint

Scapulohumeral joint

Costochondral junction

Humeroradioulnar joint

Femorotibial joint

Tarsus

Carpus

Metatarsophalangeal joint

Metacarpophalangeal joint

Proximal interphalangeal joint

Distal interphalangeal joint

Proximal interphalangeal joint

Distal interphalangeal joint

FIGURE 6–8. Comparative skeletal anatomy: Canine joints.

femorotibial joint. Distal to that joint, differences begin to appear. The horse has only a vestigial fibula, near the proximal end of the tibia. Much of the fibula has been fused to and is indiscernible from the tibia. The tarsus of the dog and the horse are very similar. They have multiple tarsal bones, including the *calcaneus* (*kal-ka′ne-us*), which is the largest, rear-most tarsal bone. Distal to the tarsus, differences between the dog and the horse are similar to those in the forelimb. The horse stands on the *third metatarsal bone.* The second and fourth metatarsal bones are vestigial and are fused to the third. The phalanges and sesamoid bones are arranged just as they are in the forelimb. The dog still bears weight on digits two through five. The first digit is frequently absent in the rear limbs of normal dogs.

6.2.6. MUSCLE ANATOMY AND ACTIVITY

Muscles in this chapter are discussed by functional muscles or muscle groups (for details regarding muscle tissue, refer to Chapter 3, section 3.2.2.3, Muscle Tissue).

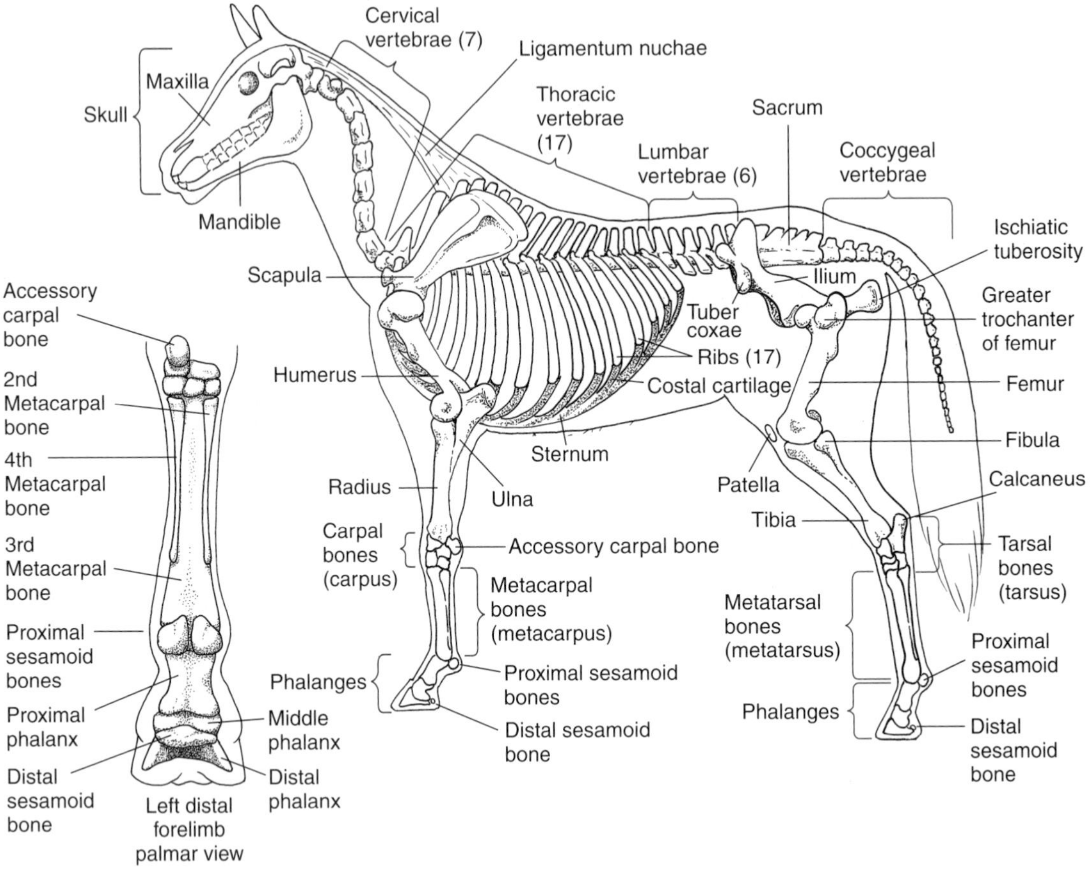

FIGURE 6–9. Comparative skeletal anatomy: Equine bones.

Because the muscles are firmly attached to the bones by *tendons*, it is by virtue of muscle activity (i.e., contraction and relaxation) that joints are moved. Refer to Figures 6–11 and 6–12 (on p. 92) for major extremity *extensor* and *flexor* muscles and muscle groups. Notice that each major joint has opposing muscles associated with it. Hence, with regard to joints and their associated muscles, for every action there is an equal and opposite reaction.

Muscle groups, shown in Figures 6–11 and 6–12, are as follows:

Biceps (*bi'seps*) muscle group: flexor of the humeroradioulnar joint; located cranial to the humerus.

Triceps (*tri'seps*) muscle group: extensor of the humeroradioulnar joint; located caudal to the humerus.

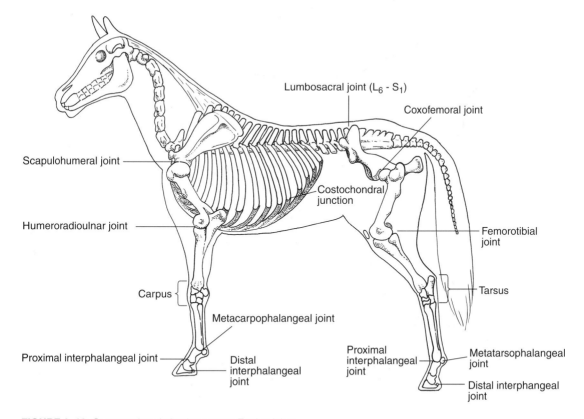

FIGURE 6–10. Comparative skeletal anatomy: Equine joints.

Digital extensor muscles of the forelimb: extend the carpus and the digits; located on the cranial antebrachium.

Digital flexor muscles of the forelimb: flex the carpus and the digits; located on the caudal antebrachium.

Gluteal (*gloo'te-al*) muscle group: serves in part for flexion of the coxofemoral joint and abduction of the hindlimb; located between the ilium, sacrum, and proximal femur.

Quadriceps (*kwod'rĭ-seps*) muscle group: extensor of the femorotibial joint; located cranial to the femur.

Semimembranosus/semitendinosus muscle group: flexor of the femorotibial joint; located caudal to the femur.

Digital extensor muscles of the hindlimb: extend the digits and flex the tarsus; located on the cranial crus.

Digital flexor muscles of the hindlimb: flex the digits and extend the tarsus; located on the caudal crus.

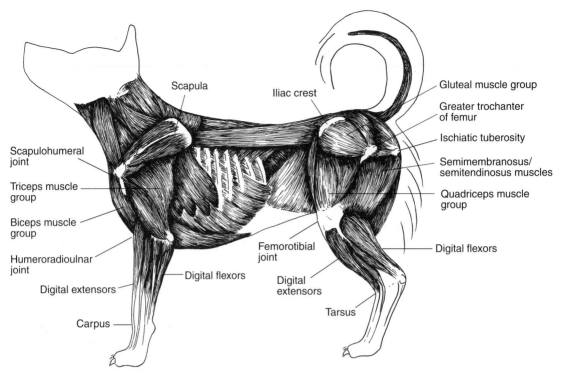

FIGURE 6–11. Canine comparative muscular anatomy.

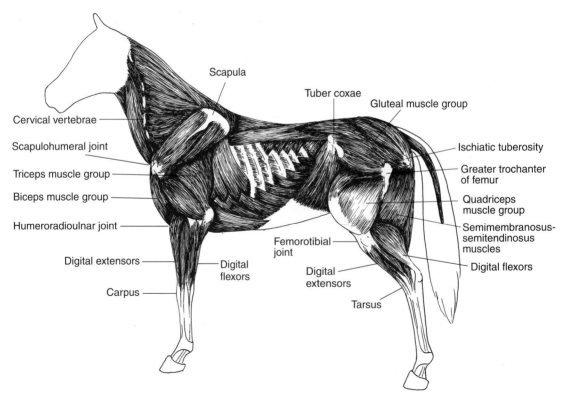

FIGURE 6–12. Equine comparative muscular anatomy.

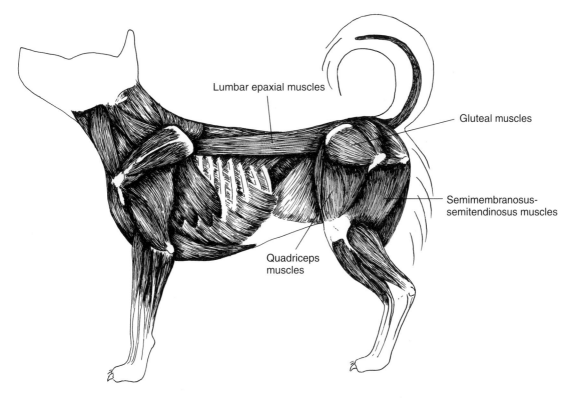

FIGURE 6–13. Common canine intramuscular injection sites.

6.2.7. COMMON INTRAMUSCULAR INJECTION SITES

Intramuscular (I.M.) injections are frequently used for medication administration. Because muscles have significant blood supply, they provide relatively rapid absorption of injected agents. It is important that students have a working knowledge of the muscle sites that provide suitable locations for intramuscular injections. Refer to Figures 6–13 and 6–14 (on p. 94) for the common intramuscular injection sites used in veterinary medicine. Compare these illustrations to the skeletal illustrations to define the osseous landmarks for each site. It is very important to locate and maintain isolation of a muscle group using its osseous landmarks whenever an I.M. injection is administered.

The following list gives each intramuscular injection site, along with its respective osseous landmarks and the species in which it is most frequently used.

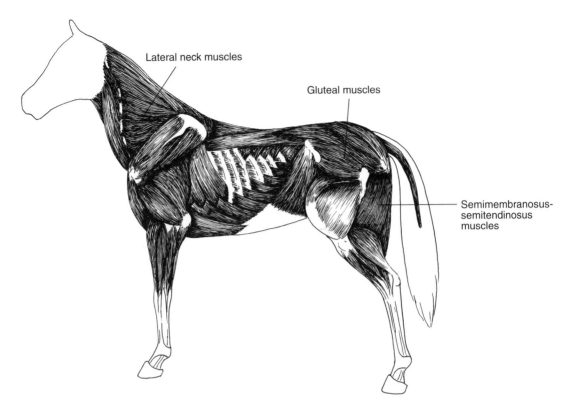

Lateral neck muscles

Gluteal muscles

Semimembranosus-
semitendinosus
muscles

FIGURE 6–14. Common equine intramuscular injection sites.

1. *Lateral neck muscles*
   Used predominantly in adult horses and cattle, the lateral neck muscles are bordered by the *ligamentum nuchae*[10] (dorsal), the *scapula* (caudal), and the *cervical vertebrae* (ventral).
2. *Lumbar epaxial muscles*
   Used predominantly in companion animals (i.e., dogs and cats), the lumbar epaxial muscles are bordered by the *caudal rib* (cranial), the spinous processes of the *lumbar vertebrae* (medial), and the *iliac crest* (caudal).

---

[10]Ligamentum nuchae (*lig"ah-men'tum nu'ka*); a large ligament found on the dorsal aspect of the neck. It is used as a dorsal border of the lateral neck intramuscular injection site in large animals.

3. *Gluteal muscles*

As used in horses and cattle, the gluteal muscles are bordered by the *sacrum* (medial), the *tuber coxae* (cranial), the *greater trochanter* of the femur (lateral), and the *ischiatic tuberosity*[11] (caudal).

As used in companion animals, the gluteal muscles are bordered by the *sacrum* (medial), the *iliac crest* (cranial), and the *greater trochanter* of the femur (lateral). The ischiatic tuberosity is often helpful in locating the greater trochanter of the femur, but otherwise is not a functional osseous landmark for this injection site in dogs and cats.

4. *Quadriceps muscles*

Used predominantly in companion animals, the quadriceps muscles are bordered by the *coxofemoral joint* (proximal), the *femur* (caudal), and *femorotibial joint* (distal).

5. *Semimembranosus/semitendinosus muscles*

Used both in large and small animal medicine, the semimembranosus and semitendinosus muscles are bordered by the *ischiatic tuberosity* (proximal), the *femur* (cranial), and the *femorotibial joint* (distal). It should be noted that a major nerve (the *sciatic nerve*[12]) passes through this muscle group just caudal to the femur. Damage to this nerve could result in paralysis of the patient. Therefore, students should not attempt to use this muscle group for I.M. injections until they have been appropriately instructed in the safe use of the site.

6.3. Self-Test

Using the previous information in this chapter, respond to each of the following questions using the most appropriate medical term(s).

1. The _____ joint (or hip joint) is a joint formed between the pelvis and the femur.

2. The ___cervical___ vertebrae are those vertebrae that are found in the neck.

3. The spaces found between the ribs are medically termed ___intercostal___ spaces.

---

[11]Ischiatic tuberosity (*is"ke-at'ik, ish"e-at'-ik; pertaining to the ischium*); the ischium is the most caudal portion of the pelvis; the ischiatic tuberosity is a caudolateral osseous protuberance of the ischium

[12]Sciatic nerve (*si-at'ik*); this nerve and its branches supply motor function to the semimembranosus/semitendinosus muscle group, the digital flexors, and the digital extensors of the hindlimb.

4. ___abduction___ is the act of drawing a limb away from the body.

5. Inflammation of a joint is medically termed ___arthritis___.

6. The ___cortex___ is a layer of connective tissue that surrounds a bone.

7. A(n) _____ muscle group is a muscle group that causes a joint to bend, reducing the angle of the joint.

8. A(n) _____ is a tough, flexible bundle of connective tissue that firmly holds two bones together.

9. Inflammation of muscle tissue is medically termed _____.

10. ___coccygeal___ vertebrae are those vertebrae found in the tail.

11. The ___knee___ joint (or stifle joint) is a joint of the hindlimb formed between the femur and the tibia.

12. A(n) ___I. M.___ injection is a form of medication administration by which drugs are placed deep within muscle tissue.

13. The ___humerus___ joint (or elbow joint) is a joint formed by the humerus and the bones of the antebrachium.

14. A(n) _____ is a joint formed between two phalanges.

15. The _____ is that region of the hindlimb that lies immediately distal to the tarsus.

16. The vertebrae associated with the chest cavity are the ___thoracic___ vertebrae.

17. The act of drawing a limb toward the body is called ___adduction___.

18. ___synovial___ fluid is a transparent, viscous fluid, like egg white, that acts as a lubricant in joints.

19. _____ surgery would be any surgical procedure intended to correct a musculoskeletal deformity.

20. A(n) _____ muscle group is one that would out-stretch a joint, increasing the angle of the joint.

21. The ___epiphysis___ of a bone is located at the end of a long bone and is covered by articular cartilage.

22. The _____ is a membrane that lines the wall of the medullary cavity.

23. A(n) _____ fracture is a type of fracture in which numerous bone fragments occur.

24. _____ discs are chondroid objects found between vertebral bodies that act as shock absorbers for the spinal column.

25. The tough, cord-like connective tissue bands that connect muscle to bones are called _____tendons_____ .

26. The _____ junction would be described as the junction formed by the end of the osseous rib and the cartilage of the rib that attaches the rib to the sternum.

27. The _epiphyseal plate_ is the growth plate of a bone, from which the bone grows in length.

28. The shoulder joint is medically referred to as the _____ joint.

29. The _____diaphysis_____ is also referred to as the shaft of a long bone.

30. The companion animal intramuscular injection site that uses the landmarks of the sacrum medially, the iliac crest cranially, and the greater trochanter of the femur laterally is the _____ muscle group.

Anatomy Challenge

On each of the diagrams provided (Figs. 6–15 and 6–16), identify as many of the bones and joints as you can within a timed period. Allow 10 minutes per diagram. Each blank has been numbered so that you may find the correct answers in the answer key for this section.

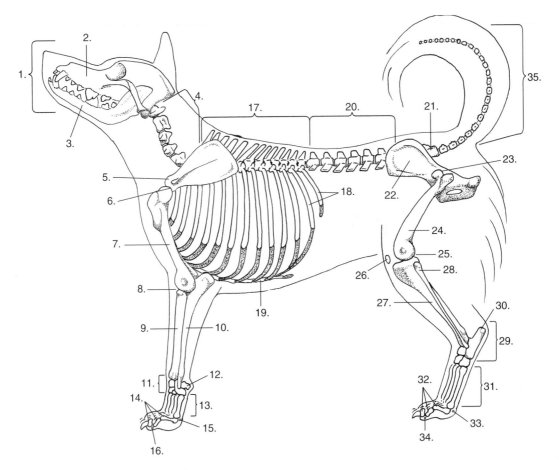

FIGURE 6–15. Canine anatomy challenge.

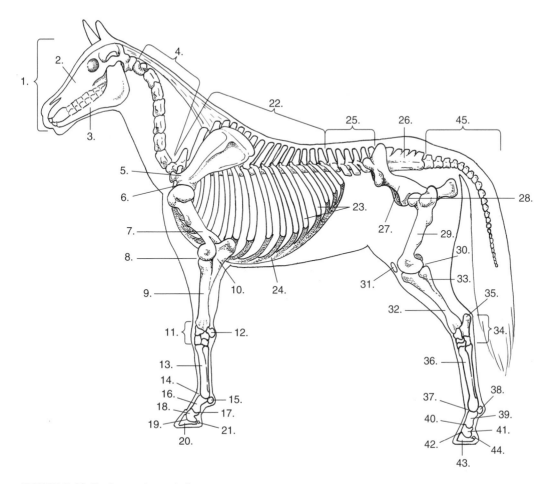

FIGURE 6–16. Equine anatomy challenge.

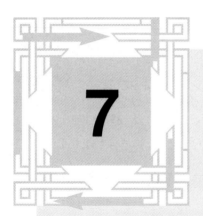

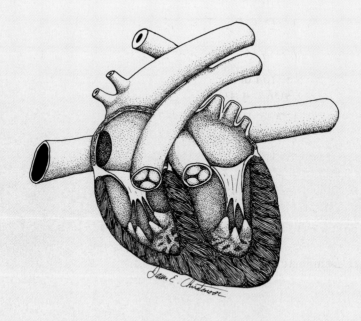

The Cardiovascular System

GOALS AND OBJECTIVES

By the conclusion of this chapter, the student will be able to:

1. Recognize common root words, prefixes, and suffixes related to the cardiovascular system.
2. Divide simple and compound words into their respective parts.
3. Recognize, correctly pronounce, and appropriately use common medical terms related to the cardiovascular system.
4. Demonstrate an understanding of cardiovascular anatomy.
5. Recognize common pulse points and phlebotomy sites in domestic animals.
6. Trace the blood flow of an adult animal sequentially through a complete cycle.
7. Demonstrate a basic understanding of cardiovascular physiology with regard to blood flow, the cardiac cycle (systole and diastole), heart sounds, and electrocardiography.

7.1. Introduction to Related Terms

Divide each of the following terms into its respective parts ("R" root, "P" prefix, "S" suffix, "CV" combining vowel).

1. **Cardiac**　　　(R) _cardi_ (S) _ac_

    cardiac (kar'de-ak; pertaining to the heart)

2. **Cardiologist**　(R) _cardi_ (CV) _o_ (R) _log_ (S) _ist_

    cardiologist (kar-de-ol'o-jist; one who specializes in heart study; a doctor specializing in heart disease and treatment)

3. **Pericardial**　　(P) _peri_ (R) _card_ (S) _al_

    pericardial (per"i-kar'de-al; pertaining to surrounding the heart; anatomically refers to the tissue membrane that surrounds the heart, called the pericardium)

4. **Epicardium**　　(P) _epi_ (R) _cardi_ (S) _um_

    epicardium (ep"i-kar'de-um; upon the heart; anatomically refers to the thin, most superficial tissue layer of the heart)

5. **Myocardial**　　(R) _my_ (CV) _o_ (R) _cardi_ (S) _al_

    myocardial (mi"o-kar'de-al; pertaining to muscle of the heart)

6. **Endocardium**　(P) _endo_ (R) _cardi_ (S) _um_

    endocardium (en"do-kar'de-um; within the heart; anatomically refers to the thin tissue layer that lines the interior of the heart)

7. **Atrial**　　　　(R) _atri_ (S) _al_

    atrial (a'tre-al; pertaining to an atrium; anatomically the atria are two of the four chambers within the heart)

8. **Ventricular**　　(R) _ventricul_ (S) _ar_

    ventricular (ven-trik'u-lar; pertaining to a ventricle; anatomically the ventricles are two of the four chambers within the heart)

9. **Atrioventricular**　(R) _atri_ (CV) _o_ (R) _ventricul_ (S) _ar_

    atrioventricular (a"tre-o-ven-trik'u-lar; pertaining to an atrium and a ventricle)

10. **Aortic**　　　　(R) _aort_ (S) _ic_

    aortic (a-or'tik; pertaining to the aorta; anatomically the aorta is the main artery leading from the heart)

11. **Pulmonic**　　　(R) _pulmon_ (S) _ic_

    pulmonic (pul-mon'ik; pertaining to the lungs)

12. **Arterial**   (R) _arter_   (CV) _i_   (S) _al_

arterial (ar-te're-al; pertaining to an artery or arteries)

13. **Arteriole**   (R) _arteri_   (CV) _o_   (S) _le_

arteriole (ar-te're-ōl; a small artery)

14. **Venous**   (R) _veno_   (S) _ous_

venous (ve'nus; pertaining to a vein or veins)

15. **Venule**   (R) _venu_   (S) _le_

venule (ven'ūl; a small vein)

16. **Phlebotomy**   (R) _phleb_   (CV) _o_   (S) _tomy_

phlebotomy (flĕ-bot'o-me; the cutting of a vein; clinically refers to the puncture of a vein with a needle for the withdrawal of blood)

17. **Phlebitis**   (R) _phleb_   (S) _itis_

phlebitis (flĕ-bi'tis; inflammation of a vein)

18. **Cardiomyopathy** (R) _cardi_   (CV) _o_   (R) _myo_   (CV) _o_   (S) _pathy_

cardiomyopathy (kar"de-o-mi-op'ah-the; a disease of heart muscle)

19. **Electrocardiogram** (R) _electr_   (CV) _o_   (R) _cardi_   (CV) _o_   (S) _gram_

electrocardiogram (e-lek"tro-kar'de-o-gram; a recording of electricity of the heart; clinically referred to as an ECG, the electrocardiogram is a graphic tracing of the heart's electrical activity)

20. **Echocardiogram** (R) _echo_   (R) _cardi_   (CV) _o_   (S) _gram_

echocardiogram (ek"o-kar'de-o-gram; a recording of echoes of the heart; clinically refers to the use of ultrasonic waves to record the anatomy and motion of the heart)

21. **Angiogram**   (R) _angi_   (CV) _o_   (S) _gram_

angiogram (an'je-o-gram; a recording of vessels; clinically refers to a radiographic procedure in which radiopaque dye is injected into the vasculature for better visualization of the vessels)

22. **Intravenous**   (P) _intra_   (R) _veno_   (S) _ous_

intravenous (in"trah-ve'nus; pertaining to within a vein; clinically often refers to a route of medication administration)

23. **Perivascular**   (P) _peri_   (R) _vascul_   (S) _ar_

perivascular (per"ĭ-vas'ku-lar; pertaining to around a vessel)

24. **Bradycardia** (P) brady (R) cardi (S) ia

bradycardia (brād"ĕ-kar'de-ah; a condition of a slow heart)

25. **Tachycardia** (P) tachy (R) cardi (S) ia

tachycardia (tak"ĕ-kar'de-ah; a condition of a rapid heart)

26. **Systolic** (R) systol (S) ic

systolic (sis-tol'ik; pertaining to contraction; clinically refers to the phase of the cardiac cycle when the heart muscle is contracting)

27. **Diastolic** (R) diastol (S) ic

diastolic (di"ah-stol'ik; pertaining to expansion; clinically refers to the phase of the cardiac cycle when the heart muscle is relaxed, allowing the chambers to expand)

28. **Asystole** (P) a (R) systole

asystole (ah"sis'to-le, a-sis'to-le; absence of contraction; clinically refers to the absence of cardiac activity)

29. **Stenosis** (R) sten (CV) o (S) is

stenosis (ste-no'sis; a condition of narrowing)

30. **Cardiomegaly** (R) cardi (CV) o (S) megaly

cardiomegaly (kar"de-o-meg'ah-le; enlargement of the heart)

31. **Hypertrophy** (P) hyper (R) trophy

hypertrophy (hi-per'tro-fe; overgrowth or above-normal development)

32. **Interatrial** (P) inter (R) artri (S) al

interatrial (in"ter-a'tre-al; pertaining to between the atria)

33. **Interventricular** (P) inter (R) ventricul (S) ar

interventricular (in"ter-ven-trik'u-lar; pertaining to between the ventricles)

34. **Arrhythmia** (P) arr a (R) rrhythm (S) ia

arrhythmia (ah-rith'me-ah, a-rith'me-ah; a condition without rhythm)

35. **Vasoconstriction** (R) vas (CV) o (R) constric (S) tion

vasoconstriction (vas"o-kon-strik'shun; the process of vessel constricting)

36. **Vasodilation** (R) vas (CV) o (R) dila (S) tion

vasodilation (vas"o-di-la'shun; the process of vessel dilating)

37. **Sphygmomanometer**
(R) ~~Sphygm~~(CV) O̲ (R) man̲ (CV) O̲ (S) meter̲

sphygmomanometer (sfig"mo-mah-nom' ĕ-ter; measurer of pulse pressure; clinically refers to an instrument used to measure blood pressure)

7.2. Cardiovascular Anatomy and Physiology

7.2.1. CARDIAC ANATOMY

The heart is located in the ventral chest cavity, between the third and seventh ribs for most domestic animals (Fig. 7–1). The heart is designed to pump blood throughout the body. It is therefore very muscular and is made up of a series of chambers and valves.

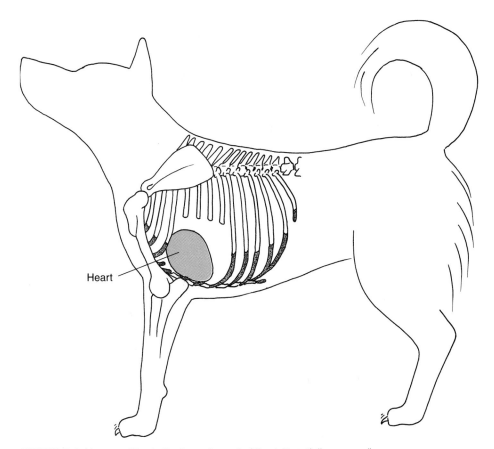

Heart

FIGURE 7–1. Heart position in the thoracic cavity (ribs 4–7 partially removed).

The heart is enveloped by the *pericardial sac*. Anatomically, when the pericardial sac is removed, the next tissue layer of the heart exposed is the *epicardium* (Fig. 7–2). The epicardium is the thin, most superficial epithelial tissue of the heart proper. It serves to produce a thin, proteinaceous fluid that prevents friction between the epicardium and the pericardial sac. Beneath the epicardium is the *myocardium* (see Chapter 3, section 3.2.2.3, Muscle Tissue, for details regarding myocardial tissue). The interior of the cardiac chambers is lined with *endocardium*, an endothelial tissue.

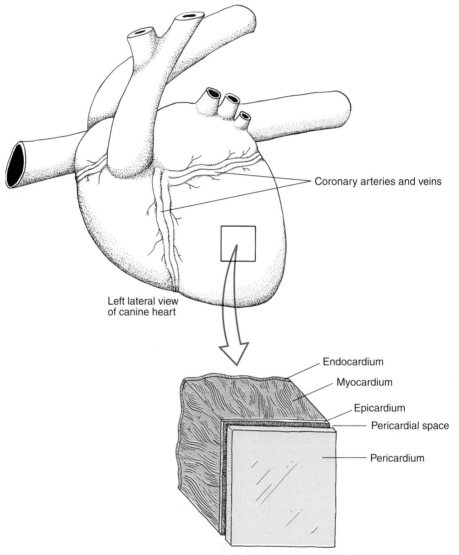

Coronary arteries and veins

Left lateral view
of canine heart

Endocardium
Myocardium
Epicardium
Pericardial space
Pericardium

Full thickness cardiac tissue specimen

FIGURE 7–2. Cardiac tissues.

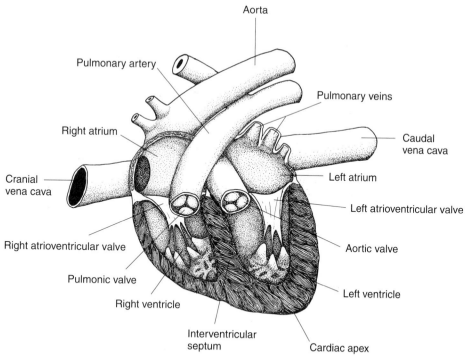

FIGURE 7–3. Cardiac chambers and valves (schematic left-lateral view of canine heart).

The heart is divided into four chambers (Fig. 7–3). The smallest, least muscular of the chambers are the *atria*. The atria are located near the base of the heart.[1] They are separated into right and left chambers by a wall, the *interatrial septum*. Venous blood returning to the heart enters the atria first.

The *ventricles* are the larger and more muscular of the cardiac chambers. They are separated from one another by the *interventricular septum*, and are separated from the atria by valves. The right chambers are separated by the *right atrioventricular valve*, whereas the left chambers are separated by the *left atrioventricular valve*. These two valves are open during the filling phase of the heart and closed during *ventricular systole* (*sis'to-le*). During ventricular systole, the blood is forced from the ventricles through two other valves. Blood from the right ventricle passes through the *pulmonic valve* and blood from the left ventricle passes

---

[1]The base of the heart is found on the dorsal aspect. The great vessels of the heart (vena cavae, aorta, pulmonary arteries, and pulmonary veins) are clustered at the base of the heart.

through the *aortic valve*. These valves close during *diastole* (*di-as'to-le*). Because blood from the left ventricle must travel farther through the body, the myocardium making up the walls of that chamber is much thicker. It is the myocardium of the left ventricle that forms the *cardiac apex* (*a'peks*).

7.2.2. ARTERIES AND VEINS

Arteries are thick-walled, muscular vessels that carry blood away from the heart to other areas of the body. The basic structure of an artery is a series of layers (Fig. 7–4). The innermost arterial layer is composed of endothelial cells. These cells, much like those that make up the endocardium, provide a very smooth intra–arterial surface for the blood to flow through. The endothelium is supported by a layer of elastic and fibrous connective tissues. Surrounding these tissues is a very thick layer of smooth muscle, which makes up the bulk of the arterial wall. This smooth muscle is very important for changing the diameter of the vessel lumen (*lu'men*). When the smooth muscle contracts, the diameter of the arterial lumen is reduced (*vasoconstriction*). Conversely, when the smooth muscle is relaxed, the diameter of the arterial lumen is increased in size (*vasodilation*). The activities of vasoconstriction and vasodilation play a significant role in the regulation of blood pressure. By either increasing or decreasing vessel lumen size, resistance to blood flow is either increased or diminished, and thereby blood pressure is increased or diminished. Enveloping the former layers of the arterial wall is a thick layer of elastic and fibrous connective tissues. The connective tissues of the arterial wall provide strength to withstand the forces of high blood pressure (inherent to arteries). They also provide great elasticity, permitting the

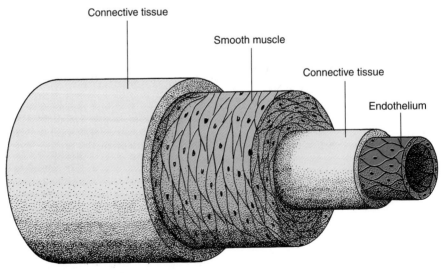

FIGURE 7–4. Arterial wall.

arteries to stretch in accommodation to the increased blood volumes associated with ventricular systole.

The largest artery of the body is the *aorta*. It originates from the left ventricle, arches shortly after leaving the heart, and then courses caudally along the dorsum of the animal. It terminates at the final arterial branches that supply the hindlimbs. All major arteries of the body originate from the aorta, with the exception of the *coronary (kor'ŏ-na're) arteries*, which supply the heart itself, and the *pulmonary arteries*, which supply the lungs. The size of the arteries progressively becomes smaller the further away from the heart they are. Many of the peripheral arteries can be used clinically as pulse points. By palpating over a peripheral artery, the pulsation created by the heart pumping the blood can be felt. For each contraction of the heart, a peripheral pulse should be felt. Figures 7–5 and 7–6 show the common pulse points in domestic animals. (If you are unfamiliar with some of the anatomic landmarks cited for these vessels, refer to Chapter 6, "The Musculoskeletal System.") Note that most peripheral vessels are bilaterally symmetrical.

The following are common pulse points of domestic animals. Each artery has been listed, with a brief description of its location and species specificity for use where applicable.

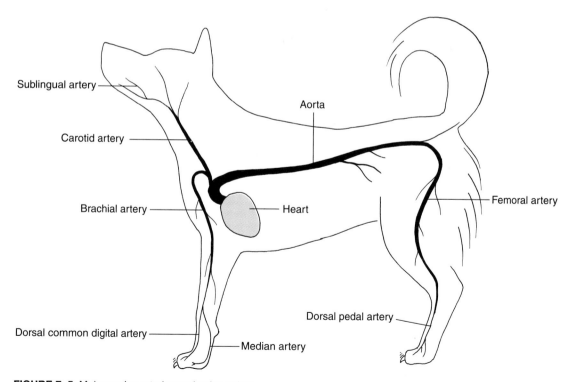

FIGURE 7–5. Major canine arteries and pulse points.

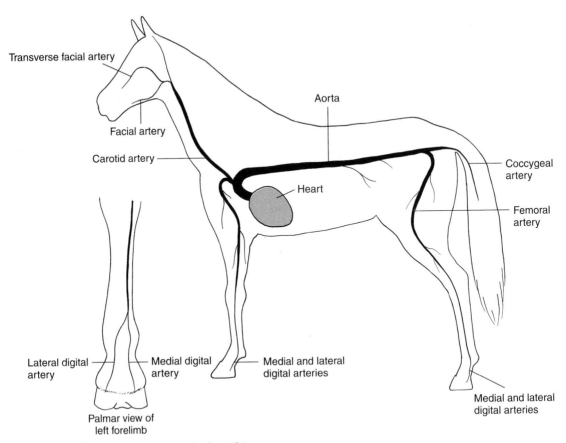

FIGURE 7–6. Major equine arteries and pulse points.

Sublingual (sub-ling'gwal) artery

The sublingual artery is located on the ventral midline of the tongue. It is a commonly used pulse point in anesthetized animals.

Facial (fa'shal) artery

The facial artery is frequently used as a pulse point in horses and cattle. Two branches are easily palpated: the transverse branch courses over the *zygomatic arch* (*zi"go-mat'ik*, cheek bone), just below the eye; the other branch courses over the ventrocaudal mandible.

Carotid (kah-rot'id) artery

The carotid artery lies in the ventrolateral neck, lateral to the trachea (windpipe). In heavily muscled animals, this artery may be difficult to palpate.

Median artery

The median artery is located near the midline of the palmar aspect of the metacarpus. It is readily palpated in dogs and cats.

Dorsal common digital (dij'ĭ-tal) artery

The dorsal common digital artery is located on the dorsal aspect of the metacarpus, coursing across the metacarpus at a mediolateral oblique angle. It is easily palpated in dogs and cats.

Medial and lateral digital arteries

The medial and lateral digital arteries are located on the palmar (plantar) aspect of the proximal phalanges. The medial branch is located near the palmaromedial (plantaromedial) aspect of the limb, whereas the lateral branch is located near the palmarolateral (plantarolateral) aspect of the limb. These arteries, found in all four limbs, are used for pulse determination in horses.

Brachial (bra'ke-al) artery

The brachial artery lies on the medial aspect of the proximal forelimb (i.e., medial to the humerus). Used in companion animals, this artery may be difficult to palpate in heavily muscled patients.

Femoral (fem'or-al) artery

The femoral artery lies on the medial aspect of the proximal hindlimb (i.e., medial to the femur). It is probably the most frequently used pulse point in dogs and cats.

Lateral dorsal metatarsal (met"ah-tar'sal) artery

The lateral dorsal metatarsal artery lies in the rear limb, on the lateral aspect of the metatarsus. It is used for pulse determination in horses.

Dorsal pedal artery

The dorsal pedal artery is located on the dorsal midline of the metatarsus. It is frequently used for pulse determination in dogs and cats.

Coccygeal (kok-sij'e-al) artery

The coccygeal artery is located on the ventral midline of the tail. It is most easily palpated in horses and cattle at the proximal portion of the tail.

Veins (*vānz*) are vessels that carry blood to the heart. Structurally, veins are much thinner and less muscular than arteries (Fig. 7–7). The interior surfaces of veins are lined with endothelium, just like the arteries. In contrast, however, because the blood flowing through veins is under far less pressure than arterial blood, *intravenous unidirectional valves* help keep the blood flowing one way. The smooth muscle and connective tissue layers are arranged similarly to arteries, but

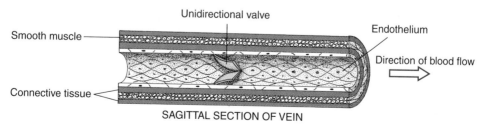

SAGITTAL SECTION OF VEIN

FIGURE 7–7. Venous wall.

with less bulk. Because smooth muscle is present in venous walls, veins too have the capacity to vasoconstrict and vasodilate, contributing to the regulation of blood pressure.

The largest vein of body is the *vena cava*, which is divided into cranial and caudal portions. The *cranial vena cava* collects blood from the head and the cranial body, whereas the *caudal vena cava* collects blood from the abdomen and caudal body. Both the cranial and caudal vena cavae deposit blood into the right atrium. Most other major veins of the body (with the exception of *coronary* and *pulmonary veins*) ultimately deposit their blood into the cranial and caudal vena cavae. Pulmonary veins carry blood from the lungs to the left atrium.

Veins have thin walls, are under less pressure than arteries, and carry blood to the heart for redistribution throughout the body. For those reasons, they are frequently used for blood collection and administration of intravenous (I.V.) medications. Some medications are too caustic to come in contact with most tissues of the body. Such medications must be given intravenously, using a large vein for quick dilution of the agent. If a portion of a caustic medication were given *perivascularly*, tissues in that area may become inflamed, die, and slough (*sluf*) from the body. Appropriate aseptic technique must be observed for *phlebotomy* and administration of intravenous medications to prevent the development of *phlebitis* or perivascular sloughing. Figures 7–8 and 7–9 show the common phlebotomy sites in domestic animals.

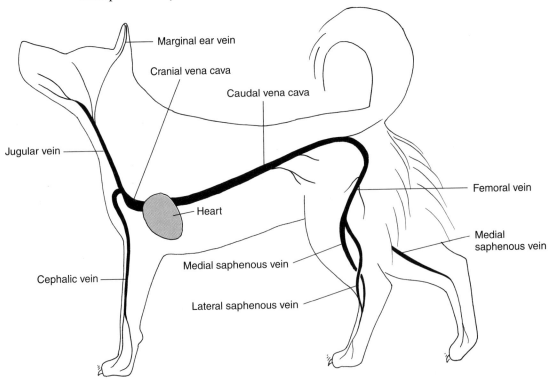

FIGURE 7–8. Major canine veins and phlebotomy sites.

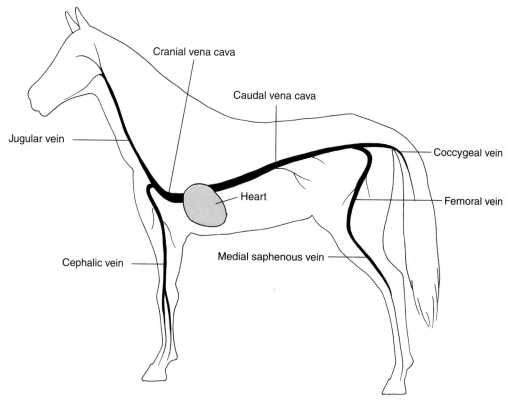

FIGURE 7–9. Major equine veins and phlebotomy sites.

The following is a list of each phlebotomy site, including anatomic landmarks and those species in which it is most frequently used.

Cephalic (sĕ-fal'ik) vein
> The cephalic vein is located on the craniomedial aspect of the forelimb, between the elbow and the carpus. It is the most frequently used phlebotomy site in dogs and cats. It is an alternative site in horses, particularly foals.

Jugular (jug'u-lar) vein
> The jugular vein is located in the ventrolateral neck, lateral to the trachea. It is frequently used for collection of large volumes of blood from all domestic animals.

Marginal ear vein
> The marginal ear vein is located at the margins of the ear pinna (flap). It is frequently used in rabbits, pigs, and flop-eared dogs.

Lateral saphenous (sah-fe'nus, sā''fĕ-nus) vein
> The lateral saphenous vein is located on the lateral aspect of the hindlimb. It courses across the distal, lateral tibia at a craniocaudal-distoproximal oblique angle. It is frequently used in dogs and cats, and is an alternative site in horses, particularly foals.

Medial saphenous vein

The medial saphenous vein is located on the medial aspect of the distal hindlimb, and courses medial to the tibia between the tarsus and the femorotibial joint. It is used frequently in cats and dogs.

Femoral vein

The femoral vein is located on the medial aspect of the proximal hindlimb, medial to the femur. It is used most frequently in cats and sometimes in dogs.

Coccygeal vein

The coccygeal vein is located on the ventral midline of the tail. It is frequently used at its proximal aspect in cattle.

7.2.3. BLOOD FLOW

It is essential that the flow of blood throughout the body be a consistent, never-ending process. The constant movement of the blood helps prevent intravascular coagulation (clotting), delivers oxygen and other nutrients to body tissues, and removes wastes from body tissues. The entire cardiovascular system was designed for one-way flow of blood. If a pair of red blood cells were followed through one circuit in an adult animal, the sequence of events would be as follows (Fig. 7–10). Let's begin in the vena cavae. We will follow one cell through the caudal vena cava and the other cell through the cranial vena cava. They will meet in the right atrium, from which they flow through the right atrioventricular valve, into the right ventricle, through the pulmonic valve, and into the pulmonary artery. (The blood at this time is carrying very little oxygen and large quantities of carbon dioxide. To make the appropriate gas exchanges in the lungs, we must go through a gradual transition of progressively smaller vessels to reach the capillaries (*kap'ĭ-lar"ēz*), where gas exchange takes place. Capillaries are the smallest, thinnest-walled vessels of the cardiovascular system.) We continue our journey traveling through branches of pulmonary arteries, into *pulmonary arterioles*, and finally squeeze through the *capillaries* of the lungs, picking up a new supply of oxygen and eliminating the carbon dioxide. We squeeze out of the capillaries into *pulmonary venules*, then into pulmonary veins and flow into the left atrium of the heart. From the left atrium we pass through the left atrioventricular valve, into the left ventricle, through the aortic valve, and into the aorta. In the systemic circulation, we carry our fresh supply of oxygen through a series of arteries, arterioles, and capillaries. In the systemic capillaries, oxygen is delivered to the tissues, carbon dioxide and other wastes are picked up, and we return by way of the systemic venules and veins to the vena cavae. Figure 7–11 (on p. 116) summarizes the blood flow circuit discussed.

7.2.4. CARDIAC CYCLE

The *cardiac cycle* is the activity in which the heart engages to create a heartbeat. It is a series of synchronous events. Throughout the cardiac cycle, pressures within the heart and in general circulation rise and fall. During *diastole*, the myocardium

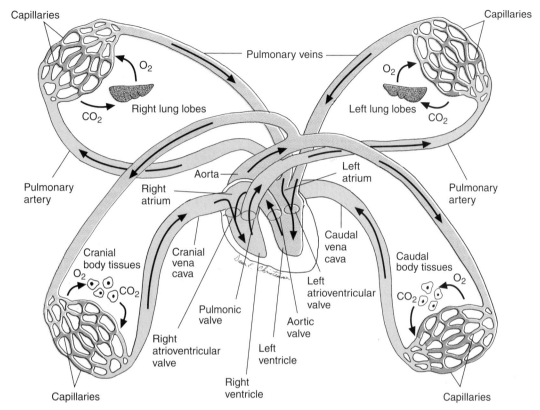

FIGURE 7–10. Adult blood flow schematic.

is relaxed, permitting the atria and the ventricles to fill with blood. The atrioventricular valves are open and pressures in the system are relatively low during diastole. Near the end of the filling phase, the atria contract (*atrial systole*), forcing as much blood as possible into the ventricles. On being engorged with blood, the ventricles contract (*ventricular systole*). At the beginning of ventricular systole, the pressure within the ventricles rises sharply. The increased pressure forces the atrioventricular valves to close and, with nowhere else to go, the blood forces open and rushes through the pulmonic and aortic valves. When ventricular systole is complete, the heart again enters into its diastolic phase and the aortic and pulmonic valves close.

Blood pressure is controlled by a number of variables, including blood volume, vasoconstriction, vasodilation, as well as *cardiac output*. Cardiac output is the sum of *cardiac rate* plus *cardiac stroke volume*.[2] Blood pressure can be measured

---

[2]Cardiac stroke volume is the volume of blood pumped (each time) during ventricular systole.

Systemic circulation

⇓

Vena cavae

⇓

Rt. atrium

⇓

Rt. atrioventricular valve

⇓

Rt. ventricle

⇓

Pulmonic valve

⇓

Pulmonary arteries

⇓

Lungs

⇓

Pulmonary veins

⇓

Lt. atrium

⇓

Lt. atrioventricular valve

⇓

Lt. ventricle

⇓

Aortic valve

⇓

Aorta

⇓

Systemic circulation

FIGURE 7–11. Adult blood flow summary.

by the use of a *sphygmomanometer*. The cuff of the sphygmomanometer is placed over a peripheral artery and inflated enough to occlude the artery completely. The air pressure within the cuff is gradually released to the point where blood begins to flow through the artery again. The reading taken at this moment is referred to as the *systolic pressure*. The air continues to be released from the cuff until blood flow through the artery can no longer be detected. The reading taken at this moment is referred to as the *diastolic pressure*. Blood pressure readings are recorded in millimeters of mercury (mm Hg), as systolic over diastolic. The two numbers reflect the pressures exerted by the blood on the vasculature during ventricular systole and diastole.

7.2.5. HEART SOUNDS

Normal heart sounds are created by the synchronous *closure* of the valves. The sounds generated are much like those created by slamming a door. The heart sounds can be divided into a *first heart sound* (*lub*) and a *second heart sound* (*dup*). The first heart sound is produced by the closure of the atrioventricular valves, and the second heart sound is created by closure of the aortic and pulmonic valves. During a single cardiac cycle, both the first and the second heart sounds are generated; they signify the beginning and the end of each cycle.

Abnormal heart sounds are usually created either by asynchronous closure of the valves, splashing of blood into a large chamber, or by turbulent blood flow creating audible vibrations. Asynchronous closure of valves may be heard as *split heart sounds* (lub-d-dup). The splashing of blood into the ventricles, when the atrioventricular valves open, may create a *third heart sound* (lub dup dup). In an animal such as the horse, whose ventricles are naturally large, generation of such a third heart sound may be normal. In most companion animals, however, a third heart sound may be indicative of *dilatory cardiomyopathy*. The abnormal heart sounds produced by turbulent blood flow are referred to as *murmurs*. Leaky (*insufficient*) valves, *stenotic valves* or vessels, and septal defects are the most frequent causes of murmurs. At times, the vibrations from the turbulence associated with murmurs can be so great that it can actually be palpated through the chest wall.

7.2.6. ELECTROCARDIOGRAPHY

All of the myocardial activity of the heart is controlled by an electrical system called the *cardiac conduction system* (Fig. 7–12 on p. 118). The electrical activity acts like a battery: it discharges electrical impulses (*depolarization*). After being discharged, the entire system must be recharged (*repolarization*) to ready itself for the next cycle of events. The electrocardiograph (ECG) machine is used to record this electrical activity.

The *sinoatrial node* (*si"no-a'tre-al*, SA node) is the pacemaker of the cardiac conduction system. It is located in the caudodorsal right atrium near the opening from the cranial vena cava. When it discharges, the SA node stimulates the cascade of events that occurs during the cardiac cycle. The electrical impulse quickly travels through the atrial myocardium, initiating atrial systole. The electrical activity recorded by the ECG machine at this time is the *P wave* (Fig. 7–13 on p. 119). The impulse continues to progress through the myocardium, rapidly concentrating at a mass of specialized tissue located in the ventral right atrium, near the interatrial septum. This specialized mass of tissue is called the *atrioventricular node* (AV node). As the impulse reaches this site, it is momentarily slowed. Slowing of the impulse at this time allows the atria to empty fully before the ventricles are stimulated to contract. The portion of the ECG tracing that corresponds to the AV node is referred to as the *P-R segment*. The impulse quickly continues through the rest of the cardiac conduction system. It first progresses to the *bundle of HIS* (*hiss*),

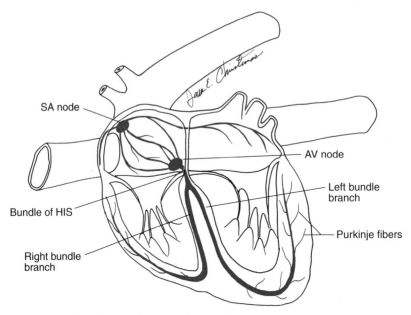

FIGURE 7–12. Cardiac conduction system anatomy.

located in the craniodorsal interventricular septum. It quickly travels through the *right and left bundle branches,* terminating in the *Purkinje fibers (per-kin'je),* and stimulates ventricular systole. The electrical activity from the bundle of HIS through ventricular depolarization is recorded on the ECG tracing as the *QRS complex.* The final electrical activity to be recorded on the ECG tracing is the *T wave,* which signifies repolarization of the ventricular myocardium. The magnitude of all of the electrical activity generated through the ventricles is so great that repolarization of the atria is not detected by the ECG.

The cardiac conduction system is important for controlling the cardiac rate and rhythm. If the electrical activity is too slow, *bradycardia* will be clinically evident. If the electrical activity is too fast, *tachycardia* will be clinically evident. *Arrhythmias* develop from abnormal and uncoordinated electrical activity. The arrhythmias may be caused by a primary disease problem in the cardiac conduction system, whereas others may be simply the result of electrolyte imbalances in the body. Regardless of the cause, some arrhythmias may be very serious and, if left untreated, may progress to *asystole.*

The *cardiologist* may elect to use other diagnostic tools to evaluate cardiac patients fully. In cases of cardiomyopathy, *echocardiography* may be useful in determining how well the heart can contract. The cardiologist may also be able to visualize abnormal chamber dilation or *myocardial hypertrophy* from the echocardiogram. Radiography is often useful for visualizing *cardiomegaly.* Other special radiographic procedures, such as the *angiogram,* help outline problem areas along the vessels. Early detection of cardiovascular problems, coupled with appropriate medical, nutritional, or surgical management, may result in happy, healthy, long-lived veterinary patients, in spite of cardiac disease.

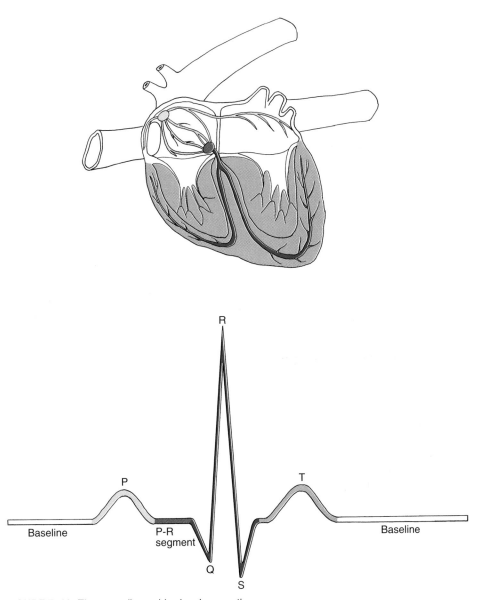

FIGURE 7–13. Electrocardiographic signal generation.

7.3. Self-Test

Using the previous information in this chapter, respond to each of the following questions using the most appropriate medical term(s). Do not use abbreviations.

1. _____Systole_____ is the phase of the cardiac cycle when the heart muscle is contracting.

2. The valve located between the left ventricle and the left atrium is the
bicuspid (mitral atrioventricular

3. The _pericardium_ sac is a thin tissue membrane that forms an envelope around the heart.

4. The medical term for heart muscle is _myocardium_.

5. Blood returns from the lungs through the pulmonary veins to the
left atrium.

6. The _aorta_ is the largest artery of the body, which originates at the left ventricle and terminates in the caudal abdomen, where it divides to supply the hindlimbs.

7. _phlebitis_ is inflammation of a vein or veins.

8. A heart rate that is slower than normal is medically termed
bradycardia.

9. A(n) _ecg_ is a diagnostic procedure in which a machine records the electrical activity of the heart.

10. The _pulmonary valve_ valve is associated with the right ventricle; blood must pass through this valve on its way to the lungs.

11. A veterinary professional who specializes in venipuncture for the collection of blood specimens is called a(n) _____.

12. A radiographic procedure in which radiopaque dye is injected intravenously to highlight vessels within the body is called a(n) _____.

13. A(n) _arteriole_ is a tiny vessel carrying blood away from the heart, leading directly to the capillaries.

14. A veterinary professional who specializes in the study of the heart and heart disease is referred to as a(n) _____.

15. The absence of any cardiac contraction is medically termed
asystole.

16. The phase of the cardiac cycle during which the heart is at rest is
diastole.

17. _____ is the medical term meaning "enlargement of the heart."

18. Abnormal heart sounds created by blood turbulence are called murmurs. Some may be caused by abnormally narrow vessels or valves. This condition of narrowing is medically termed _____.

19. The _____ is the specific electrical impulse recorded on the ECG tracing that is directly associated with firing of the SA node and atrial depolarization.

20. The _____ is the wall that separates the right atrium from the left atrium.

21. The __pulmonic__ and the __aortic__ valves are closed during the diastolic phase of the cardiac cycle. Closure of these two valves creates the second heart sound.

22. A condition in which the heart is beating more rapidly than normal is medically termed __tachycardia__ .

23. A(n) __capillaries__ is the smallest type of blood vessel in the body, through which gas exchange (oxygen and carbon dioxide) takes place.

24. Trace the blood flow of an adult animal through one complete circuit. Beginning with the systemic circulation returning to the heart, sequentially list each of the major structures through which the blood passes.

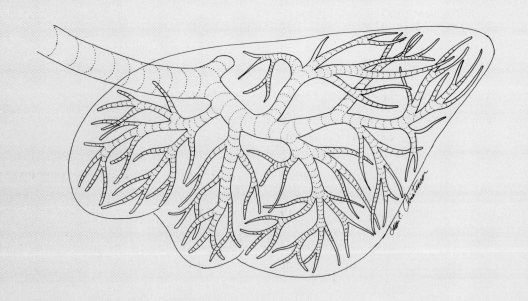

The Respiratory System

GOALS AND OBJECTIVES

By the conclusion of this chapter, the student will be able to:

1. Recognize common root words, prefixes, and suffixes related to the respiratory system.
2. Divide simple and compound words into their respective parts.
3. Recognize, correctly pronounce, and appropriately use common medical terms related to the respiratory system.
4. Demonstrate an understanding of respiratory and thoracic cavity anatomy.
5. Demonstrate an understanding of respiratory physiology with regard to breathing mechanisms, respiratory volumes, gas exchange, and protective mechanisms.

8.1. Introduction to Related Terms

Divide each of the following terms into its respective parts ("R" root, "P" prefix, "S" suffix, "CV" combining vowel).

1. **Pleural**   (R) _pleur_ (S) _al_

   pleural (ploor'al; pertaining to the pleura[1])

2. **Pneumonia**   (R) _pneumon_ (S) _ia_

   pneumonia (nu-mo'ne-ah; [Gr. pneumonia] a condition of the lungs; clinically refers to inflammation of the lungs with consolidation)

3. **Tracheobronchitis**   (R) _trache_ (CV) _o_ (R) _bronch_ (S) _itis_

   tracheobronchitis (tra"ke-o-brong-ki'tis; inflammation of the trachea and bronchi)

4. **Endotracheal**   (P) _endo_ (R) _trache_ (S) _al_

   endotracheal (en"do-tra'ke-al; pertaining to within the trachea)

5. **Tracheotomy**   (R) _trache_ (CV) _o_ (S) _tomy_

   tracheotomy (tra"ke-ot'o-me; to incise [cut into] the trachea; clinically refers to a surgical procedure in which an incision is made into the trachea)

6. **Tracheostomy**   (R) _trache_ (CV) _o_ (S) _stomy_

   tracheostomy (tra"ke-os'to-me; to create a "mouth" in the trachea; clinically refers to an artificial opening created in the trachea as well as the apparatus used to maintain patency of the opening)

7. **Laryngitis**   (R) _laryng_ (S) _itis_

   laryngitis (lar"in-ji'tis; inflammation of the larynx)

8. **Rhinitis**   (R) _rhin_ (S) _itis_

   rhinitis (ri-ni'tis; inflammation of the nose)

9. **Rhinopneumonitis**   (R) _rhin_ (CV) _o_ (R) _pneumon_ (S) _itis_

   rhinopneumonitis (ri"no-nu"mo-ni'tis; inflammation of the nose and the lungs)

10. **Pneumothorax**   (R) _pneum_ (CV) _o_ (R) _thorax_

    pneumothorax (nu"mo-tho'raks; air of the chest; clinically refers to free air in the pleural space)

---

[1]Pleura (pleurae—pl., derived from [Gr. *pleura*, rib, side]) is the tissue lining the thoracic cavity and covering the thoracic viscera.

11. **Hemothorax**   (R) hemo   (CV) o   (R) thorax

hemothorax (he-mo-tho'raks; blood of the chest; clinically refers to blood in the pleural space)

12. **Pyothorax**   (P) py   (CV) o   (R) thorax

pyothorax (pi"o-tho'raks; pus of the chest; clinically refers to pus in the pleural space)

13. **Atelectasis**   (R) atelect   (S) asis

atelectasis (at"ĕ-lek'tah-sis; imperfect/incomplete expansion; clinically refers to "collapse" of the lungs)

14. **Tachypnea**   (P) tachy   (R) pnea

tachypnea (tak"ip-ne'ah; rapid breathing)

15. **Bradypnea**   (P) brady   (R) pnea

bradypnea (brad"e-pne'ah, brād"ip'ne-ah; slow breathing)

16. **Hyperpnea**   (P) hyper   (R) pnea

hyperpnea (hi"perp-ne'ah; above-normal breathing; clinically refers to a breathing pattern characterized by increased rate and depth)

17. **Dyspnea**   (P) dys   (R) pnea

dyspnea (disp'ne-ah; difficult breathing)

18. **Apnea**   (P) a   (R) pnea

apnea (ap-ne'ah, ap'ne-ah; absence of breathing)

19. **Hypercapnia**   (P) hyper   (R) capn   (S) pnia ia

hypercapnia (hi"per-kap'ne-ah; a condition of above-normal carbon dioxide)

20. **Hypoxia**   (P) hypo   (R) ox   (S) ia

hypoxia (hi-pok'se-ah; a condition of below-normal oxygen)

21. **Alveolar**   (R) alveol   (S) ar

alveolar (al-ve'o-lar; pertaining to an alveolus[2] or alveoli)

22. **Sinusitis**   (R) sinus   (S) itis

sinusitis (si"nŭ-si'tis; inflammation of a sinus)

---

[2]Alveolus [L. dim. of *alveus*, hollow]; alveoli are the small air sacs within the lungs.

23. **Intercostal** (P) _inter_ (R) _cost_ (S) _al_

    intercostal (in"ter-kos'tal; pertaining to between the ribs)

24. **Bronchiole** (R) _bronch_ (CV) _i_ (S) _ole_

    bronchiole (brong'ke-ōl; a small bronchus; anatomically refers to the tiny airways that lead to the alveoli)

25. **Inspiration** (P) _in_ (R) _spira_ (S) _tion_

    inspiration (in"spĭ-ra'shun; the act of breathing in)

26. **Expiration** (P) _ex_ (R) _pira_ (S) _tion_

    expiration (eks"pĭ-ra'shun; the act of breathing out)

27. **Aspiration** (P) _a_ (R) _spira_ (S) _tion_

    aspiration (as"pĭ-ra'shun; the act of breathing to [in]; a- is derived in this case from the prefix "ad-" meaning "to" or "toward"; clinically frequently refers to the inspiration of foreign materials into the lungs)

28. **Cyanosis** (R) _cyan_ (CV) _o_ (S) _sis_

    cyanosis (si"ah-no'sis; a condition of blueness; clinically refers to blue coloration of the mucous membranes)

29. **Hemoptysis** (R) _hem_ (CV) _o_ (S) _ptysis_

    hemoptysis (he-mop'tĭ-sis; to spit blood; clinically refers to coughing up blood)

30. **Antitussive** (P) _anti_ (R) _tuss_ (S) _ive_

    antitussive (an"tĭ-tus'iv; pertaining to being against coughing; clinically refers to an agent used to suppress coughing)

31. **Epiglottis** (P) _epi_ (R) _glottis_

    epiglottis (ep"ĭ-glot'is; upon the glottis[3])

32. **Intranasal** (P) _intra_ (R) _nas_ (S) _al_

    intranasal (in"trah-na'zal; pertaining to within the nose)

33. **Achondral** (P) _a_ (R) _chondr_ (S) _al_

    achondral (a-kon'dral; pertaining to no cartilage)

34. **Nasopharynx** (R) _nas_ (CV) _o_ (R) _pharynx_

    nasopharynx (na"zo-far'inks; the nose and pharynx[4])

---

[3]Glottis [Gr. *glottis*], the vocal apparatus; the epiglottis is the cartilaginous flap that covers the opening to the glottis (larynx).

[4]Pharynx is derived from [Gr. *pharynx*], meaning "throat."

35. **Nasogastric**   (R) _nas_   (CV) _o_   (R) _gastr_   (S) _ic_

nasogastric (na"zo-gas'trik; pertaining to the nose and stomach)

8.2. Respiratory Anatomy and Physiology

The respiratory system, working in conjunction with the cardiovascular and hematopoietic systems, provides the body with the necessary exchange of gases (oxygen and carbon dioxide). A fully functional respiratory system is necessary for cellular respiration throughout the body to be accomplished.

Structurally, the respiratory system is a series of tubes and sacs (Fig. 8–1). Air enters the system during *inspiration* and exits during *expiration*. As air first enters through the *nares*,[5] it passes through numerous folds of tissue called the *nasal turbinates*. The nasal turbinates are covered with highly vascular mucous membranes that serve to warm, humidify, and filter the inspired air. They are covered with ciliated pseudostratified columnar epithelium. The epithelium not only produces mucus to entrap particles from the inspired air, but the cilia provide a constant caudad sweeping motion. This activity helps to ensure that foreign particles

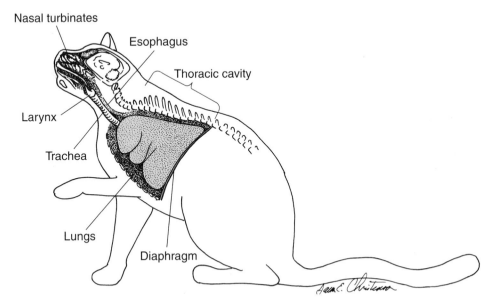

FIGURE 8–1. Feline respiratory tract.

---

[5]Nares (*na'rēz*; naris, singular) denotes the nostrils of domestic animals.

and organisms are constantly being removed from the nose to the *pharynx*, so that they may be swallowed. Through this protective mechanism and sneezing, veterinary patients are able to rid foreign materials from the nasal passages to protect the lower airways. Much of this protection may be lost by open-mouth breathing. Air inspired through the mouth is not warmed, humidified, or filtered as efficiently as that through the nasal turbinates. *Aspiration* of foreign materials and dehydration (drying) of lower airways are more likely to occur with open-mouth breathing. Open-mouth breathing sometimes has advantages, however. Many domestic animals (especially dogs) use a specialized form of rapid, shallow, open-mouth breathing called *panting*. Panting provides these animals with a means of dissipating heat from their bodies. The rapid movement of air over the moist mucous membranes of the mouth (especially the tongue) dissipates heat primarily through evaporation. Unlike the horse, dogs and cats do not have the capacity to sweat profusely for regulating body heat. Panting is by far their best natural defense against overheating.

Two major passageways are associated with the nasal turbinates, the *dorsal nasal meatus*[6] and *ventral nasal meatus* (Fig. 8–2). These two passages are merely that, large passages. The ventral nasal meatus is clinically relevant because it is used for the *intranasal* placement of *endotracheal* tubes or *nasogastric* tubes. The dorsal nasal meatus dead-ends in the nasal turbinates. If a nasogastric tube were mistakenly passed forcefully into the dorsal nasal meatus, *epistaxis*[7] would likely result. Other structures associated with the nasal passages are the *sinuses*. The sinuses are considered dead space because air tends to stagnate in these chambers. Although sinuses do not aid in the ventilatory activity, they provide resonance during vocalization and reduce the overall weight of the head.

Air from the nasal passages eventually passes through the *nasopharynx*, the pharynx, and into the *larynx* (Fig. 8–3 on p. 130). To gain entry to the larynx, the *epiglottis* and *arytenoid cartilages*[8] must be withdrawn from the opening (Fig. 8–4 on p. 131). The larynx is constructed of smooth muscle and *chondral* plates, and lined with mucous membranes. It is supported in the throat by a delicate bony structure called the *hyoid* (*hi'oid*) *apparatus*. The *vocal folds* are housed by the larynx. Vocalization occurs when muscles associated with the arytenoid cartilages place tension on the vocal folds. As air (generally expiratory air) passes by the taut vocal folds, they vibrate, creating audible sounds.

Next, the inspired air passes through the *trachea*. The trachea is composed of fibrous connective tissue, smooth muscle, and a series of chondral C-shaped rings (Fig. 8–5 on p. 131). The chondral rings provide semirigid support for the trachea,

---

[6]Meatus (*me-a'tus*, [L. *meatus*, a way, a path, a course]) means an opening or passage.

[7]Epistaxis (*ep"ĭ-stak'sis*) is derived from [Gr. *epistaxis*] meaning "nosebleed."

[8]Arytenoid (*ar"ĕ-tĕ'noid, ar"ĕ-te'noid*; [Gr. *arytaina*, ladle + *-oid*, resembling]); refers to the pitcher-shaped cartilages associated with the larynx.

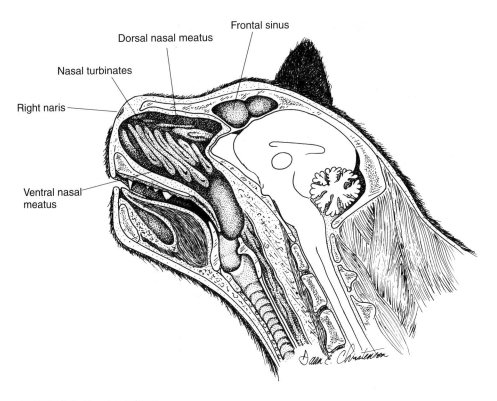

Frontal sinus

Dorsal nasal meatus

Nasal turbinates

Right naris

Ventral nasal
meatus

FIGURE 8–2. Nasal passages.

helping to maintain a patent[9] airway. The dorsal border of the trachea, which lies next to the *esophagus*,[10] is *achondral*. This allows for expansion of the esophagus during the passage of food. Otherwise, if the trachea were a completely rigid structure, large boluses of food would probably become lodged in the esophagus. The endotracheal mucosa is made up of ciliated pseudostratified columnar epithelium. Like the nasal turbinates, the trachea (and *bronchi*) have a *mucociliary escalator* to remove mucus and debris from the caudal/lower airways. This moves mucus and debris to a point in the larger airways where it may be coughed out. At the caudal end of the trachea is the *tracheal bifurcation* (a fork in the road, if you will). This marks the end of the trachea and the beginning of the bronchi.

---

[9]Patent (*pa'tent*; [L. *patens*]) means "open," "unobstructed."

[10]The esophagus (*e-sof'ah-gus*) is the muscular passage through which food travels from the mouth to the stomach.

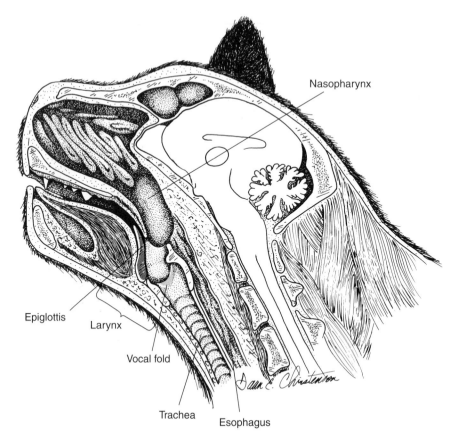

FIGURE 8–3. The pharynx and larynx.

The *primary bronchi* are the first branches off the trachea. From that point, the bronchi continue to branch, like a tree, becoming smaller as they progress (Fig. 8–6 on p. 132). The primary bronchi are quite large airways, with C-shaped chondral rings like the trachea. The *secondary bronchi*, the next branches from the primary bronchi, are covered with small, irregularly shaped chondral plates that provide structural support to the complete circumference of the secondary bronchi. As we progress to the *tertiary bronchi*,[11] the airways become even smaller and lose more cartilage. The chondral plates in the tertiary bronchi do not com-

---

[11]Tertiary (*ter'she-er-e*) is derived from [L. *tertiarius*], meaning "third in order."

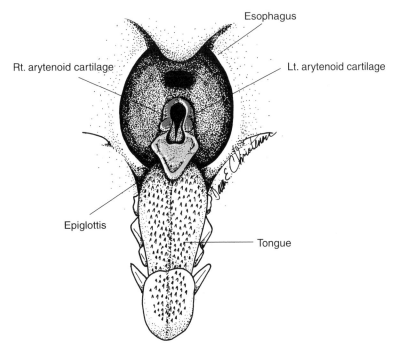

FIGURE 8–4. Laryngeal opening.

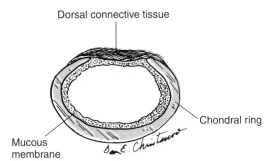

FIGURE 8–5. Transverse section of trachea.

pletely surround the airways. As we progress even further, the *bronchioles* are devoid of any cartilage (Fig. 8–7 on p. 132). The bronchioles are composed entirely of smooth muscle and connective tissue, with cuboidal epithelium for their mucous membranes. The *terminal bronchioles* lead to the *alveolar ducts*, which are basically portals to the *alveoli.*

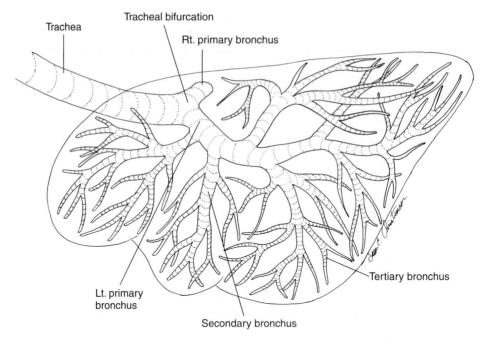

FIGURE 8–6. Bronchi.

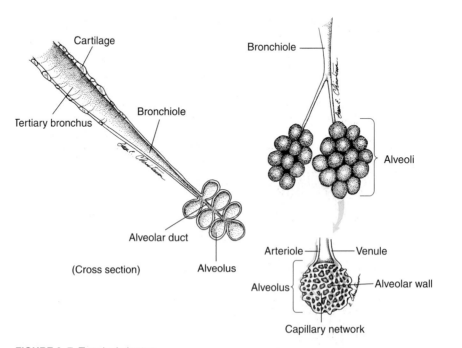

FIGURE 8–7. Terminal airways.

132

The alveoli are delicate clusters of sacs, composed of simple squamous epithelium. Each alveolus is surrounded by a dense network of *capillaries*[12] (see Fig. 8–7). It is through the *respiratory membrane* (alveolar and capillary walls) that gas exchange takes place. The alveoli make up the bulk of the pulmonary tissue. There is species variation regarding lung lobe configuration. Most domestic animals have a configuration resembling that of the cat's lungs, with cranial, middle, and caudal lung lobes bilaterally and an accessory lung lobe dorsocaudal to the heart (see Fig. 8–1). The horse is the one major exception to this arrangement, because horses have only right, left, and accessory lung lobes.

The *pleural cavity* is another term for the thoracic cavity. It is called the pleural cavity by virtue of the tissue that lines the cavity and covers the viscera (i.e., pleura). *Parietal pleura*[13] lines the chest wall and *visceral pleura* covers the lungs and other organs. The pleura is a continuous tissue layer. The pleural tissue actually meets in the middle of the thoracic cavity to form a thin tissue wall that envelops the thoracic viscera and serves to separate the right from the left side of the chest cavity. This centrally located tissue is called the *mediastinum* (me"de-as-ti'num). All of the pleural tissue secretes small amounts of fluid into the thoracic cavity, just enough to coat the pleura with a very thin film. This fluid minimizes friction between the visceral and parietal pleurae and provides surface tension between the chest wall and the lungs. This latter attribute is discussed in the next section.

8.2.1. MECHANISMS OF BREATHING

Breathing is both an involuntary and a voluntary act. The involuntary act is regulated by control centers in the brain stem. Voluntary respiratory actions involve conscious thought from higher levels in the brain. There are respiratory actions, however, both voluntary and involuntary, that do not serve to ventilate the animal (i.e., provide for gas exchange). Good examples of this type of voluntary action would be barking, meowing, whinnying, or mooing. Vocalization is a necessary form of communication, but it does not play a role in pulmonary ventilation, just as panting does not. Involuntary respiratory actions, such as sneezing and coughing, also do not contribute to pulmonary ventilation, but are necessary protective mechanisms.

Mechanically, breathing occurs easily and passively because of differences in air pressure. Air follows the path of least resistance. In fact, the entire act of breathing is analogous to the operation of a bellows used in a fireplace. When not in motion, air pressure inside and outside of the bellows is equal, at *atmospheric pressure* (760 pounds per square inch [psi] at sea level). The bellows draws air in

---

[12]Capillaries (*kap-ĭ-lar'ēz*) are the smallest blood vessels of the body.

[13]Parietal (*pah-ri'ĕ-tal*, [L. *parietalis*]) refers to the walls of a cavity.

when it is opened up. By opening up the bellows, the size of the space inside has been increased rapidly. The volume of air that filled the bellows before it was enlarged can no longer fill the new space. In essence, the air pressure inside the bellows has been lowered. Therefore, air rushes in until the air pressure inside the bellows is equal to the atmospheric pressure outside. The air will not leave the bellows until it is compressed. By reducing the size of the bellows, the new volume of air can no longer fit. The force of compression increases the air pressure inside the bellows, and therefore it rushes out into the surrounding air.

Ventilation in animals occurs in the same way as in the bellows. To increase the size of the pleural cavity, muscles of respiration are used. The *intercostal muscles* expand the rib cage. The size of the pleural cavity is further increased by the *diaphragm* (*di'ah-fram*) moving caudally. *Abdominal muscles* are relaxed to expand the abdominal cavity, making room for the diaphragm. Once the size of the pleural cavity and the size of the lungs have been significantly increased, air rushes into the airways and alveoli. The lungs expand with the pleural cavity because of the *surface tension* between the parietal and visceral pleurae. The thin film of fluid between the pleural tissues makes them stick together, just like a wet glass sticks to a table top on a hot summer day. This surface tension can be maintained only if no extraneous substances/pressures come between the pleural tissues. For all practical purposes, the pleural cavity itself exists in a vacuum and must be maintained in such a state for pulmonary ventilation to be accomplished. Normal expiration is a purely passive motion. Most of the tissues of the lungs and the pleural cavity are elastic. Like a rubber band, these tissues spring back when stretched. This reduces the available space for air in the alveoli, increasing alveolar pressure, and so forcing the air out of the lungs. This ventilatory process is repeated over and over again.

8.2.2. RESPIRATORY VOLUMES

During every normal respiratory motion (i.e., a breath; inspiration and expiration), a certain amount of air is moved. That volume of air that is moved during a complete respiratory motion is called the *tidal volume*. The tidal volume is adequate to meet a normal animal's needs at rest. But what if an animal is stressed? For example, what if a cat was suddenly awakened from its nap and chased by a large dog? The tidal volume is no longer enough to provide the additional oxygen needed by the cat's muscles to be able to escape. He needs pulmonary space in reserve to get him through this crisis. If normal, the cat has the ability to expand his chest further than he routinely would at rest. The additional volume of air that he can take in, over and above his normal tidal volume, is called the *inspiratory reserve volume*. If the cat is running, his muscles produce much more CO_2 than they did at rest. That CO_2 ultimately makes its way to his lungs to be exchanged for more oxygen. He needs the ability to expire more air to facilitate taking in the larger volumes of oxygen required by his body. The volume of air that he can expire, beyond that of his tidal volume, is called the *expiratory reserve volume*. The sum of the tidal volume, the inspiratory reserve volume, and the expiratory reserve volume is called the *vital capacity*. The vital capacity is vital to this cat, if he expects to escape the jaws of the vicious dog. If, while he was running away, he fell into a pond right after expiring a breath, there would be enough air remaining in his alveoli (the *residual volume*) to get him back to the surface. Then, by continuing to use his vital capacity, he would be able to swim to safety. The residual volume is a volume of air that cannot be expired, under any circumstances. It is there to keep gas exchange going for brief periods of time, no matter what. The residual volume also helps prevent *atelectasis* during normal respiratory activity.

8.2.3. GAS EXCHANGE

Average room air contains approximately 78% nitrogen, 21% oxygen, and 0.04% carbon dioxide. Each of these gases exerts a certain amount of weight (pressure), contributing to atmospheric pressure. Because the pressure exerted by each element is only part of what makes up the total gaseous mixture of room air, it is referred to as *partial pressure*. For example, if atmospheric pressure is 760 mmHg and carbon dioxide is 0.04% of room air, then the partial pressure of carbon dioxide in room air is approximately 0.3 mmHg ($pCO_2 = 0.3$ mmHg). Partial pressures are exerted by gases in the body, too. In general, we are concerned with the pO_2 and the pCO_2 in the circulating blood. The net difference in the partial pressures of these gases in the bloodstream versus the alveolar spaces influences diffusion across the respiratory membrane.

Oxygen is an essential element for life for all body tissues. Through normal cellular activities, oxygen is used and carbon dioxide is produced. The oxygen arrives at the tissues via the blood. *Hemoglobin* (he-mo-glo'bin; a compound found in red blood cells) binds with the oxygen (forming *oxyhemoglobin*) to transport it to the tissues. Approximately 98 percent of O_2 is transported as oxyhemoglobin, a compound that imparts the red color to the blood. On arrival in the alveolar capillaries, the red blood cells are O_2 deprived. The pO_2 of blood entering the lungs is approximately 35 to 45 mmHg in most domestic animals. The pO_2 of the alveoli is approximately 104 mmHg. Because the pO_2 of the capillary blood is much less than the pO_2 of the alveolar lumen, diffusion from the alveoli to the blood takes place. Blood leaving the lungs and arriving at the tissue capillaries typically has a pO_2 of about 90 to 95 mmHg. The tissues have a pO_2 of approximately 40 mmHg. So, on arrival at the tissue capillaries, the oxygen naturally diffuses from the blood into the tissues. The opposite effect takes place concurrently with CO_2. The CO_2 diffuses from the tissues to the blood, where some (15–25%) of it is bound to hemoglobin (forming *carbaminohemoglobin*, a compound that imparts a blue coloration to the blood.) A large portion of CO_2 is combined with H_2O, creating compounds such as carbonic acid (H_2CO_3) and bicarbonate (HCO_3^-). These latter compounds play integral roles in the acid–base balance of the body. The CO_2 is carried to the lungs, where it diffuses out of the bloodstream into the alveoli. It should be noted that CO_2 diffuses approximately twenty times faster than O_2. This gas exchange process is and must be never-ending. If gas exchange is compromised in any way, the whole body suffers.

8.2.4. PATHOPHYSIOLOGY

There are many respiratory diseases that are commonplace in veterinary practice. It is not unusual to see cats, especially young cats, presenting clinically with infectious upper respiratory diseases. Many of the pathogenic agents are viral, like the feline *rhinopneumonitis* virus. Dogs have their share of upper respiratory diseases as well. Infectious *tracheobronchitis* (kennel cough) is probably the most common. Most of the upper respiratory diseases of domestic animals have very high *morbidity* and very low *mortality*. That is to say, the animals appear quite clinically ill, with nasal discharges, sneezing, coughing, and depression, but most of the animals eventually recover from the diseases, just as people do from the common cold. In animals who are immune suppressed, particularly the very young and geriatric patients, more serious respiratory complications may develop. If an upper respiratory disease is able to progress and cause inflammation in the pulmonary airways and tissues, gas exchange will likely be affected. Frequently, secondary bacterial *pneumonia* develops in debilitated animals who contract viral upper respiratory diseases. As the alveolar membranes become inflamed, they swell, creating a much thicker respiratory membrane. Gas exchange can still take place, but it is significantly hindered (especially O_2 uptake). As the pneumonia develops further, with excessive amounts of mucus and pus accumulating in the alveolar spaces, gas exchange becomes severely impaired if not nearly impossible and may lead to life-threatening *hypoxia* and *hypercapnia*. The animal must use its reserve volumes just to maintain the body at rest. Visibly such an animal is *dyspneic*. The *tachypnea* or the use of reserve volumes (manifested by *hyperpnea*) may still not be sufficient to facilitate adequate gas exchange. These patients are usually *cyanotic*, because their red blood cells contain more carbaminohemoglobin than oxyhemoglobin. In highly vascular areas, such as the mucous membranes of the mouth, cyanosis is easily seen. Some pneumonias may progress to *pleuritis* as well. Inflamed pleural tissues are very painful. Try to imagine intense pain associated with *every* respiratory movement. Undoubtedly, you would try to minimize movement of the chest. By minimizing respiratory movement, as patients with pleuritis do, gas exchange is further reduced. The *hypercapnia* with the accompanying tissue *hypoxia* worsens and has deleterious effects on the body. Intense nursing care is required for pneumonia and *pleuropneumonia* patients, if they are to have any chance of survival.

Other noninfectious diseases such as feline *asthma* (*az'mah*) and equine pulmonary *emphysema* (*em"fĭ-se'mah*) can have similar effects on gas exchange. With these diseases, air becomes trapped in the alveoli. Although the animals attempt to use their expiratory reserve to try to eliminate the trapped air, hypercapnia and tissue hypoxia still develop. Pleural cavity disorders, many of which are caused by trauma, can also compromise gas exchange in the lungs. The most common traumatic injuries seen in companion animal practice result from patients being hit by automobiles. Frequently, a *pneumothorax* or a *hemothorax* develops after severe trauma to the chest. The free air/blood in the pleural cavity interferes with the surface tension between the visceral and parietal pleurae. If the mediastinum is intact, this effect might be secluded to the affected side only. Atelectasis may occur on the affected side if sufficient intrapleural pressures are present. Atelectasis is nearly guaranteed if a perforating injury occurs to the chest wall. In the event of such an injury, surface tension is lost. With such a wound, every time the chest is expanded with a respiratory movement, air rushes into the pleural cavity instead of the lungs. Obviously, any of these traumatic incidents reduces the amount of available pulmonary tissue for gas exchange to take place. In addition, a perforating wound to the chest may lead to the development of pleuritis or a *pyothorax.*

Some veterinary patients have structural defects in their respiratory tracts that compromise their ventilatory abilities. For example, English bulldogs have excessive amounts of soft tissue in the pharyngeal area. The excessive tissue significantly interferes with normal respiratory activities, especially inspiration, and is often surgically removed. Unfortunately, the surgical trauma may temporarily cause so much swelling in the pharynx that the larynx becomes completely obstructed, resulting in *apnea.* In such a case, an emergency *tracheotomy* must be performed to maintain a patent airway. Once the pharyngeal swelling has diminished, the *tracheostomy* tube can be removed, and the patient should be able to respire normally.

There are many ways in which the body's homeostasis can be disturbed through the respiratory system. The physiology of the respiratory system in health and disease needs to be fully understood to make appropriate medical decisions regarding patient care. For example, *antitussives* may be appropriate for some disease conditions and inappropriate in others. To suppress a productive cough in a tracheobronchitis patient could lead to consolidation of airway secretions deep in the lungs, potentially causing airway obstruction and pneumonia. It is also imperative that the patient be kept adequately hydrated, so that the mucociliary escalator can keep pushing the mucus and other secretions forward to be coughed out. On the other hand, a patient coughing nonproductively to the point of *hemoptysis* must be given some relief for the airways to heal. We, as veterinary professionals, must work in harmony with the body's natural defense mechanisms to properly maintain the well-being of respiratory patients.

8.3. Self-Test

Using the previous information in this chapter, respond to each of the following questions using the most appropriate medical term(s).

1. The medical term for difficulty with breathing is ___dyspenia___.

2. Inflammation of the trachea and bronchi is medically termed ___trachiobronchitis___.

3. _____ is a condition of the lungs in which they cannot expand. Such a condition often develops after a penetrating wound to the thorax.

4. _____ will be seen in the mucous membranes of a patient who has more carbon dioxide than oxygen bound to hemoglobin in his bloodstream.

5. _____, or inflammation of the nose, is frequently seen in cats with infectious upper respiratory diseases.

6. The _____ are folds of tissue in the nasal passages that are intended to warm, humidify, and filter inspired air.

7. The _____ is the combined total of the tidal volume, inspiratory reserve volume, and the expiratory reserve volume.

8. Coughing up blood is medically termed _____.

9. A(n) _____ is a drug used to suppress coughing.

10. The ___alveoli___ are tiny, grape-like clustered sacs within the lungs that are composed of simple squamous epithelium. They, with the pulmonary capillaries, form the respiratory membrane.

11. The ___epiglottis___ is a chondral tissue flap that, when closed over the laryngeal opening, prevents aspiration of foreign material into the lungs.

12. An abnormal respiratory pattern in which the patient is breathing very rapidly is medically termed ___terdypenia pnea___.

13. Absence of breathing is medically termed ___apnea___.

14. The _____ volume is the normal volume of air moved during a single breath.

15. The surgical procedure in which an incision is made into the trachea is medically termed a(n) ___trachiostomy___.

16. Trauma to the nasal mucosa through placement of a nasogastric tube could result in bleeding. Bleeding from the nose is medically termed _____.

17. _bronchios_ are tiny, achondral airways that lead to the alveoli.

18. Inflammation of the lining of the thoracic cavity is medically termed
pleuralitis .

19. The condition in which pus accumulates in the thoracic cavity is medically termed a(n)
_____ .

20. The diaphragm, abdominal muscles, and _intercostal_ muscles all contribute to normal respiratory motions.

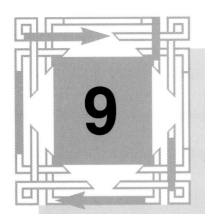

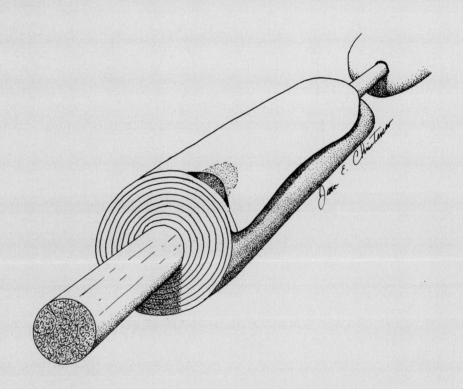

The Neurologic System

GOALS AND OBJECTIVES

By the conclusion of this chapter, the student will be able to:

1. Recognize common root words, prefixes, and suffixes related to the neurologic system.

2. Divide simple and compound words into their respective parts.

3. Recognize, correctly pronounce, and appropriately use common medical terms related to the neurologic system.

4. Demonstrate an understanding of neuroanatomy.

5. Demonstrate an understanding of neurophysiology, with regard to neurotransmission, motor and sensory pathways, autonomic pathways, and olfaction.

6. Demonstrate an understanding of the reflex arc with regard to spinal reflexes.

7. Demonstrate an understanding of and compare a pure reflex action to a response to pain.

8. Demonstrate an understanding of the blood–brain barrier.

9.1. Introduction to Related Terms

Divide each of the following terms into its respective parts ("R" root, "P" prefix, "S" suffix, "CV" combining vowel).

1. **Neuritis**   (R) _____   (S) _____

    neuritis (nu-ri'tis; inflammation of a nerve or nerves)

2. **Cerebral**   (R) _____   (S) _____

    cerebral (ser'ĕ-bral, ser-e'bral; pertaining to the cerebrum [L. "brain"])

3. **Cerebellar**   (R) _____   (S) _____

    cerebellar (ser"ĕ-bel'ar; pertaining to the cerebellum)

4. **Afferent**   (P) _____   (R) _____

    afferent (af'er-ent, a'fer-ent; to carry to/toward; af- derived from ad- , "to")

5. **Efferent**   (P) _____   (R) _____

    efferent (ef'er-ent, e'fer-ent; to carry out; ef- derived from ex- , "out")

6. **Sympathetic**   (R) _____   (S) _____

    sympathetic (sim"pah-thet'ik; pertaining to sympathy; anatomically refers to the sympathetic portion of the autonomic nervous system)

7. **Parasympathetic**   (P) _____   (R) _____   (S) _____

    parasympathetic (par"ah-sim"pah-thet'ik; pertaining to "beyond" sympathy; anatomically refers to the parasympathetic portion of the autonomic nervous system)

8. **Autonomic**   (P) _____   (CV) ____   (R) _____   (S) _____

    autonomic (aw"to-nom'ik; pertaining to self-control; anatomically refers to the autonomic nervous system)

9. **Cholinergic**   (R) _____   (R) _____   (S) _____

    cholinergic (ko"lin-er'jik; pertaining to choline work; physiologically refers to function with the neurotransmitter acetylcholine)

10. **Sympathomimetic** (R) _____   (CV) ____   (R) _____   (S) _____

    sympathomimetic (sim"pah-tho-mi-met'ik; pertaining to sympathy imitation; clinically refers to any agent that mimics the sympathetic activity of the autonomic nervous system)

11. **Synaptic**   (R) _____   (S) _____

    synaptic (sĭ-nap'tik; pertaining to a synapse [Gr. "connection"])

12. Neuroglial   (R) _____   (CV) ___   (S) _____

neuroglial (nu-rog'le-al; pertaining to nerve "glue"; anatomically refers to the accessory, supportive structures of neural tissue)

13. Astrocyte   (R) _____   (CV) ___   (S) _____

astrocyte (as'tro-sīt; a star cell)

14. Oligodendrocyte   (P) _____   (CV) ___   (R) _____   (CV) ___   (S) _____

oligodendrocyte (ol"ĭ-go-den'dro-sīt; a little "tree" cell; anatomically refers to a cell with few dendritic branches)

15. Ependymal   (R) _____   (S) _____

ependymal (e-pen'dĭ-mal; pertaining to the ependyma [Gr. "upper garment," "tunic"]; anatomically the ependyma lines the ventricles of the brain and the central canal of the spinal cord)

16. Microglial   (P) _____   (CV) ___   (S) _____

microglial (mi-krog'le-al, mi-kro-gle'al; pertaining to small "glue"; anatomically refers to the smallest of the neuroglial cells)

17. Bipolar   (P) _____   (R) _____   (S) _____

bipolar (bi-po'lar; pertaining to two poles)

18. Unipolar   (P) _____   (R) _____   (S) _____

unipolar (u"nĭ-po'lar; pertaining to one pole)

19. Multipolar   (P) _____   (R) _____   (S) _____

multipolar (mul"tĭ-po'lar; pertaining to many poles)

20. Axonal   (R) _____   (S) _____

axonal (ak'so-nal; pertaining to an "axle"; in neurology, refers to an axon)

21. Meningitis   (R) _____   (S) _____

meningitis (men"in-ji'tis; inflammation of a meninx or meninges)

22. Cerebrospinal   (R) _____   (CV) ___   (R) _____   (S) _____

cerebrospinal (ser"ĕ-bro-spi'nal, sĕ"re'-bro-spi-nal; pertaining to the cerebrum and spine [i.e., spinal cord])

23. Hemisphere   (P) _____   (R) _____

hemisphere (hem'ĭ-sfēr; half a ball or globe)

24. **Brachial**   (R) _____   (S) _____

   brachial (bra'ke-al; pertaining to the brachium [L. "arm"])

25. **Lumbosacral**   (R) _____   (CV) ___   (R) _____   (S) _____

   lumbosacral (lum"bo-sa'kral; pertaining to the lumbus [i.e., lumbar vertebrae] and the sacrum)

26. **Intervertebral**   (P) _____   (R) _____   (S) _____

   intervertebral (in"ter-ver'tĕ-bral, in"ter-ver-te'bral; pertaining to between vertebrae)

27. **Electroencephalogram**
   (R) _____   (CV) ___   (R) _____   (CV) ___   (S) _____

   electroencephalogram (e-lek"tro-en-sef'ah-lo-gram; a recording of electricity of the brain)

28. **Analgesia**   (P) _____   (R) _____   (S) _____

   analgesia (an"al-je'ze-ah; a state without pain)

29. **Anesthesia**   (P) _____   (R) _____   (S) _____

   anesthesia (an"es-the'ze-ah; a state without sensation)

30. **Paralysis**   (P) _____   (R) _____   (S) _____

   paralysis (pah-ral'ĭ-sis; a state beyond loose [Gr. lyein, to loosen]; that is, immobility; loss of motor function)

31. **Paraplegia**   (P) _____   (S) _____

   paraplegia (par"ah-ple'je-ah; paralysis "beyond"; clinically refers to paralysis of the caudal body/limbs)

32. **Tetraplegia**   (P) _____   (S) _____

   tetraplegia (tet"ră-ple'je-ah; paralysis of four; clinically refers to paralysis of all four limbs; cf. quadriplegia)

33. **Quadriplegia**   (P) _____   (S) _____

   quadriplegia (kwod"rĕ-ple'je-ah; paralysis of four; clinically refers to paralysis of all four limbs; cf. tetraplegia)

34. **Hemiplegia**   (P) _____   (S) _____

   hemiplegia (hem"e-ple'je-ah; paralysis of half; clinically refers to paralysis of one side of the body)

35. **Monoplegia**   (P) _____   (S) _____

   monoplegia (mon"o-ple'je-ah; paralysis of one; clinically refers to paralysis of one limb)

36. **Hemiparesis**   (P) _____   (R) _____

   hemiparesis (hem"e-par'e-sis; half weakness; clinically refers to weakness or partial loss of function of one side of the body)

37. **Ataxia**   (P) _____   (R) _____   (S) _____

   ataxia (ah-tak'se-ah, a-tak'se-ah; a condition without order; clinically refers to muscular incoordination/stumbling)

38. **Olfactory**   (R) _____   (S) _____

   olfactory (ol-fak'to-re; pertaining to smell)

39. **Myelogram**   (R) _____   (CV) ___   (S) _____

   myelogram (mi'ĕ-lo-gram; a recording of the spinal cord)

40. **Zoonosis**   (R) _____   (R) _____   (S) _____

   zoonosis (zo"o-no'sis; a disease of animals; clinically refers to disease of animals that may be transmitted to humans)

9.2. Neuroanatomy and Physiology

The neurologic system is a complex network of interconnecting components that work together to maintain homeostasis in the body. Many body functions and actions take place because of neural stimulation. The components of the nervous system are much like the circuits of a telegraph system. Lines, transmitters, receivers, relays, and electrical current are what make a telegraph system work. For clarity, some of the following sections compare the components of the nervous system to those of the telegraph, as well as using other analogies.

9.2.1. NEURONS

9.2.1.1. Cell Types

The nervous system has numerous types of nerve cells (*neurons*), each with a specific place and function within the circuit. Each cell type is described in the following list, including where it is found and what its primary function is.

1. *Unipolar neuron* (Fig. 9–1)
   A *unipolar neuron* has what appears to be a single pole (*axon*). The cell body is eccentrically located at a midpoint along the "*axonal* fiber." Actually, one end of the fiber serves as a *dendrite*, to receive and relay impulses toward the cell body. The other end of the fiber serves as a true axon, carrying impulses away from the cell body. Unipolar neurons are found predominantly in sensory nerve fibers. Their dendrites make up the *sensory nerve fibers* of the pe-

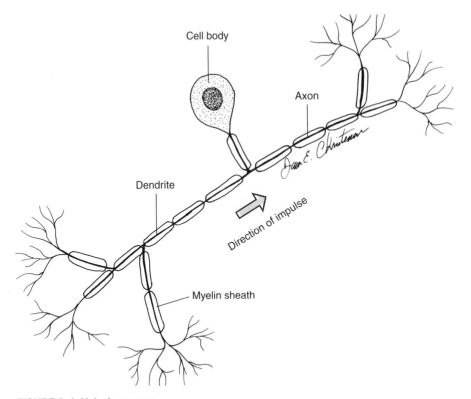

FIGURE 9–1. Unipolar neuron.

ripheral nerves. The cell bodies of unipolar neurons are found collected in masses of neural tissue called *ganglia*. The axons of unipolar neurons continue the sensory pathway from the ganglia into the central nervous system.

2. *Bipolar neuron* (Fig. 9–2)

A *bipolar neuron* has a cell body located between two poles. Actually, one end serves as a dendrite (receiver) and the other end serves as an axon (transmitter). Most bipolar neurons are associated with specialized sensory tissue, like that associated with vision, hearing, and olfaction.

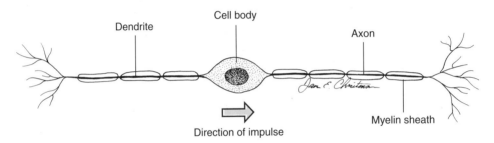

FIGURE 9–2. Bipolar neuron.

3. *Multipolar neuron* (Fig. 9–3)

   A *multipolar neuron* has many projections (poles). The cell body of a multipolar neuron is at the receiving end of the neuron, with numerous dendritic processes projecting from it. Impulses are received by the dendrites, travel through the cell body, and exit by way of the axon. Multipolar neurons make up the bulk of the motor neurons of the central and peripheral nervous systems.

4. *Schwann cell* (Fig. 9–4 on p. 148)

   Schwann cells are *neuroglial* cells of the peripheral nervous system. Schwann cells wrap themselves around the axons of peripheral nerve fibers, forming a *myelin sheath*. The myelin sheath provides insulating characteristics for the nerve fibers.

5. *Astrocyte* (Fig. 9–5 on p. 149)

   Astrocytes are neuroglial cells of the central nervous system. They have many cellular processes protruding from them, giving them a star-like appearance. They wrap their numerous appendages around neurons as well as blood vessels in the brain. They give structural support to the brain tissues, and form scar tissue after injuries. The cellular processes that wrap around the blood vessels in the brain create the *blood–brain barrier*.

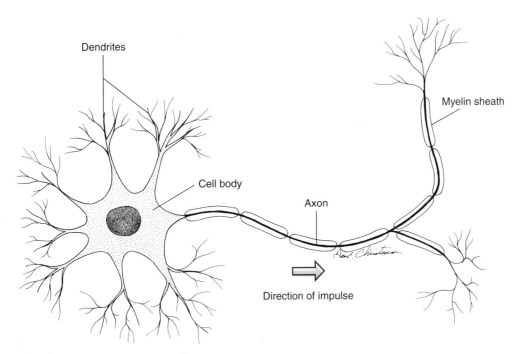

Dendrites

Myelin sheath

Cell body

Axon

Direction of impulse

FIGURE 9–3. Multipolar neuron.

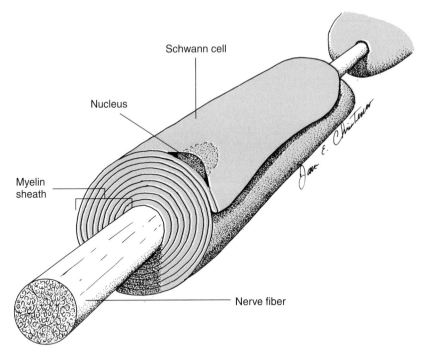

FIGURE 9–4. Schwann cell.

6. *Oligodendrocyte* (Fig. 9–6 on p. 150)
   Oligodendrocytes are also neuroglial cells of the central nervous system. They look very much like astrocytes, but with fewer processes. Oligodendroglial cells produce the myelin found in the brain and spinal cord. Unlike Schwann cells, oligodendroglial cells have numerous processes that wrap around separate axons. Therefore, a single oligodendrocyte can provide myelin for many axonal fibers.

7. *Microglial cell* (Fig. 9–7 on p. 150)
   Microglial cells are the smallest of the neuroglial cells of the central nervous system. They provide support for neurons, and phagocytize organisms and debris from the tissues of the brain.

8. *Ependymal cell* (Fig. 9–8 on p. 151)
   Ependymal cells are neuroglial cells found lining the ventricles of the brain and the central canal of the spinal cord. They are actually a type of simple cuboidal epithelium.

9.2.1.2. Afferent and Efferent Neurons

Afferent neurons are those that carry impulses from the peripheral nervous system toward the central nervous system. They provide the sensory pathways from peripheral nerves to the spinal cord and to the brain. *Efferent* neurons are those

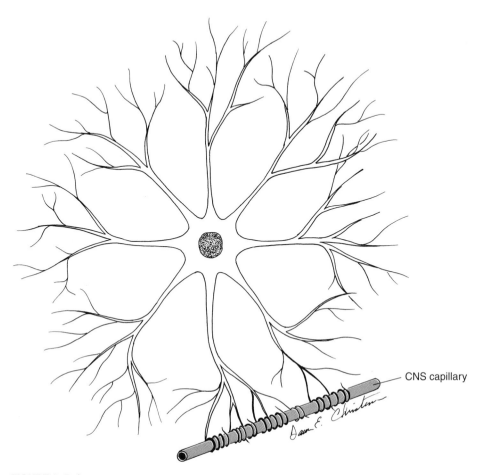

FIGURE 9–5. Astrocyte.

that carry impulses from the central nervous system to the peripheral nervous system. They provide the motor pathways from the brain and spinal cord to the peripheral nerves and ultimately to the target organs.

Each nerve is made up of a bundle of neuronal fibers, much like electrical cords and telephone lines. Each nerve has both afferent and efferent fibers, providing pathways for sending to and receiving from the central nervous system. Nerves could be likened to expressways. They have lanes (neural fibers) set aside for strictly "northbound" traffic and other lanes designated for strictly "southbound" traffic. The afferent pathway is designed more like a toll-way, because there are very few exits. In fact, along the afferent pathway only two exits are available for most nerves. One exit leads just to the spinal cord; this path is discussed with reflex arcs. The other exit leads to the brain. Once in the brain, there

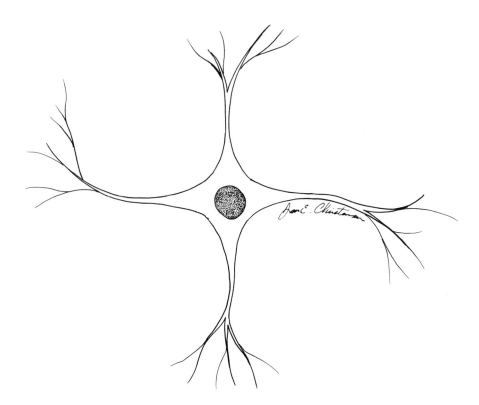

FIGURE 9–6. Oligodendrocyte.

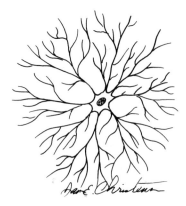

FIGURE 9–7. Microglial cell.

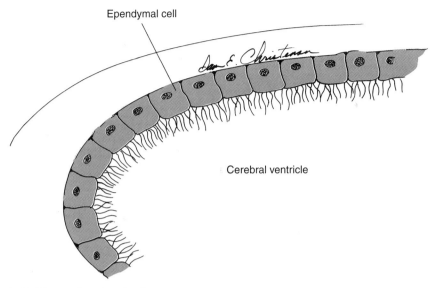

FIGURE 9–8. Ependymal cell.

are many divided highways and side-streets leading to specific areas of the brain. Along the efferent pathway there are many exits, just like the interstate system throughout the United States. Ultimately, a series of exits carries the nerve impulses to a specific destination at an effector organ or tissue.

9.2.1.3. Upper Motor and Lower Motor Neurons

Upper motor and lower motor neurons are simply subdivisions or subclassifications of efferent neurons, based on location. For the most part, those efferent pathways of the central nervous system (primarily the brain) are considered *upper motor neurons* (UMN). Upper motor neurons ultimately control lower motor neuron activity. The *lower motor neurons* (LMN) are those efferent pathways of the peripheral nervous system. Disturbances of either the UMNs or the LMNs result in abnormal motor activity.

9.2.2. CENTRAL NERVOUS SYSTEM (CNS) ANATOMY

The *central nervous system* comprises the brain and spinal cord. The brain serves as the central supercomputer for the body. However, unlike most computers, the brain has an almost inexhaustible amount of access and operating memory, as well as storage space. The spinal cord provides a telecommunication superhighway between the brain and the massive network of peripheral nerves.

9.2.2.1. Brain

The brain, housed in the cranial vault, provides ultimate control over most activities of the body, both voluntary and involuntary. The largest portion of the brain is composed of the *cerebral hemispheres* (Fig. 9–9). The right and left cerebral hemispheres are separated by a longitudinal fissure or groove. To increase the functional surface area of the cerebrum, its tissue has been made into a series of "folds." The depressions or grooves of the cerebrum are called *sulci*.[1] The bulging ridges of the cerebrum are called *gyri*.[2] The large amount of surface area is important because all of the *gray matter* (composed of cell bodies) is spread in a thin layer over the surface of the cerebrum. The bulk of the cerebrum is composed of *white matter* (myelinated fibers). The white matter provides all of the telecommunication links for rapid transfer of information between the processing centers in the gray matter and those in the other portions of the brain and spinal cord. All conscious thought takes place in the cerebrum. The cerebrum is responsible for data processing, systems management, and data storage, much like a computer. It receives sensory information from various places in the body, analyzes the data, controls motor responses, and then commits all related information to memory.

Rostroventral to each cerebral hemisphere is an *olfactory bulb* (see Fig. 9–9). These bulbs lie in close proximity to the porous (*ethmoid*[3]) bone that separates the

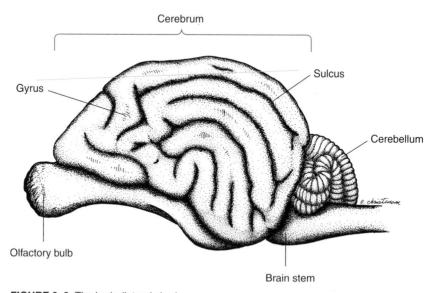

FIGURE 9–9. The brain (lateral view).

---

[1]Sulci (*sul'ki*), plural of sulcus; from [L. *sulcus*, groove, trench].

[2]Gyri (*ji'ri*), plural of gyrus; from [Gr. *gyrus*, ring, circle].

[3]Ethmoid (*eth'moid*); from [Gr. *ethmos*, sieve + *-oid*, resembling].

cranial vault from the nasal passages. The olfactory bulbs are well developed in most domestic animals. Receptors of the olfactory nerves pass through the ethmoid bone into the nasal passages. When olfactory receptors are stimulated in the nasal passages, the nerve impulse travels along the afferent fibers of the olfactory nerves to the olfactory bulbs. The olfactory tracts continue to carry the impulse into the cerebrum for analysis.

The *cerebellum* is small in comparison to the cerebrum. It lies caudal to the cerebral hemispheres and dorsal to the brain stem (see Fig. 9–9). Similar to the cerebrum, the cerebellum has numerous, small convolutions and folds. A sagittal section of the cerebellum renders an arborizing appearance, somewhat like cauliflower (Fig. 9–10). The composition of the cerebellum, with regard to gray and white matter, is much like that of the cerebrum. The bulk of the cerebellum is composed of white matter, with a thin layer of gray matter on the surface. The cerebellum is responsible for involuntary control of balance, posture, and coordination of movement. It attempts to maintain equilibrium and balance on receiving sensory information from portions of the inner ear, as well as visual and tactile input. Equilibrium is discussed in detail in Chapter 11, "The Ear."

The interbrain (*diencephalon*[4]) includes the *thalamus* and *hypothalamus*[5] (see Fig. 9–10). The diencephalon provides connections between the cerebral hemi-

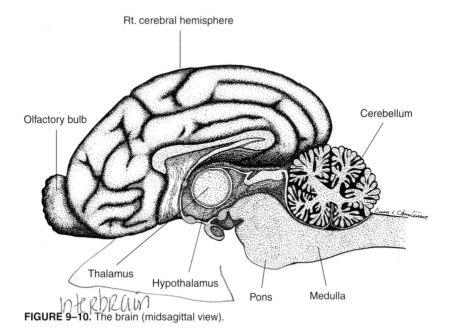

Rt. cerebral hemisphere

Olfactory bulb

Cerebellum

Thalamus

Hypothalamus

Pons

Medulla

FIGURE 9–10. The brain (midsagittal view).

---

[4]Diencephalon (*di"en-sef'ah-lon*); from [*dia-* , between + *encephal(o)-* , brain].

[5]Hypothalamus (*hi"po-thal'ah-mus*); from [*hyp(o)-* below + Gr. *thalamos*, inner chamber].

spheres and the brain stem. The thalamus serves primarily as a relay station ("traffic cop"), routing all sensory information (except olfactory input) to appropriate areas of the brain. The hypothalamus provides for many of the body's basic homeostatic maintenance needs. For example, body temperature as well as cardiac rate and blood pressure are controlled through the hypothalamus.

The *brain stem* is composed of the midbrain (*mesencephalon*[6]), the *pons* (*ponz*), and the *medulla*[7] (see Fig. 9–10). The midbrain, for all practical purposes, connects the diencephalon with the rest of the brain stem. The pons is a rounded protrusion on the ventral aspect of the brain stem that forms a bridge between the midbrain and the medulla; the word *pons* in Latin literally means "bridge." The medulla forms the caudal part of the brain stem that lies ventral to the cerebellum, between the pons and the *foramen magnum*.[8] Both the pons and the medulla contain many control centers for functions such as respiratory rate and rhythm. In addition, 11 of the 12 pairs of cranial nerves arise from the brain stem (Fig. 9–11). The first cranial nerve (olfactory nerve) arises from the cerebrum.

9.2.2.2. Spinal Cord

The *spinal cord* (Fig. 9–12) begins where the brain stem leaves off, as it passes through the foramen magnum. The spinal cord passes caudally through the *vertebral foramina* to approximately the level of the lumbar vertebrae. Adipose and other connective tissues fill any space in the vertebral canal between the spinal cord and the vertebral bone. In the lumbar/lumbosacral area, the spinal cord begins to branch excessively, giving it a "horse's tail" appearance—hence the name *cauda equina* (*kaw'dah e-kwi'nah*) for this portion of the cord. Because the spinal cord serves as the telecommunication superhighway between the brain and the peripheral nerves, it is composed largely of myelinated tracts (white matter). The myelinated tracts of the spinal cord give rise to the *spinal nerves*, which pass through the *intervertebral foramina* and branch into various peripheral nerves. Because of this arrangement, the white matter of the spinal cord is the most superficial portion of it. The gray matter is centrally located in the spinal cord, which, in a transverse section, looks somewhat like a butterfly (Fig. 9–13 on p. 156).

9.2.2.3. Meninges

The entire brain and spinal cord are encased in three membranes (*meninges*). Each *meninx* is somewhat different structurally and functionally. Minute spaces separate the meninges from one another.

---

[6]Mesencephalon (*mes"en-sef'ah-lon*); from [*mes(o)-* , middle + *encephal(o)-* , brain].

[7]Medulla (*me-dul'ah, me-du'lah*); derived from [L. "inmost part"].

[8]Foramen magnum (*for-a'men mag'num*); a foramen (*foramina*, pl.) is a natural opening or passage; the foramen magnum is the hole at the base of the skull through which the spinal cord passes.

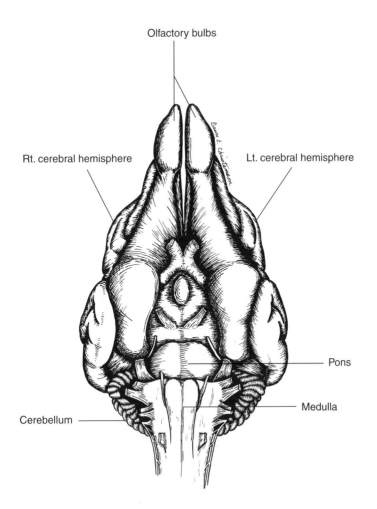

Olfactory bulbs

Rt. cerebral hemisphere

Lt. cerebral hemisphere

Pons

Medulla

Cerebellum

FIGURE 9–11. The brain (ventral view).

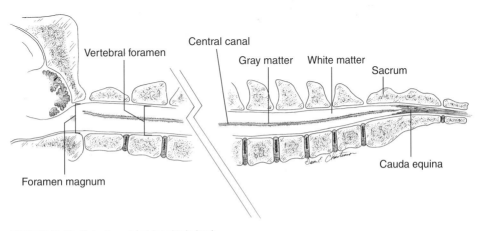

Vertebral foramen

Central canal

Gray matter

White matter

Sacrum

Foramen magnum

Cauda equina

FIGURE 9–12. Spinal cord (midsagittal view).

155

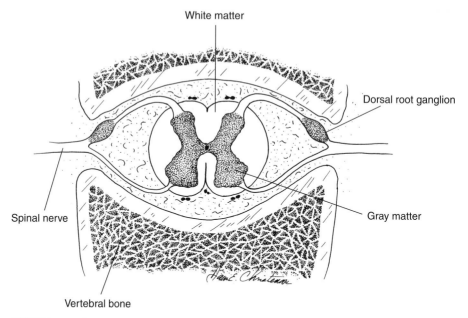

White matter

Dorsal root ganglion

Spinal nerve

Gray matter

Vertebral bone

FIGURE 9–13. Spinal cord (tranverse section).

The *dura mater* (*du'rah ma'ter; du'rah mah'ter*) literally means "tough mother." It is the most superficial of the three membranes (Fig. 9–14), and is composed of tough, protective, fibrous connective tissue. In the cranial vault, the dura mater is attached to the skull, but in the vertebral canal, there is space surrounding the dura. The space between the dura mater and the rest of the vertebral canal is called the *epidural*[9] *space*. This space is frequently used for regional *anesthesia*, particularly in companion animal medicine.

The middle meninx is the *arachnoid mater* (*ah-rak'noid*; see Fig. 9–14). It is called the "arachnoid mater" because its net-like structure resembles a spider's web. Numerous strands of the arachnoid attach it to the innermost meningeal layer, the pia mater.

The *pia mater* (*pi'ah ma'ter; pe'ah mah'ter*), meaning "soft mother," is the thinnest and most delicate of the meninges. It lies closest to the brain and spinal cord (see Fig. 9–14). It is highly vascular and closely follows the contour of the brain

---

[9]Epidural (*ep"ĭ-du'ral*); [*epi-* , upon]; pertaining to upon the dura.

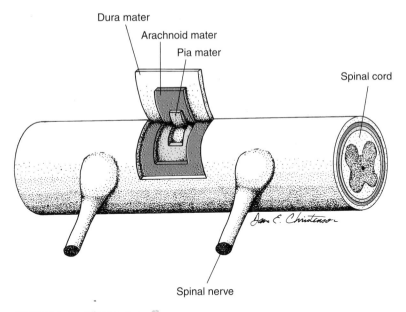

Dura mater
Arachnoid mater
Pia mater
Spinal cord
Spinal nerve

FIGURE 9–14. The meninges.

and spinal cord. It is therefore important for providing nutritional support by way of the bloodstream to the underlying neural tissues.

9.2.2.4. Cerebrospinal Fluid

Cerebrospinal fluid (CSF) flows in the *subarachnoid space*. It is produced in the ventricles of the brain by specialized clusters of capillaries and ependymal cells. Most of the CSF is produced by the *lateral ventricles* (one lateral ventricle is found per cerebral hemisphere). From there it trickles into the *third ventricle*, which is located in the area of the diencephalon. The fluid must pass through the *mesencephalic aqueduct*[10] to reach the *fourth ventricle*, which is located in the brain stem, rostroventral to the cerebellum. From the fourth ventricle it flows into the central canal of the spinal cord and into the subarachnoid space around the brain and spinal cord, in essence floating these structures (Fig. 9–15). This provides a cushioning effect for everyday movement and minor trauma. Production and flow of CSF is continuous. A mechanism for reabsorption of the fluid is provided through the arachnoid mater. Although the arachnoid mater is avascular, specialized projections of the arachnoid bring the CSF close to vessels associated with the dura mater so that it may be reabsorbed.

---

[10]Mesencephalic aqueduct (*mes"en-sĕ-fal'ik ak'wĕ-dukt"*); aqueduct comes from [L. "water canal"].

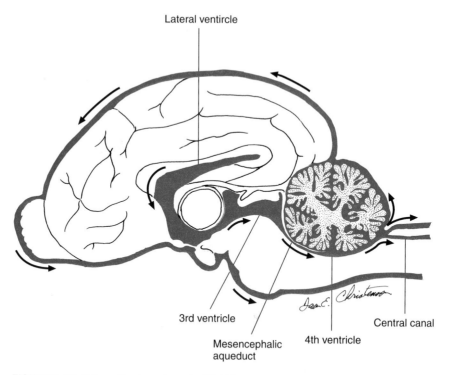

Lateral ventircle

3rd ventricle

Mesencephalic
aqueduct

4th ventricle

Central canal

FIGURE 9–15. Schematic of cerebrospinal fluid flow.

Cerebrospinal fluid is characteristically a transparent, colorless, acellular liquid. It provides an ionic balance for the neural tissues it bathes. Changes in the character of the CSF generally reflect pathologic changes in the meninges, brain, and spinal cord. Disease conditions such as *meningitis, encephalitis,* and *myelitis* may be detected through microscopic examination of the CSF. The fluid is collected by a CSF tap, in which a needle is inserted into the subarachnoid space and fluid withdrawn. Sites for CSF taps in domestic animals include the joint between the skull and first cervical vertebra, the joint between the fourth and fifth lumbar vertebrae, and the joint between the fifth and sixth lumbar vertebrae. These same sites are also used for *myelography.* During a myelogram, radiopaque dye is injected into the subarachnoid space. As the dye flows in conjunction with the CSF, abnormalities in the vertebral canal can be detected radiographically.

9.2.2.5. Blood–Brain Barrier

The *blood–brain barrier* protects the tissues of the brain from potentially harmful substances. It is formed by the *astroglial cells* that wrap their appendages around the capillaries in the brain. The "safety net" formed by these cells selectively permits passage only of some substances into the brain tissue. Molecular size is probably one of the biggest factors influencing the selectivity of the blood–brain barrier. Unfortunately, this barrier is so efficient in its function that it often does not permit passage of therapeutic agents, like certain antibiotics, into the brain.

9.2.3. PERIPHERAL NERVOUS SYSTEM (PNS) ANATOMY

The *peripheral nervous system* provides the body with a complex network of nerves, much like the telephone lines that stretch around the world. The peripheral nervous system includes everything outside of the brain and spinal cord. This includes cranial nerves, spinal nerves, nerves of the limbs, and nerves supplying the viscera. The entire peripheral nervous system is designed to receive sensory input, transmit it to the central nervous system, and then transmit appropriate response information from the central nervous system to the organs and tissues of the body.

9.2.3.1. Peripheral Nerves   need to Know.

The *cranial nerves* consist of 12 pairs of nerves originating from various regions of the brain and brain stem. The following list of cranial nerves includes a brief description of the respective nerve's function.

1. The *olfactory nerve* is the first cranial nerve. It provides for the sense of smell, as discussed in section 9.2.2.1.
2. The *optic nerve*[11] is the second cranial nerve. It provides sensory fibers for vision.
3. The *oculomotor nerve*[12] (cranial nerve III) provides primarily motor input for eye and eyelid movement.
4. The *trochlear (trok'le-ar) nerve* (cranial nerve IV) provides primarily motor input for eye movement.
5. The *trigeminal (tri-jem'ĭ-nal) nerve* (cranial nerve V) provides sensory fibers for parts of the face, mouth, and head. It also provides motor fibers for muscles associated with chewing.
6. The *abducens (ab-du'senz) nerve* (cranial nerve VI) provides primarily motor input for eye movement.
7. The *facial (fa'shal) nerve* (cranial nerve VII) provides motor input to facial muscles as well as some of the glands associated with the face and mouth. It also branches to some sensory nerve fibers associated with the face and head, providing for perception of things such as taste. The facial nerve is easily damaged in animals whose faces are insufficiently padded when laterally recumbent for long periods of time.
8. The *vestibulocochlear (ves-tib"u-lo-ko'kle-ar) nerve* (cranial nerve VIII) provides sensory fibers to areas of the inner ear associated with equilibrium and hearing.

---

[11]Optic (*op'tik*); from [*opt(o)-* , sight + *-ic*, pertaining to].
[12]Oculomotor (*ok"u-lo-mo'tor*); from [*ocul(o)-* , eye + *motor*, mover].

9. The *glossopharyngeal nerve*[13] (cranial nerve IX) provides motor input for muscles associated with swallowing, as well as for salivary gland secretions. It also provides some sensory fibers for the tongue (i.e., taste) and the throat.

10. The *vagus (va'gus) nerve* (cranial nerve X) is a very important nerve associated largely with the parasympathetic branch of the autonomic nervous system. Its fibers are primarily motor, providing for functions such as vocalization and swallowing. Its motor input also provides autonomic control for much of the thoracic and abdominal viscera. Stimulation of the vagus nerve slows the heart rate and accelerates gut motility. Its sensory fibers are also associated with areas of the throat and the thoracic and the abdominal viscera. It is important to note that the location of each vagus nerve as it passes through the neck is closely associated with the carotid artery and the jugular vein (see Chapter 7).

11. The *accessory nerve* (cranial nerve XI) provides motor input for muscles of the throat, neck, and cranial back/shoulder.

12. The *hypoglossal nerve*[14] (cranial nerve XII) provides motor input for tongue movement.

There are a multitude of peripheral nerves throughout the body. Only a few other nerves are discussed here, in keeping with those that are the most clinically relevant. The *brachial plexus*[15] is a bundle of spinal nerves that supplies all sensory and motor fibers for the forelimb (Fig. 9–16). Major blood vessels supplying the forelimb are closely associated with the brachial plexus as it enters the proximal forelimb. Severe damage to the brachial plexus results in paralysis of the affected limb. A single nerve arising from the brachial plexus and of particular importance in the forelimb is the *radial nerve*. It is a large nerve that at one point passes over the lateral aspect of the humerus (see Fig. 9–16). It is easily damaged here by a severe blow to the lateral brachium or by prolonged pressure over the area (e.g., as in a recumbent animal). The radial nerve provides motor input to most of the extensor muscles of the forelimb. Damage to the radial nerve results in *monoparesis* as well as significant sensory loss. Also of significance in the forelimb are the *digital nerves*. Many of the digital nerves (front and rear limbs) are of clinical importance in equine medicine when one is trying to isolate the location and cause of lameness.

The *lumbosacral plexus* is a bundle of spinal nerves that supply the hindlimb. Arising from the lumbosacral plexus is the *sciatic nerve* (si-at'ik; Fig. 9–17 on p. 162). The sciatic nerve is one of the most important nerves of the hindlimb. The sciatic nerve and its branches provide motor input to most of the muscles of the hindlimb, except those of the cranial and medial thigh. It lies caudal to the femur. When using the caudal thigh muscles for injection of medication, particularly in companion animals, improper technique or irritating medications could damage

---

[13]Glossopharyngeal (*glos"o-fah-rin'je-al, glos"o-far-in-je'al*); from [*gloss(o)-* , tongue + *pharyng(o)-* , throat + *-al*, pertaining to].

[14]Hypoglossal (*hi"po-glos'al*); from [*hyp(o)-* , below + *gloss(o)-* , tongue + *-al*].

[15]Plexus (*plek'sus*); pl. plexus or plexuses; from [L. *plexus*, braid].

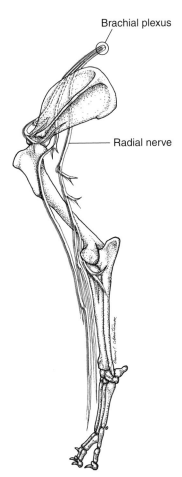

Brachial plexus

Radial nerve

FIGURE 9–16. Brachial plexus (lateral view).

the sciatic nerve. Varying degrees of paresis or paralysis could result. Another nerve of the hindlimb that is of clinical importance is the *obturator nerve (ob'tu-ra"tor*; see Fig. 9–17). It provides motor input for muscles of the medial thigh (i.e., adductors). It is most frequently damaged during difficult calving (birth of a calf). This is because the nerve passes over the pelvis, in the "birth canal," before it passes through the obturator foramen and courses down the limb. Obturator nerve paralysis leaves the cow unable to support her hindquarters.

9.2.4. AUTONOMIC NERVOUS SYSTEM

The *autonomic nervous system* helps control vital functions of the body automatically. Most of the autonomic nervous system is composed of motor neurons. Functions like breathing, cardiac rate, and digestion are controlled, in part, by the autonomic nervous system. It has its own methods of checks and balances

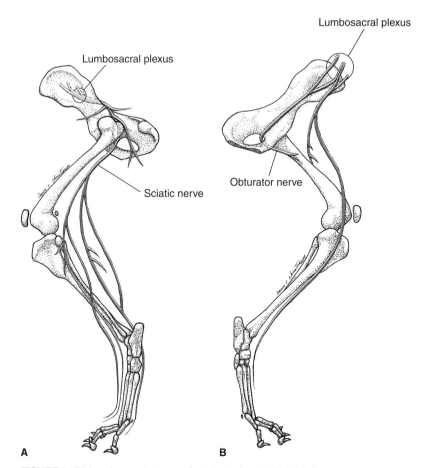

FIGURE 9–17. Lumbosacral plexus. **A,** Lateral view; **B,** Medial view.

provided through its *sympathetic* and *parasympathetic* branches. Both branches are continually working, in kind of a tug-of-war arrangement. Which branch dominates at any given moment depends on the needs of the body at the time. Centers in the brain help determine which type of activity is needed at a given moment.

9.2.4.1. Sympathetic System

The sympathetic branch of the autonomic nervous system provides for *"fight-or-flight"* responses. If a cat mistakenly wandered into a yard guarded by two large, fractious dogs, this portion of the autonomic nervous system would have "sympathy" for the poor cat. It stimulates various areas of the cat's body, making it possible for the cat to escape. The cat's cardiac and respiratory rates increase. Blood is redirected to vital organs (heart, lungs, and brain). His muscles too are given an ample supply of blood so that he can run away. Areas that do not need large amounts of blood at this time are the skin and the digestive tract. Sympathetic fibers also stimulate the adrenal glands to cause them to produce larger amounts of adrenalin (*epinephrine*) than normal. Adrenalin has a *sympathomimetic* effect on many of these same areas of the body. The sympathetic nervous system initiates the fight-or-flight response, and the epinephrine keeps it going as long as the cat needs to flee (or fight, if he's foolish).

9.2.4.2. Parasympathetic System

The body must have a way to counter the effects of the sympathetic system. The parasympathetic branch of the autonomic nervous system provides just that. Whatever the sympathetic branch stimulates in a given organ, the parasympathetic branch has the opposite effect. The only exception to this occurs with the adrenal glands, because they have only sympathetic innervation. So, as soon as that poor cat is out of danger, the parasympathetic system begins to overpower the sympathetic system to slow the cardiac and respiratory rates. Blood no longer is conserved for the vital organs. The cat can relax. That is precisely the type of activity that is stimulated by the parasympathetic system, *"rest and repose."* Most of the peak activity of the digestive tract is stimulated by the parasympathetic system—rightly so, because digestion is facilitated best when an animal is quietly resting. Cows and other ruminant animals demonstrate this best when they lay around for hours on end chewing their cud.

9.2.5. NEUROTRANSMISSION

Neurotransmission is nothing more than a means of sending electrochemical messages throughout the body, along nerve fibers. This occurs in a way much like Morse code being transmitted over telegraph lines. A message is transmitted from a distant point and is received at another point. If a reply is needed, a message is transmitted back to the point of origin.

9.2.5.1. Unmyelinated Nerve Fibers

Unmyelinated nerve fibers do not have an insulating myelin sheath surrounding them. They are exposed, in their entirety, to interstitial fluids. Chemically, the intracellular fluids are different from the extracellular fluids. Although both fluids contain a mixture of ions, the intracellular fluid of a neuron at rest (*polarized*) contains large amounts of potassium ions. The extracellular fluids surrounding this neuron contain large amounts of sodium ions (Fig. 9–18). When a nerve fiber is stimulated, through active transport the Na^+ is taken into the neuron, while concurrently the K^+ is sent to the extracellular fluid (*depolarization*). The net exchanges of ions generates an electrical charge (impulse). The ionic exchange begins at the receptor end of the neuron, and continues in a systematic, sequential way along the length of the neuron. Before the impulse has even reached the

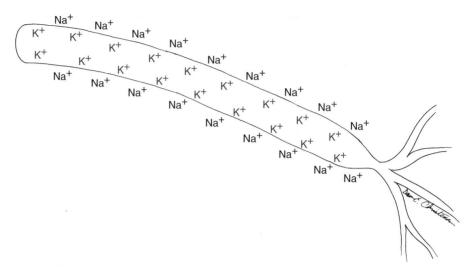

FIGURE 9–18. Polarized unmyelinated neuron.

other end of the neuron, ions at the receptor end of the cell begin reverting to their original positions (*repolarization*). Neurons "recharge" (repolarize) themselves, just as nickel–cadmium batteries must be recharged when they have been depleted. During depolarization and repolarization, ions are *actively* being exchanged across the cell membrane. Therefore, the total period during which ionic exchange occurs is referred to as the *action potential* (Fig. 9–19). *Resting potential* refers to a neuron at rest, when the ions are "in the starting blocks" awaiting "firing of the starting gun" (neuronal stimulation).

9.2.5.2. Myelinated Nerve Fibers

Comparing the rate of transmission of unmyelinated nerve fibers to that of myelinated nerve fibers is like comparing the pony express to the telegraph. The pony express was fast, but the telegraph was so much faster that it put the former out of business. Of course, this is not to say that the telegraph did not have its share of problems. For instance, on long stretches of telegraph lines, especially in damp weather, much of the current traveling in the lines would "leak." Plus, some of the strength of the signal would be lost because of natural resistance in the line itself. This would result in a weak signal at its destination. To maintain the strength of the signal, the telegraph system incorporated components called relays along the lines. The relays would provide a "boost" to the telegraph signal. In addition, telegraph lines, particularly those placed underground, were insulated to minimize leakage of current. Fortunately, most of the nerve fibers in the body are myelinated. Consequently, very little of the nerve impulse "leaks" from

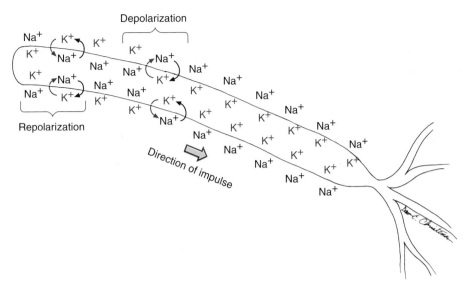

FIGURE 9–19. Action potential of an unmyelinated neuron.

the nerve fiber. Resistance along the nerve fiber could still weaken the impulse, however. Like the telegraph, myelinated nerve fibers are equipped with relays (*nodes of Ranvier*; Fig. 9–20). The nodes of Ranvier (*rahn-ve-a'*) are the only areas along a myelinated fiber at which ionic exchange takes place. The rest of the nerve fiber is insulated by myelin. The myelin prevents "leakage" of the impulse from the nerve fiber and the nodes of Ranvier provide the impulse with a boost to maintain its strength. As a myelinated nerve fiber is stimulated, action potential occurs only at the nodes of Ranvier. The electrical charge then shoots through the myelinated portion of the fiber to the next node of Ranvier. This continues se-

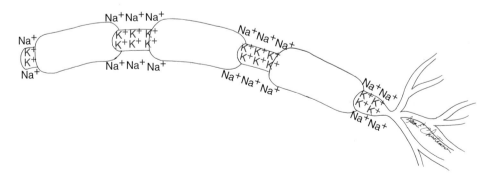

FIGURE 9–20. Polarized myelinated neuron.

quentially until the impulse reaches its destination, creating a *saltatory*[16] form of transmission (Fig. 9–21). This system provides for an extremely efficient, rapid mode of transmission of neural impulses.

9.2.5.3. Synapse

The *synapse* is another type of relay that provides a connection between two neurons or between a neuron and a target organ. Structurally, an interneuronal synapse is formed by the axon (transmitting end) of the *presynaptic nerve fiber*, a small space (the *synaptic cleft*), and the dendrites (receiving end) of the *postsynaptic nerve fiber* (Fig. 9–22). The end of the presynaptic nerve fiber contains small vesicles filled with a chemical *neurotransmitter* substance. As the nerve impulse reaches the *synaptic vesicles*, they release the neurotransmitter substance into the synaptic cleft. As the neurotransmitter comes in contact with the receiving end of the postsynaptic neuron, depolarization of that neuron is stimulated (Fig. 9–23). The most common neurotransmitter substance found in the body is *acetylcholine* (*as"ĕ-til-ko'lēn*; *ah-se"til-ko'lēn*). The parasympathetic branch of the autonomic nervous system uses acetylcholine almost exclusively as its neurotransmitter substance. Consequently, parasympathetic nerve fibers are referred to as *cholinergic* nerve fibers.

9.2.5.4. Reflexes and the Reflex Arc

Reflexes are protective mechanisms, reactions to stimuli, that occur independently of the will. For instance, if one were to make a menacing gesture with a finger, as if to poke a dog's eye, that dog by pure reflex action would close the eyelids and

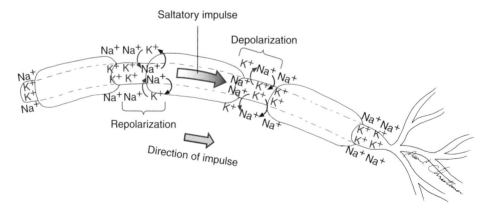

FIGURE 9–21. Action potential of a myelinated neuron.

---

[16]Saltatory (*sal'tah-to"re*); from [L. *saltatio*, to jump].

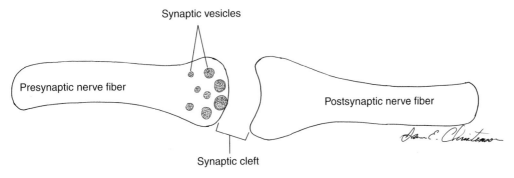

FIGURE 9–22. Interneuronal synapse.

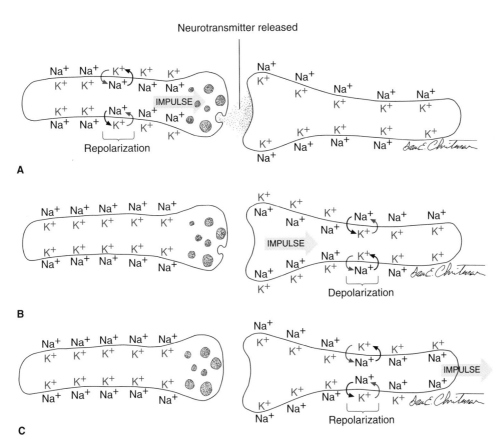

FIGURE 9–23. Synaptic neurotransmission.

retract the eye back into the orbit. This type of action occurs independent of the conscious mind. Reflexes are designed to give rapid responses to potentially dangerous stimuli. They are intended to protect the body before the brain has a chance to process sensory input about the situation.

A *reflex arc* provides rapid turnaround of sensory to motor impulses. The simplest example of a reflex arc is that of the *patellar reflex*. With an animal in lateral recumbency and the stifle semiflexed, the patellar tendon is struck with a reflex hammer. Striking the tendon stretches it slightly. The stretching action stimulates receptors in the cranial thigh muscles, generating a nerve impulse. The impulse quickly travels along the afferent pathway through the dorsal root ganglion to the spinal cord. The impulse slingshots from the spinal cord back down an efferent pathway to the cranial muscles of the thigh. The muscles are stimulated to contract, causing extension of the stifle joint. The entire process takes a split second and occurs completely independent of the brain.

A response to *pain* combines reflex actions with conscious thought. Applying a painful stimulus, such as pinching a dog's toe, immediately initiates a reflex arc. The sensory impulse travels along an afferent pathway, through the dorsal root ganglia to the spinal cord, rapidly switches to an efferent pathway, and travels back down to the limb where the muscles are stimulated to contract. All the joints of the limb are flexed, and as a result the limb is withdrawn. While this protective reflex is in progress, some of the sensory input from the toe pinch travels along afferent pathways to the brain. On reaching the brain, the information is analyzed and a command sent by efferent pathways to an appropriate target. As a result, the dog's conscious response to the pain may be vocalization, turning toward or away from the stimulus, biting the individual who applied the stimulus, or a combination thereof. Lower motor neurons control the *withdrawal reflex* and upper motor neurons control the conscious reaction. The nerve impulses initiated by the toe pinch are transmitted so rapidly that both the withdrawal reflex and the conscious response may appear to occur simultaneously.

9.2.6. PATHOPHYSIOLOGY

Damage to components of the nervous system may occur as a result of trauma or disease. Depending on the cause and severity of the damage, the resultant effects may range from minor sensory loss to death. Severed nerves cannot regenerate. However, if a portion of a nerve remains intact it may be possible for it to repair itself. Such repair takes a long time. The damaged nerve may never again provide completely normal transmission, but it may provide for functional use of the affected body part that it innervates.

One of the most common traumatic spinal cord injuries in dogs occurs because of rupture of one or more of the *intervertebral discs*. The intervertebral discs lie between the vertebral bodies, ventral to the vertebral canal and the spinal cord. The discs are composed of two different types of tissue. The outer portion (thick shell) of the disc is made of layers of a type of fibrous, cartilaginous, connective tissue. The center of the disc contains a gelatinous substance. The discs are designed to absorb the compressive forces placed on the spinal column. Unfortunately, the design of the discs is flawed. The cartilage portion of the discs is thin on the dorsal border. Deterioration of the discs, due to age or disease, weakens this already weak link. Now, with even the normal force generated by jumping off of a chair, the gelatinous center of the deteriorating disc may not be contained, and it bulges or ruptures through the weak dorsal border. This compresses the spinal cord dorsally against the vertebral bone. The length of time postinjury, the degree of compression of the spinal cord, and the ensuing myelitis determine the degree of paresis or paralysis present in the patient. The onset of clinical signs with protrusion of an intervertebral disc may be very sudden (*acute*), or progressive. The first thing an owner might notice is *ataxia* in his or her pet. Rupture of cervical discs usually results in *tetraplegia*. Rupture of discs in the caudal thoracic area usually results in *paraplegia*. Sometimes protrusion of the disc material is unilateral in the canal, exerting pressure on the spinal nerve roots and ganglia. This may result in *monoparesis* or *hemiplegia*. Myelography is generally used to isolate the specific disc(s) involved. The *prognosis*[17] of a paralyzed patient depends on the length of time postinjury and the degree of *analgesia* present, particularly in the extremities. For example, a paraplegic animal is tested for superficial pain and possibly deep pain in the hindlimbs. A mild painful stimulus is applied to the toes (i.e., a toe pinch). If the patient responds to the mild pain, his prognosis is good; the afferent tracts to the brain are still functional. If, however, a patient shows signs of complete analgesia when tested for both superficial and deep pain shortly after the injury, his prognosis is poor. Prompt surgical intervention to decompress the spinal cord in areas of disc protrusion, along with medications to reduce inflammation, may restore a paralyzed patient's mobility. No guarantees can be made. The recovery period for these patients is typically quite long. Owner patience and cooperation are important during the recovery period.

Damage to the brain manifests itself in many ways. Frequently, cerebral trauma results in abnormal neurotransmission patterns. Such activity is clinically observed as seizures (*epilepsy*[18]). To try to isolate the area of the brain involved with the seizure activity, a veterinarian may order an *electroencephalogram* (EEG). The EEG records electrical activity of the brain. There are numerous causes of seizures and all avenues must be explored to arrive at a definitive diagnosis. For many veterinary patients, epileptic activity can be controlled through medications.

Many of the infectious neurologic diseases of domestic animals are preventable through routine immunizations. Adherence to appropriate vaccination protocols is imperative to ensure the well-being of the animals, as well as to protect public health. *Equine encephalomyelitis* is a preventable viral disease of horses that is *zoonotic*. It is transmitted by mosquitoes and can be very debilitating or even fatal to people. A viral disease like rabies is deadly to both animals and hu-

---

[17]Prognosis (*prog-no'sis*); from [Gr. *prognosis*, foreknowledge] to forecast; clinically refers to the forecast of the probable outcome of a patient's response to a disease.

[18]Epilepsy (*ep'ĭ-lep"se*); from [Gr. *epilepsia*, seizure].

mans. Vaccination of domestic animals against this killer is of the utmost importance. In recent years, reported cases of rabies in the United States have been
steadily rising.

9.3. Self-Test

*Using the previous information in this chapter, respond to each of the following questions using the
most appropriate medical term(s). Do not use abbreviations.*

1. The _____ is the largest part of the brain and is responsible for
   all conscious thought.

2. A(n) _____ neural pathway is one that carries impulses toward
   the central nervous system.

3. The _____ prevents the movement of potentially harmful substances into the brain. It is formed by astroglial cells.

4. The _____ is the portion of the brain responsible for controlling
   balance and coordinating movement.

5. Spinal nerves originate at the spinal cord and pass through
   _____ foramina to form peripheral nerves.

6. Epinephrine is a(n) _____ hormone because its effects simulate
   those of the sympathetic nervous system.

7. _____ fluid is produced in the ventricles of the brain and flows
   through the subarachnoid space.

8. _____ is the absence of pain.

9. In the central nervous system, the neural cell bodies compose the
   _____ matter.

10. The meningeal layer that is highly vascular and lies closest to the brain and spinal cord is
    the _____.

11. Motor or _____ nerve fibers transmit neural impulses from the
    central nervous system to peripheral nerves and target organs.

12. A(n) _____ is a radiographic procedure in which radiopaque
    dye is injected into the subarachnoid space.

13. A(n) _____ disease is one that may be transmitted from animals
    to people.

14. _____ and _____ both are conditions in which all four limbs are paralyzed.

15. Nerve fibers that use acetylcholine as their neurotransmitter substance are said to be _____ fibers.

16. _____ are cells of the central nervous system that provide myelin for the nerve fibers. Their many appendages make them look like "little trees."

17. Inflammation of the brain and spinal cord is medically termed

_____.

18. The _____ is the bundle of nerves that supplies the entire fore-limb.

19. The _____ of a neuron refers to depolarization and repolariza-tion, collectively.

20. The _____ are the only portions of a myelinated neuron at which depolarization and repolarization take place.

21. Myelinated neural fibers compose the _____ matter of the cen-tral nervous system.

22. The _____ is the most superficial meninx, composed of tough, fibrous connective tissue.

23. _____ is a state in which all sensation is absent.

24. _____ is a condition in which one side of the body is paralyzed.

25. Muscular incoordination, such that an animal cannot walk without weaving and stum-bling, is medically termed _____.

26. A(n) _____ is a diagnostic procedure that records brain waves.

27. The principal portion of the autonomic nervous system that is responsible for "rest and re-pose" activities is the _____ branch.

28. _____ is a condition in which an animal is paralyzed in the hindquarters only.

29. The _____ branch of the autonomic nervous system is responsi-ble for "fight-or-flight" reactions to stimuli.

30. The _____ nerve is a major nerve of the hindlimb that provides motor pathways to all hindlimb muscles except the cranial and medial thigh.

31. A condition in which an animal is weak in a single limb, exhibiting signs of partial sensory and motor deficits, is medically termed _____.

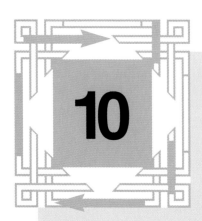

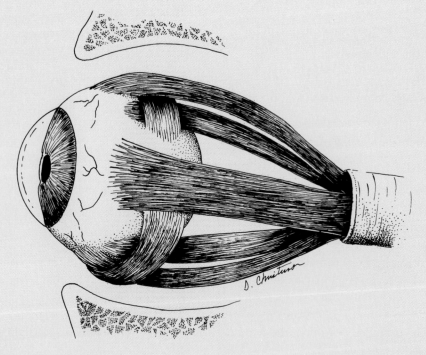

The
Eye

GOALS AND OBJECTIVES

By the conclusion of this chapter, the student will be able to:

1. Recognize common root words, prefixes, and suffixes related to ophthalmology.
2. Divide simple and compound words into their respective parts.
3. Recognize, correctly pronounce, and appropriately use common medical terms related to ophthalmology.
4. Demonstrate an understanding of ocular anatomy.
5. Demonstrate an understanding of ocular physiology with regard to aqueous production, flow, and drainage.
6. Demonstrate an understanding of the visual pathway.

10.1. Introduction to Related Terms

Divide each of the following terms into its respective parts ("R" root, "P" prefix, "S" suffix, "CV" combining vowel).

1. **Ophthalmology**   (R) _____ (CV) ___ (S) _____

   ophthalmology (of"thal-mol'o-je; study of the eye)

2. **Intraocular**   (P) _____ (R) _____ (S) _____

   intraocular (in"trah-ok'u-lar; pertaining to inside the eye)

3. **Periocular**   (P) _____ (R) _____ (S) _____

   periocular (per"e-ok'u-lar; pertaining to around the eye)

4. **Extraocular**   (P) _____ (R) _____ (S) _____

   extraocular (eks"trah-ok'u-lar; pertaining to outside the eye)

5. **Optic**   (R) _____ (S) _____

   optic (op'tik; pertaining to sight/vision)

6. **Palpebral**   (R) _____ (S) _____

   palpebral (pal'pĕ-bral, pal-pe'bral; pertaining to the palpebra [L. "eyelid"])

7. **Conjunctival**   (R) _____ (S) _____

   conjunctival (kon"junk-ti'val; pertaining to the conjunctiva)

8. **Corneal**   (R) _____ (S) _____

   corneal (kor'ne-al; pertaining to the cornea)

9. **Keratoconjunctivitis** (R) _____ (CV) ___ (R) _____ (S) _____

   keratoconjunctivitis (ker"ah-to-kon-junk"tĭ-vi'tis; inflammation of the cornea and the conjunctiva)

10. **Iridocorneal**   (R) _____ (CV) ___ (R) _____ (S) _____

    iridocorneal (ir"ĭ-do-kor'ne-al; pertaining to the iris and the cornea)

11. **Scleral**   (R) _____ (S) _____

    scleral (sklĕ'ral; pertaining to the sclera [Gr. "hard"])

12. **Miosis**   (R) _____ (CV) ___ (S) _____

    miosis (mi-o'sis; a condition of smallness; clinically refers to pupillary constriction)

13. **Mydriatic**   (R) _____ (S) _____

mydriatic (mid"re-at'ik; pertaining to mydriasis [mid"ri'ah-sis; Gr.]; clinically refers to pupillary dilation)

14. **Anisocoria**   (P) _____ (CV) ___ (R) _____ (S) _____

anisocoria (an"ĭ-so-ko're-ah, an-e"so-ko're-ah; a condition of unequal pupils)

15. **Nasolacrimal**   (R) _____ (CV) ___ (R) _____ (S) _____

nasolacrimal (na"zo-lak'rĭ-mal; pertaining to the nose and lacrima [L. "tears"])

16. **Photophobia**   (R) _____ (CV) ___ (R) _____ (S) _____

photophobia (fo"to-fo'be-ah; a condition of light "fear"; clinically refers to abnormal visual intolerance of light)

17. **Uveitis**   (R) _____ (S) _____

uveitis (u"ve-i'tis; inflammation of the uvea)

18. **Blepharospasm**   (R) _____ (CV) ___ (S) _____

blepharospasm (blef'ah-ro-spazm"; spasm of an eyelid; clinically refers to tonic [rigid] muscular spasm of the eyelids, generally in a closed position)

19. **Distichiasis**   (R) _____ (CV) ___ (S) _____

distichiasis (dis"tĭ-ki'ah-sis; a state of a double line [Gr. distichia, double line]; clinically refers to a double row of eyelashes)

20. **Ectropion**   (P) _____ (R) _____ (CV) ___ (S) _____

ectropion (ek-tro'pe-on; an outward turning [Gr.]; clinically refers to eversion, outward rolling of an eyelid)

21. **Entropion**   (P) _____ (R) _____ (CV) ___ (S) _____

entropion (en-tro'pe-on; an inward turning; clinically refers to inversion, inward rolling of an eyelid)

22. **Retinopathy**   (R) _____ (CV) ___ (S) _____

retinopathy (ret"ĭ-nop'ah-the; a disease of the retina)

23. **Ophthalmologist**   (R) _____ (CV) ___ (R) _____ (S) _____

ophthalmologist (of"thal-mol'o-jist; one who specializes in eye study; i.e., a doctor of ophthalmology)

24. **Contralateral**   (P) _____ (R) _____ (S) _____

contralateral (kon"trah-lat'er-al; pertaining to the opposite side)

25. Unilateral   (P) _____   (R) _____   (S) _____

unilateral (u"nĭ-lat'er-al; pertaining to one side)

26. Buphthalmos   (R) _____   (R) _____

buphthalmos (buf-thal'mos; an ox eye; clinically refers to abnormal enlargement of the eye)

10.2. Ocular Anatomy and Physiology

10.2.1. PERIOCULAR ANATOMY

There are many accessory structures surrounding the eye, most of which serve to protect the eye itself. The *orbit* of most domestic animals and humans is a bony structure that surrounds the globe. The orbit of the dog and cat is incomplete along its dorsolateral border (Fig. 10–1). This makes *proptosis*[1] of the globe much easier in the dog and the cat. In other animals, the orbit would have to be fractured to facilitate proptosis. Within the orbit is much adipose and loose connective tissue to provide support and cushioning for the globe.

The *palpebrae* provide protection for the exposed surfaces of the anterior globe (Fig. 10–2). The exposed, outer surface of the palpebrae of domestic animals is covered with fine hairs. At the edges of each lid is a row of eyelashes. The remaining surfaces of the palpebrae are lined with a delicate epithelial mucous membrane called the *conjunctiva*. The *palpebral conjunctiva* is continuous with the *ocular conjunctiva*, forming a "sac" associated with each palpebra. (Ocular conjunctiva covers the exposed portion of the sclera up to but not on the cornea.) The *dorsal conjunctival sac* is associated with the upper eyelid and the *ventral conjunctival sac* is associated with the lower eyelid. The palpebral muscles permit opening and closure of the eyelids. Most domestic animals also have a "third eyelid," called the *nictitating membrane*.[2] It is most easily visualized near the *medial canthus*[3] of the eye. With gentle pressure applied to the dorsolateral palpebra and globe, the nictitating membrane elevates and covers the globe. The *gland nictitans* associated with this structure contributes to tear film production.

---

[1]Proptosis (*prop-to'sis*); from [Gr. *proptosis*, a fall forward]; clinically refers to displacement of the eye from the orbit.

[2]Nictitating membrane (*nik"tĭ-ta'ting*); from [L. *nictitare*, to wink].

[3]Canthus (*kan'thus*); from [Gr. *kanthos*, angle]; clinically a canthus is the angle formed by the eyelids; each eye has a medial and a lateral canthus.

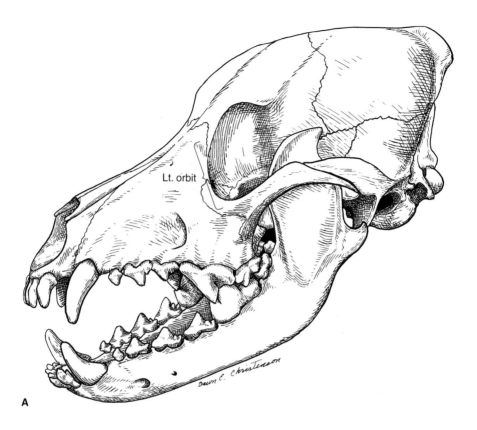

Lt. orbit

A

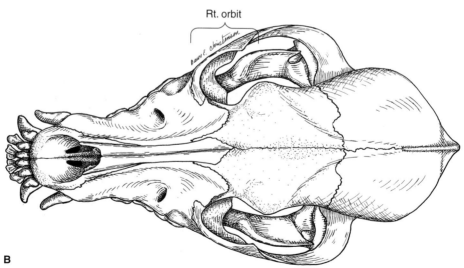

Rt. orbit

B

FIGURE 10–1. Canine orbit. **A,** Lateral view; **B,** Dorsal view.

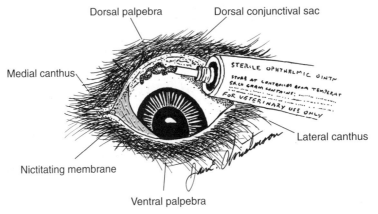

FIGURE 10–2. Palpebrae and associated structures.

10.2.2. LACRIMATION AND THE NASOLACRIMAL APPARATUS

The *lacrimal gland* (Fig. 10–3), which produces most of the tear film, is associated with the dorsal palpebra near the *lateral canthus*. Near the medial canthus on each palpebra is a *punctum*, which is the opening to the *nasolacrimal duct*. The nasolacrimal duct is designed to drain excess tears into the nose. That is why when a person cries, his or her nose tends to run.

Tears consist of two distinct components. The watery portion of the tears provides a constant bathing or flushing action; the viscous, oily portion of the tear

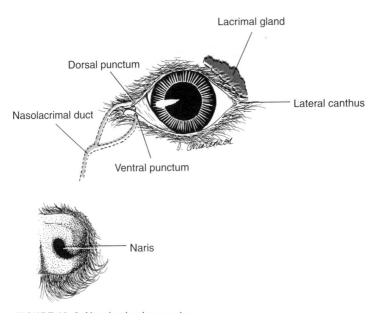

FIGURE 10–3. Nasolacrimal apparatus.

film provides a longer-lasting protective coating for the eye. Collectively, tears lubricate, moisturize, and protect the delicate tissues of the cornea and conjunctiva. Blinking provides a repetitive sweeping action that continually spreads the tear film over the eye.

Tears, particularly the watery component, are produced predominantly by the lacrimal gland. Other periocular glands secrete more of the viscous component. The tears flow down over the eye and eventually drain out through the nasolacrimal duct. Once in the nasal passages, the tears flow with the rest of the nasal secretions, eventually to be swallowed. *Epiphora*[4] may develop with excessive production of the tears or as a result of obstruction of the nasolacrimal duct. *Chronic* (*kron'ik*; long-term) epiphora is easily detected in white and light-colored animals, because the tears tend to stain the *periocular* fur brown. At the opposite end of the spectrum, *keratoconjunctivitis sicca*[5] results from minimal or absent production of the watery portion of the tears. The viscous portion of the tear film continues to be produced (excessively, to compensate), but it cannot by itself protect the delicate tissues of the cornea and the conjunctiva. It merely builds up around the eyes, creating a thick, stringy ocular discharge.

10.2.3. OCULAR ANATOMY

The globe of the eye is supported and moved by *extraocular muscles* (Fig. 10–4 on p. 180). They are attached to the toughest portion of the eye, the *sclera*. The sclera is often referred to as the "white of the eye." It is made of thick, tough, fibrous connective tissue. It actually forms and lends shape to the bulk of the globe, providing support for extraocular as well as intraocular structures.

The most anterior structure of the globe is the *cornea* (Fig. 10–5 on p. 180). The cornea is a dome-shaped, transparent, avascular structure, formed of layers of tissue (Fig. 10–6 on p. 181). The outermost layer is made of a type of stratified squamous epithelium. The thickest layer is called the *stroma*, which is made of a type of connective tissue. The innermost layer, *Descemet's membrane*,[6] is made of a type of simple squamous epithelium. The intraocular chamber, formed in part by the cornea, is the *anterior chamber*. The anterior chamber is filled with a watery fluid called *aqueous humor*. The caudal border of the anterior chamber is formed by the *iris*.

The iris is an intraocular muscle that forms a central hole called the *pupil* (Fig. 10–7 on p. 181). When looking at an animal's eyes, the iris is the colored part. The color varies from animal to animal, depending on species and breed. The smooth muscle fibers of the iris are oriented in a radiating as well as a circular manner. This orientation permits the iris to function like the aperture of a camera. When the circular muscle fibers contract, the pupil is constricted (*miosis*). Conversely, when the radiating muscle fibers contract, the pupil dilates (*mydriasis*).

---

[4]Epiphora (*e-pif'o-rah*); from [Gr. *epiphora*, sudden burst]; means an overflow of tears onto the face.
[5]Sicca (*sik'ah*); from [L. *siccus*, dry].
[6]Descemet's membrane (*des-ĕ-māz'*); named after the French anatomist Jean Descemet.

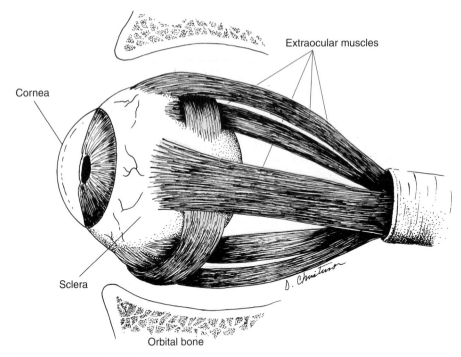

FIGURE 10–4. Extraocular muscles.

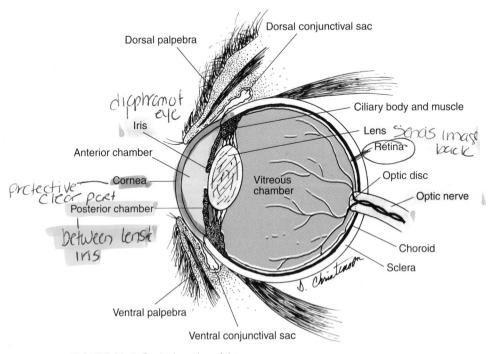

Extraocular muscles

Cornea

Sclera

Orbital bone

Dorsal palpebra

Dorsal conjunctival sac

diaphramt eye

Iris

Ciliary body and muscle

Anterior chamber

Lens *Sends image back*

Retina

Cornea

Vitreous chamber

Protective clear part

Optic disc

Posterior chamber

Optic nerve

between lens & iris

Choroid

Sclera

Ventral palpebra

Ventral conjunctival sac

FIGURE 10–5. Sagittal section of the eye.

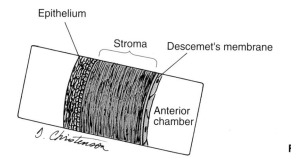

Epithelium

Stroma   Descemet's membrane

Anterior
chamber

O. Christenson

FIGURE 10–6. Corneal tissue layers.

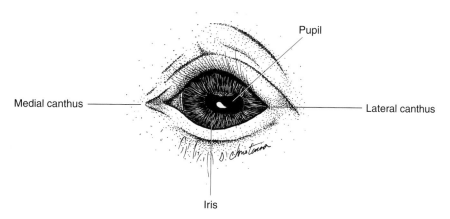

Pupil

Medial canthus

Lateral canthus

O. Christenson

Iris

FIGURE 10–7. Anterior view of the equine eye.

Directly behind the iris is the *lens*. The lens is a biconvex structure formed in layers, much like an onion. It is normally a transparent, semifirm structure. The *lens capsule* is attached to the *muscles of accommodation*, the *ciliary (sil'e-er"e) muscles*, by tough strands of connective tissue fibers. As the muscles of accommodation contract and relax, they effect changes in the shape of the lens. In so doing, light passing through the lens is focused on different areas in the back of the eye. Closely associated with the muscles of accommodation is the *ciliary body*. The ciliary body is responsible for aqueous humor production, which is discussed in a later section. The small space formed by iris, lens, and the ciliary tissues is called the *posterior chamber* (see Fig. 10–5).

Behind all of the previously mentioned structures lies the largest of all the intraocular chambers, the *vitreous (vit're-us) chamber*. The vitreous chamber is filled with a gelatinous substance called *vitreous humor* or the *vitreous body*. The vitreous humor helps maintain the shape of the globe. The walls of the vitreous chamber are lined by a series of tissue layers. The innermost of these layers is the *retina*.

The retina is a thin, transparent structure composed of specialized neural tissue. The specialized sensory receptor cells (*rods* and *cones*) of the retina are embedded in the pigmented tissue layer of the *choroid*. The importance of this connection between the pigmented tissue layer and the rods and the cones is discussed in the section on the visual pathway. The pigmented tissue found in the eyes of domestic animals is unique. It actually contains two distinctly different pigments. The black pigment is called the *tapetum nigrum*,[7] and the brightly colored (green and blue), iridescent pigment is called the *tapetum lucidum*.[8] The tapetum lucidum is found predominantly near the *fundus*[9] (Fig. 10–8), whereas the tapetum nigrum covers the remaining area up to the ciliary process. The tapetum lucidum is found in abundance in predatory animals, such as dogs and cats. It is designed to "amplify" or enhance incoming light in low-light situations. This quality is a result of the tapetum lucidum's reflective characteristics, and provides excellent night vision to those animals bearing it. It is the tapetum lucidum that vividly reflects the headlights of an oncoming car, giving a green-blue, shining appearance to the eyes. Sandwiched between the retina and the sclera is the choroid. The choroid is part of the vascular tunic of the eye, or the *uvea*, and provides vascular, nutritive support to the retina. The other two parts of the uvea are the aforementioned ciliary process (body and muscle) and the iris. Finally, the *optic disc* is a small area of the fundus where vessels enter the eye and where the *optic nerve* is attached.

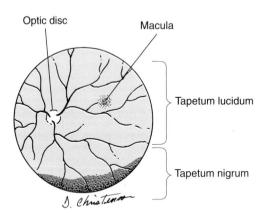

Optic disc

Macula

Tapetum lucidum

Tapetum nigrum

D. Christensen

FIGURE 10–8. Normal canine fundus.

---

[7]Tapetum nigrum (*tah-pe'tum ni'grum*); derived from [L. "black carpet"].

[8]Tapetum lucidum (*tah-pe'tum lu'sid-um*).

[9]Fundus (fun'dus); in ophthalmology the fundus refers to the back of the interior of the eye. Structures usually associated with the fundus are the optic disc, intraocular blood vessels, the macula, and the rear portion of the retina.

10.2.4. AQUEOUS PRODUCTION, FLOW, AND DRAINAGE

The production, flow, and drainage of aqueous humor can be likened to the workings of a kitchen sink. Water flows out of the faucet into the sink and flows out through the drain of the sink. The aqueous humor is an intraocular fluid produced by the ciliary body (faucet). As it is produced, it flows into the posterior chamber. From the posterior chamber, the aqueous flows through the pupil into the anterior chamber. The aqueous eventually drains through small portals found around the entire circumference of the *iridocorneal angle* (Fig. 10–9). From there it is picked up by blood vessels associated with the sclera. Aqueous humor is constantly being produced and drained within the eye, and plays an important role in providing nutrients to avascular structures like the cornea.

Just like the kitchen sink, aqueous can become "backed up." We can cause water to back up in the sink by plugging the drain, or by turning the water on so high that the drain cannot keep up. Aqueous can back up in a similar fashion. The ciliary body can overproduce the aqueous humor at such a rate that the iridocorneal drainage angle cannot accommodate the volume. On the other hand, the drainage angle can become obstructed, impeding or stopping the drainage of aqueous altogether. Either way, excess aqueous builds up within the eye. *Intraocular pressure* increases as the aqueous volume increases. Excessive intraocular pressure is clinically referred to as *glaucoma* (*glaw-ko'mah*). Left unchecked, glaucoma can cause significant damage to intraocular structures and eventually results in blindness. *Acute* (sudden) glaucoma is usually presented as a unilateral disorder. Grossly, such patients typically have *anisocoria* and *unilateral buphthalmos*. The pupil of the affected eye is usually mydriatic. Treatment of acute glaucoma must be aggressive, if vision in the affected eye is to be saved. Whether progressive or acute, if the fluid accumulations and intraocular pressure cannot

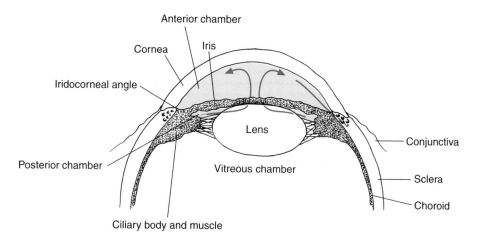

FIGURE 10–9. Schematic of aqueous flow.

be controlled medically or surgically, part or all of the affected eye may have to be removed.

10.2.5. VISUAL PATHWAY

Light entering the eye first passes through the cornea and anterior chamber (Fig. 10–10). Both the cornea and the aqueous humor refract or bend the light, concentrating it at the pupil. The light passes through the pupil and the lens. The lens, by virtue of the muscles of accommodation, focuses the light at a point on the fundus. The *macula* (*mak'u-lah*) is the most sensitive point of the fundus. The light passes through the transparent retina and strikes the pigmented tissue layer (Fig. 10–11 on p. 186). It is at the interface of the sensory cells (rods and cones) and the pigmented tissue that the sensory cells are stimulated. In cases of retinal detachment, the sensory cells of the retina detach from the pigmented tissue of the choroid, rendering that area of the retina incapable of transmitting visual information. The sensory cells, when attached to the pigmented tissue layer and exposed to light, experience a *photochemical* reaction. It is the photochemical reaction at the retinal-pigmented tissue interface that initiates a neural impulse. This impulse follows neural fibers of the retina and ultimately concentrates at the optic disc (Fig. 10–12 on p. 186). The optic disc is the portal to the optic nerve. Because there are so many nerve fibers and vessels entering at the optic disc, it has no room for sensory receptor cells. Therefore, light focused directly on the optic disc does not stimulate visual pathways; it is a blind spot in the eye. To continue, the neural impulse is transmitted by the optic nerve to the brain for interpretation. Because most animals possess binocular vision, the visual information being transmitted from each eye enters the brain *contralateral* to the respective eye.

It has been stated by many that animals see only in black and white. If this were true, then animals would not be equipped with both types of sensory receptor cells in the retina. Rods transmit black and white images, whereas cones transmit images of color. Rods require less light to be stimulated than do cones. Although the retinas of most domestic animals contain more rods than cones, they do contain both. Therefore, in appropriately lighted situations, animals can perceive color. The distribution of numbers of rods versus cones varies tremendously among the different species of the animal world. Many species of birds have particularly abundant cones in their retinas. It only stands to reason that this should be so: why else would so many birds have such brilliantly colored plumage? If they were unable to perceive it visually, it would not be very helpful for identifying potential mates and enemies.

10.2.6. PATHOPHYSIOLOGY

Veterinary *ophthalmologists* see a variety of ocular problems. Some are structural disorders, like *entropion*, *distichiasis*, or *ectropion*, which require surgical correction. Failure to correct abnormalities like entropion or distichiasis will most likely

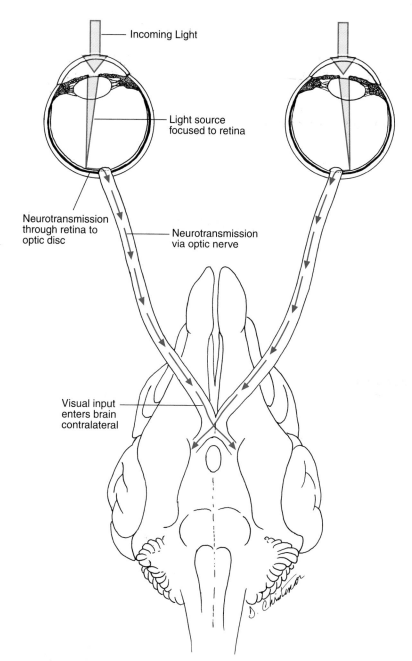

Incoming Light

Light source
focused to retina

Neurotransmission
through retina to
optic disc

Neurotransmission
via optic nerve

Visual input
enters brain
contralateral

FIGURE 10–10. Visual pathway schematic.

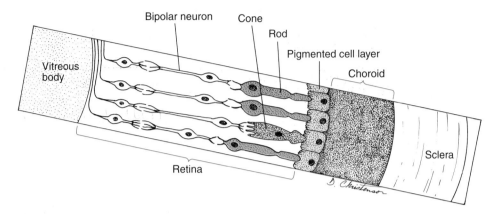

FIGURE 10–11. Retinal cross-section.

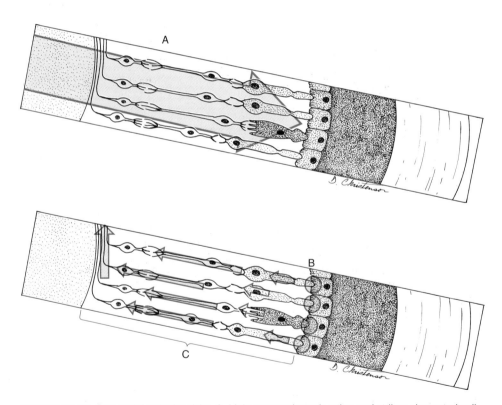

FIGURE 10–12. Sequential retinal activity. **A,** Light passes through retina and strikes pigmented cell layer. **B,** Photochemical reaction stimulated at sensory cell–pigmented epithelium interface. **C,** Neurotransmission to optic disc.

result in *keratitis* and *corneal ulceration*. Ectropion usually predisposes the animal to *conjunctivitis* and ocular trauma from foreign bodies (e.g., plant seeds).

Cataracts (lens opacity) are the most common lens abnormality seen. Some can be removed surgically. Most cataracts in veterinary patients develop over a long period of time, slowly diminishing the animal's visual acuity. These types of patients adjust so well to the gradual visual loss that the owners do not notice the visual deficit. The owner may complain of sudden blindness in the pet, when in actuality the long-term blind patient was getting along just fine until the furniture was rearranged.

Many other ocular disorders can result in blindness. Obviously, *retinopathies* have a direct impact on the visual acuity of an animal. Diseases like *chronic recurrent uveitis* cause visual loss indirectly by slowly, progressively destroying visual receptors. As the name implies, the disease is a long-term, repeated, inflammatory disorder. A horse suffering an episode of chronic recurrent uveitis is in obvious pain. The pain is manifested by *photophobia, miosis, blepharospasm,* and *epiphora*. These patients must be treated aggressively with medications to reduce the intraocular inflammation. In addition, mydriatics are often used to reduce pain and to prevent the iris from adhering to the lens (called *synechia; sǐ-nek'e-ah, sin-ēk'e-ah*). During the recovery period, for comfort and protection, the patient must be kept in a dark stall or barn. Each time the uveitis returns, the horse suffers further visual loss.

Veterinary ophthalmologists have numerous diagnostic tests and therapeutic regimens at their disposal to try to maintain healthy vision in their patients. Early recognition of possible ocular pathologic changes is paramount to maintaining the eyes in working condition. It is important to educate owners of high-risk patients about the early signs of the particular ophthalmic disease. Then, in cooperation, we may be able to thwart deterioration of that animal's vision.

10.3. Self-Test

Using the previous information in this chapter, respond to each of the following questions using the most appropriate medical term(s).

1. A(n) _____ is a veterinary professional who specializes in the examination and treatment of the eyes.

2. _____ is dilation of the pupils.

3. The _____ optic _____ nerve is the nerve that transmits visual information to the brain.

4. An outward rolling or turning of an eyelid is medically termed

   _____.

5. _____ is the name of the disease of the eye in which intraocular pressure is abnormally high.

6. The __*unclear* retina__ is a delicate, thin mucous membrane that covers the unexposed surfaces of the eyelids and the exposed portion of the sclera.

7. The __sclera *unclear*__ is a thin, transparent intraocular tissue that contains numerous specialized sensory receptor cells and nerve fibers.

8. The _____ apparatus drains tears away from the medial canthus of the eye to the nose.

9. Collectively the iris, ciliary body and muscle, and the choroid comprise the vascular tunic of the eye, or the _____.

10. An extra, second row of eyelashes on the same eyelid is medically termed

_____.

11. The __cornea__ is a transparent, dome-shaped anterior structure of the eye that is composed of epithelium, stroma, and Descemet's membrane.

12. Adherence of the iris to the lens is medically termed _____.

13. The __*unclear* sclera__ is the tough, white fibrous connective tissue that forms and supports most of the globe.

14. The angle that is formed by the iris and the cornea and that provides drainage for aqueous humor is called the _____ angle.

15. The small space formed by the iris, lens, and ciliary process is called the

_____.

16. Constriction of the pupils is medically termed _____.

17. Inflammation of the cornea and conjunctiva is medically termed

_____.

18. An abnormal intolerance of light is medically termed _____.

19. _____ is a state in which the pupils are unequal in size.

20. The _____ is referred to as the blind spot of the eye.

21. The third eyelid is the common name for the _____.

22. Overflow of tears onto the face, due to overproduction or obstruction of the drainage duct, is medically termed _____.

23. _____ is a state in which the palpebral muscles are engaged in tonic contraction, holding the eyelids tightly closed. This often results from ocular pain.

24. The _____ is the gelatinous substance that occupies the largest intraocular chamber.

25. Excessive enlargement and distention of an eye is medically termed _____.

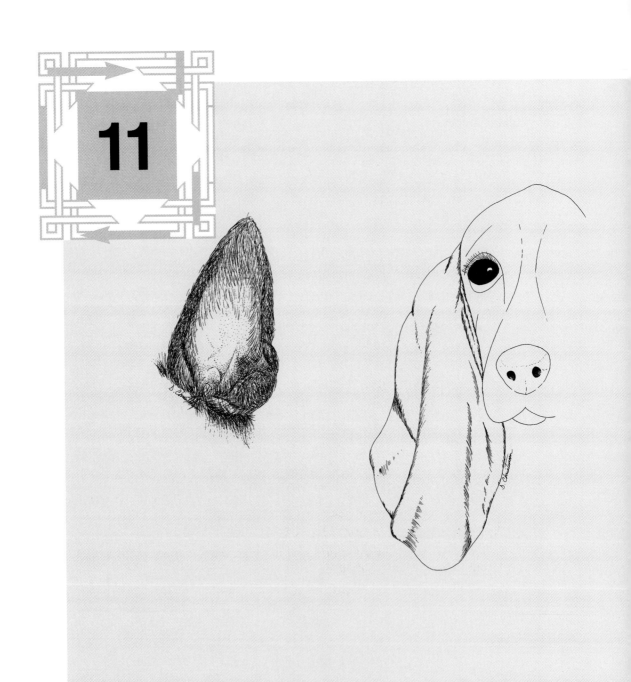

The Ear

GOALS AND OBJECTIVES

By the conclusion of this chapter, the student will be able to:

1. Recognize common root words, prefixes, and suffixes related to the ear.
2. Divide simple and compound words into their respective parts.
3. Recognize, correctly pronounce, and appropriately use common medical terms related to the ear.
4. Demonstrate an understanding of otic anatomy.
5. Demonstrate an understanding of otic physiology with regard to the auditory pathway and equilibrium.

11.1. Introduction to Related Terms

Divide each of the following terms into its respective parts ("R" root, "P" prefix, "S" suffix, "CV" combining vowel).

1. **Otic**   (R) _____   (S) _____

   otic (o′tik; pertaining to the ear; cf. aural)

2. **Otitis**   (R) _____   (S) _____

   otitis (o-ti′tis; inflammation of the ear; clinically otitis is subdivided into otitis externa [inflammation of the external ear], otitis media [inflammation of the middle ear], and otitis interna [inflammation of the inner ear])

3. **Acoustic**   (R) _____   (S) _____

   acoustic (ah-koos′tik; pertaining to sound)

4. **Audiology**   (R) _____   (CV) ___   (S) _____

   audiology (aw″de-ol′o-je; the study of hearing)

5. **Vestibular**   (R) _____   (S) _____

   vestibular (ves-tib′u-lar; pertaining to a vestibule [L. "chamber"])

6. **Semicircular**   (P) _____   (R) _____   (S) _____

   semicircular (sem″ĭ-ser′ku-lar; pertaining to a partial circle)

7. **Cochlear**   (R) _____   (S) _____

   cochlear (kok′le-ar; pertaining to the cochlea [L. "snail shell"])

8. **Tympanic**   (R) _____   (S) _____

   tympanic (tim-pan′ik; pertaining to the tympanum [Gr. "drum"])

9. **Aural**   (R) _____   (S) _____

   aural (aw′ral; pertaining to the ear; cf. otic)

10. **Otoscope**   (R) _____   (CV) ___   (S) _____

    otoscope (o′to-skōp; to examine the ear; clinically refers to an instrument used to examine the external ear)

11. **Ototoxic**   (R) _____   (CV) ___   (R) _____   (S) _____

    ototoxic (o″to-tok′sik; pertaining to ear poison; clinically refers to any agent that may be toxic to components of the inner ear or auditory nerve)

12. **Ceruminal**   (R) _____   (S) _____

    ceruminal (sĕ-roo′mĭ-nal; pertaining to cerumen [L. cera, wax]; i.e., ear wax)

13. Retrograde   (R) _____ (CV) ___ (S) _____

   retrograde (ret'ro-grād; going backward)

14. Otolith   (R) _____ (CV) ___ (R) _____

   otolith (o'to-lith; an ear stone)

15. Dynamic   (R) _____ (S) _____

   dynamic (di-nam'ik) from [Gr. dynamis, power]; pertaining to power or motion)

11.2. Otic Anatomy and Physiology

11.2.1. OTIC ANATOMY

The *external ear* (Figs. 11–1 and 11–2 on p. 194) is composed of the *pinna* (ear flap), *external acoustic meatus*,[1] and the *tympanic membrane* (ear drum). Ear pinnae come in a variety of shapes and sizes, depending on the species and breed of animal (see Fig. 11–1). Those animals with large, erect pinnae have very sharp hearing. The external acoustic meatus in most domestic animals is relatively long, with a slight "L" shape. The shape of the ear canal helps prevent perforation of the tympanic membrane by foreign objects. However, the "L" shape also tends to contribute to accumulations of *cerumen* and other secretions near the tympanic membrane.

The *middle ear* is housed by the *tympanic bulla*[2] (Fig. 11–3 on p. 195). Contained within the tympanic bullae are the *otic ossicles:*[3] the *malleus*,[4] the *incus*,[5] and the *stapes*[6] (see Fig. 11–2; Fig. 11–4 on p. 196). The malleus is attached to the inner surface of the tympanic membrane. All of the otic ossicles are interconnected, like other bones, by ligaments. They also have small muscles associated with them. The muscles are primarily there to temper the movement of the ossicles when subjected to loud sounds. This protective reflex helps to prevent damage to portions of the inner ear. The tympanic bullae are connected to the throat by the *eustachian tubes*.[7] The eustachian tubes equalize pressures and drain the middle ear. The drainage is important to keep the middle ear free of fluid accumulations. Unfortunately, the eustachian tubes also provide routes for *retrograde* bacterial infections of the middle ear.

---

[1]Meatus (*me-a'tus*); from [L. *meatus,* a way, a path, a course]; meaning an opening or passage; the external acoustic meatus is also referred to as the "ear canal."

[2]Bulla (*bul'ah*); bullae plural; from [L. *bulla,* a large vesicle]; the tympanic bullae are osseous chambers found at the base of the skull; they house the middle ear.

[3]Ossicle (*os'sĭ-kl*); from [L. *ossiculum,* a small bone].

[4]Malleus (*mal'e-us*); from [L. *malleus,* hammer].

[5]Incus (*ing'kus*); from [L. *incus,* anvil].

[6]Stapes (*sta'pēz*); from [L. *stapes,* stirrup].

[7]Eustachian (*u-sta'ke-an*); the eustachian tubes are named after an Italian anatomist, Bartolommeo Eustachio.

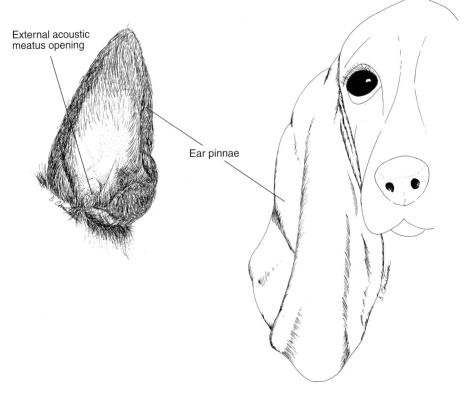

External acoustic
meatus opening

Ear pinnae

FIGURE 11–1. Pinnae.

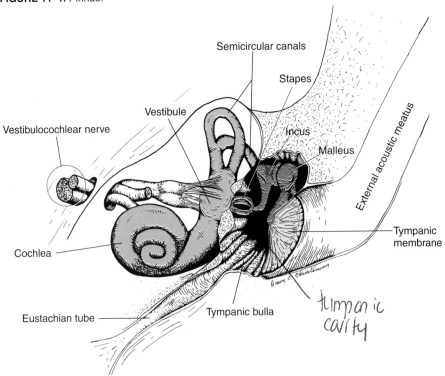

Semicircular canals

Stapes

Vestibule

Incus

Malleus

Vestibulocochlear nerve

External acoustic meatus

Cochlea

Tympanic
membrane

Eustachian tube

Tympanic bulla

tumpanic
cavity

194   **FIGURE 11–2.** Schematic cross-section of the ear.

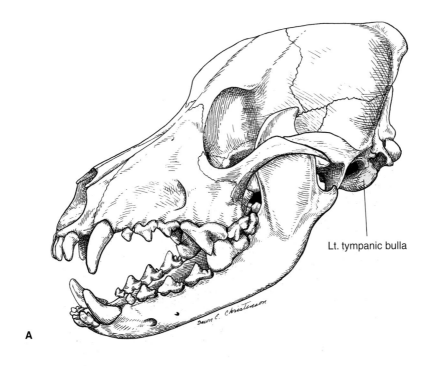

A

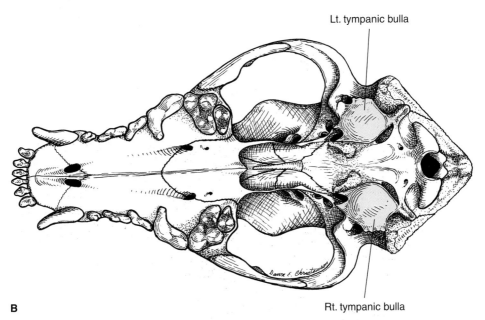

B

Lt. tympanic bulla

Lt. tympanic bulla

Rt. tympanic bulla

FIGURE 11–3. Tympanic bullae. **A**, Lateral view; **B**, Ventral view

The *inner ear* (see Fig. 11–2; Fig. 11–5) is composed of the *cochlea* and the *vestibular apparatus* (i.e., *vestibule* and *semicircular canals*). The components of the inner ear are encased in the temporal bone of the skull. Very little bone and tissue separate the inner ear from the cranial vault. The inner ear is separated from the middle ear by the *oval window*. The cochlea is so named because it resembles a snail shell. Within the hard outer shell of the cochlea are labyrinths or passages filled with fluid. Membranes separate the passages from one another; however, they are flexible enough to transmit movement between the passages (i.e., from fluid waves). In certain passages there are many specialized sensory receptor cells that are crucial to transmission of *auditory* sensory information to the brain. Such sensory input is transmitted to the brain by the cochlear branch of the *vestibulocochlear (auditory) nerve.* At the base of the cochlea is a small tissue-covered opening called the round window. Its importance is discussed in the section on Audiology (11.2.2).

The vestibule is fluid filled and also contains two smaller chambers within it. These chambers are discussed further in the section regarding *static*[8] *equilibrium.* The semicircular canals are rigid tubes that connect to and openly communicate with the vestibule. They are also fluid filled. Each semicircular canal (there are three in each inner ear) is oriented so that it is associated with a body plane. This orientation makes sensory input for *dynamic equilibrium* possible and relative to the body planes, no matter what the direction of movement of the head is. Dynamic equilibrium is discussed in greater detail in a subsequent section.

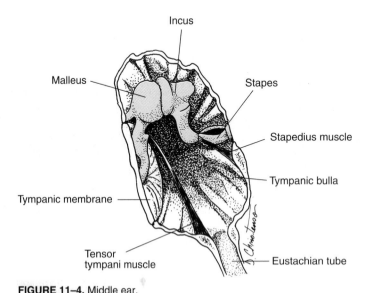

FIGURE 11–4. Middle ear.

---

[8]Static (*stat'ik*); from [L. *staticus*]; meaning at rest or not in motion.

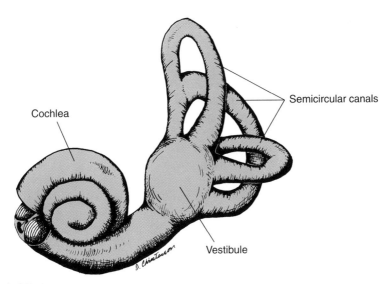

FIGURE 11–5. Inner ear.

11.2.2. AUDIOLOGY

The *auditory pathway* is a delicate, intricate path by which sound waves are converted to mechanical energy, ultimately resulting in stimulation of neural impulses. Disruption of the pathway anywhere in the sequence of events results in some form of hearing loss.

Sound waves are collected by the pinna and directed to the external acoustic meatus. The sound waves, on reaching the tympanic membrane, cause it to vibrate. Because the malleus is attached to the tympanic membrane, it and the other otic ossicles begin to move. The stapes moves through the oval window and strikes the cochlea. Each strike on the cochlea creates a fluid wave inside it. As the fluid waves pass through the winding passages of the cochlea, special sensory receptor cells are hit by the waves and stimulated. Once stimulated, the neural impulse is rushed to the brain for interpretation of the sound, via the vestibulo-cochlear nerve. The fluid waves continue to pass through the entire length of the cochlear passages and ultimately strike the *round window*. The round window is covered by a fibrous connective tissue membrane that dissipates the waves, thus preventing rebounding of the waves. Interestingly, the frequency or pitch of the original sound wave corresponds to the size of the fluid waves created in the cochlea. The waves of *low-frequency sounds* could be likened to the ring of large waves created by throwing a large rock into a pond, whereas a little pebble, like *high-frequency sounds*, creates tiny, close-set waves in the pond. Each different pitch strikes specific sensory receptor cells. Any sensory receptor cells destroyed by trauma or disease are not replaced.

Deafness and partial hearing losses can be caused by many different disruptions of the auditory pathway. Excessive ceruminal accumulations in the external acoustic meatus impair sound waves from reaching the tympanic membrane. Fluid accumulations in the tympanic bullae, due to an otitis media, impair movement of the tympanic membrane and the otic ossicles, thereby diminishing the intensity of sound transmitted. Damage or destruction of cochlear receptor cells results in hearing loss of specific frequencies. Such damage can easily occur from exposure to excessively loud noises or *ototoxic* drugs. Damage to the vestibulo-cochlear (auditory) nerve impairs or prevents transmission of sensory input to the brain; this too may result from *ototoxicity*. Audiology in routine veterinary practice is not as sophisticated as in human medicine. Auditory testing usually involves creating a loud noise (e.g., hand clap) out of sight of the patient and watching for a response to that sound. Unilateral hearing losses are difficult to detect because animals compensate so well with the remaining ear and other senses.

11.2.3. EQUILIBRIUM

There are two types of equilibrium associated with the inner ear: static equilibrium and dynamic equilibrium. Each uses a different portion of the vestibular apparatus, and both send their sensory input to the brain (specifically, the cerebellum).

Static equilibrium utilizes the two chambers within the vestibule of the inner ear (Fig. 11–6). Each chamber is lined with specialized sensory receptor cells. On top of the sensory cells is a layer of gelatinous material, and stuck to the surface of the gelatinous material are tiny *otoliths*. The remainder of each chamber is filled with fluid. The function of this portion of the vestibular apparatus is based entirely on gravity: however the head is positioned, gravity causes the otoliths to slide along the gelatinous material to the lowest point within the chamber. Wherever the otoliths fall to rest, the pressure exerted by their weight stimulates the associated sensory receptors. This initiates a neural impulse that is sent to the brain for interpretation of head and body position.

Dynamic equilibrium uses the semicircular canals of the inner ear (Fig. 11–7). Each semicircular canal is filled with fluid and has a specialized sensory receptor cell associated with its opening into the vestibule. Whenever the head is turned rapidly, the semicircular canal associated with the plane of movement moves around the fluid contained within it. To demonstrate a solid object moving around its liquid contents, fill a bowl with water and place a few ice cubes in it. Make sure that everything is sitting perfectly still before proceeding. Then, spin the bowl on the table top. Notice that initially the bowl moves but the ice cubes remain stationary; they have remained stationary because the *bowl*, not the water, has moved. Now, if the semicircular canals move around the fluid within them, what effect does this have on the sensory receptor cells positioned at their openings? The receptor cells are dragged through the fluid. Because the fluid creates resistance against the receptor cells, they are forced to bend. The bending action

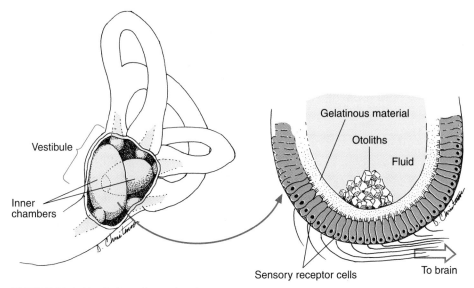

FIGURE 11–6. Vestibule and associated structures.

is just like a hand being dragged through the water while swimming. The hand bends pointing in a direction opposite the direction of movement of the arm through the water. The same is true for the sensory receptor cells. As they are bent, they are stimulated and initiate a neural impulse that is transmitted to the brain, via the vestibulocochlear nerve. The brain interprets the direction of move-

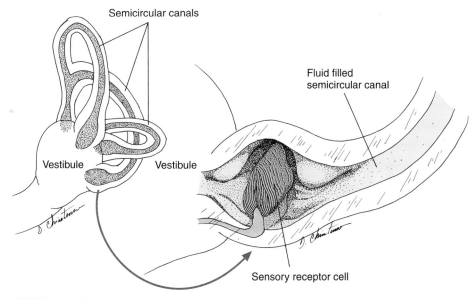

FIGURE 11–7. Semicircular canals.

ment, and stimulates appropriate motor responses elsewhere in the body to maintain balance.

Neither static nor dynamic equilibrium alone or collectively are enough to maintain balance and equilibrium. Sensory input from visual and tactile senses must also be used for the brain to determine accurately body position, direction of movement, and how to make corrections to maintain balance.

11.2.4. OTITIS

One of the most common causes of *otitis externa* in dogs and cats is the *ear mite* (*Otodectes cynotis*[9]). These tiny surface-dwelling creatures enjoy the warmth and protection of the external acoustic meatus. Unfortunately, they can cause tremendous irritation and inflammation of the external ear. Clinically, patients with ear mites are presented with excessive accumulations of dark, black-brown ceruminal debris. At times there is so much ceruminal build-up that the canal is completely occluded. The animals typically have evidence of digging and scratching at the ears in the form of scratches and abrasions of the head, neck, and pinnae. Some patients will have engaged in such vigorous head shaking to cause *aural hematoma*[10] formation. *Otoscopic* examination of the external ear reveals the tiny white creatures crawling on the dark cerumen and debris. Treatment of otitis externa due to ear mites is a twofold process. First, the external ear must be thoroughly cleaned. Care must be taken to avoid perforation of the tympanic membrane while cleaning. Second, the external acoustic meatus must be treated with medication that will kill the mites and their offspring and reduce inflammation. Antibiotics may be necessary if a secondary bacterial otitis has developed.

Otitis externa is common in animals with heavy, floppy pinnae, such as cocker spaniels and basset hounds. The large, heavy pinna tends to keep the external acoustic meatus dark, warm, and moist, providing a perfect environment for numerous types of bacteria and fungi to live and grow. Proliferation of such organisms causes severe inflammation of the external ear. Medical management of these patients is often frustrating because it is so difficult to keep the external ear clean and dry. Because of the *chronic*[11] nature of otitis externa in these types of animals, surgery is sometimes warranted. The surgical procedure usually used is called a *lateral ear ablation.*[12] In essence, the external acoustic meatus is permanently opened to the environment. The lateral ear ablation promotes drainage and aeration of the external ear, minimizing further episodes of otitis externa.

Regardless of the cause of otitis externa, it must be managed. Failure to do so could permit progression of the disease to *otitis media* or *otitis interna*. Certainly, progression to otitis interna may result not only in hearing deficits, but equilibrium and balance problems as well.

---

[9]*Otodectes cynotis* (*o″to-dek′tēz sĭ-no′tis*); from (oto- + [Gr. *dēktēs*, a biter]) "ear mite" of the dog and cat.

[10]Hematoma (*he-mah-to′mah*); from [*hemat(o)-* , blood + *-oma*, swelling]; a hematoma is an accumulation of blood under the skin.

[11]Chronic (*kron′ik*); from [Gr. *chronos*, time]; means to persist over a long period of time.

[12]Ablation (*ab-la′shun*); from [L. *ablatio*, detachment, removal].

11.3. Self-Test

Using the previous information in this chapter, respond to each of the following questions using the most appropriate medical term(s).

1. The tympanic bulla houses the middle ear, containing the _____ ossicles.

2. The external _____ or ear canal in domestic animals is relatively long and resembles an "L" in shape.

3. _____ is inflammation of the inner ear.

4. A(n) _____ is an instrument used to examine the external ear.

5. The _____ is the portion of the inner ear associated with hearing, and is shaped like a snail shell.

6. The _____ tubes are passages that connect the middle ear with the throat.

7. A(n) _____ hematoma is an accumulation of blood beneath the skin of the ear pinna. It usually results from the trauma of excessive head shaking.

8. The scientific name for the "ear mite" of dogs and cats is _____.

9. The ear drum or _____ is a flexible tissue that separates the external ear from the middle ear.

10. The _____, contained within the chambers of the vestibular apparatus, slide on the gelatinous material by virtue of gravity. They play a large role in static equilibrium.

11. The individual names of the three tiny bones of the middle ear (in sequence) are the

    _____, _____, and

    _____.

12. The _____ of the inner ear are oriented with the various body planes, and contribute sensory information for dynamic equilibrium.

13. Otitis media sometimes develops because of _____ or backward movement of bacteria from the throat to the middle ear.

14. _____ is the study of hearing.

15. The _____ at the base of the cochlea is designed to dissipate the fluid waves after they have traveled through the labyrinths.

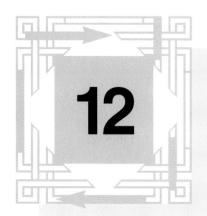

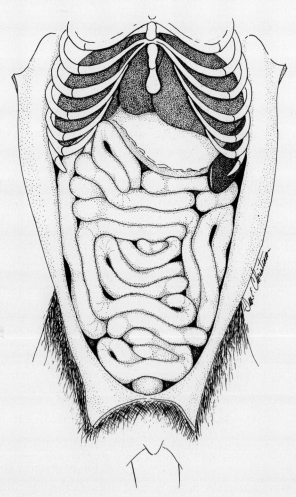

The Alimentary System

GOALS AND OBJECTIVES

By the conclusion of this chapter, the student will be able to:

1. Recognize common root words, prefixes, and suffixes related to the alimentary system.
2. Divide simple and compound words into their respective parts.
3. Recognize, correctly pronounce, and appropriately use common medical terms related to the alimentary system.
4. Demonstrate an understanding of alimentary anatomy of the simple monogastric animal.
5. Demonstrate an understanding of digestive physiology with regard to the simple monogastric animal.
6. Demonstrate an understanding of basic nutrients and nutrition.

12.1. Introduction to Related Terms

Divide each of the following terms into its respective parts ("R" root, "P" prefix, "S" suffix, "CV" combining vowel).

1. **Glossal**   (R) _____   (S) _____

   glossal (glos'al; pertaining to the tongue; cf. lingual)

2. **Lingual**   (R) _____   (S) _____

   lingual (ling'gwal; pertaining to the tongue, cf. glossal)

3. **Buccal**   (R) _____   (S) _____

   buccal (buk'al; pertaining to the cheek)

4. **Labial**   (R) _____   (S) _____

   labial (la'be-al; pertaining to the lip)

5. **Periodontal**   (P) _____   (CV) ___ (R) _____   (S) _____

   periodontal (per"e-o-don'tal; pertaining to around the teeth)

6. **Gingival**   (R) _____   (S) _____

   gingival (jin'jĭ-val, jin-ji'val; pertaining to the gingiva ["gums"])

7. **Oropharynx**   (R) _____   (CV) ___ (R) _____

   oropharynx (o"ro-far'inks; the mouth and the throat)

8. **Hypersialosis**   (P) _____   (R) _____   (CV) ___ (S) _____

   hypersialosis (hi"per-si"ah-lo'sis; a condition of excessive saliva)

9. **Esophageal**   (R) _____   (CV) ___ (S) _____

   esophageal (e-sof"ah-je'al, e-so-fa'je-al; pertaining to the esophagus)

10. **Gastric**   (R) _____   (S) _____

    gastric (gas'trik; pertaining to the stomach)

11. **Pyloric**   (R) _____   (S) _____

    pyloric (pi-lor'ik; pertaining to the pylorus; from [Gr. pyle, gate])

12. **Enteric**   (R) _____   (S) _____

    enteric (en-ter'ik; pertaining to the intestines)

13. **Duodenal**   (R) _____   (S) _____

    duodenal (du"o-de'nal, du"od'en-al; pertaining to the duodenum)

14. **Jejunal** (R) _____ (S) _____

jejunal (jĕ-joo'nal, je-joo'nal; pertaining to the jejunum)

15. **Ileocecal** (R) _____ (CV) ___ (R) _____ (S) _____

ileocecal (il"e-o-se'kal; pertaining to the ileum and the cecum)

16. **Hepatic** (R) _____ (S) _____

hepatic (hĕ-pat'ik; pertaining to the liver)

17. **Biliary** (R) _____ (S) _____

biliary (bil'e-a-re; pertaining to bile)

18. **Icteric** (R) _____ (S) _____

icteric (ik'ter-ik; pertaining to icterus [jaundice])

19. **Pancreatic** (R) _____ (S) _____

pancreatic (pan"kre-at'ik; pertaining to the pancreas)

20. **Gastroenteritis** (R) _____ (CV) ___ (R) _____ (S) _____

gastroenteritis (gas"tro-en-ter-i'tis; inflammation of the stomach and intestines)

21. **Colitis** (R) _____ (S) _____

colitis (ko-li'tis; inflammation of the colon)

22. **Peritoneal** (R) _____ (S) _____

peritoneal (per"ĭ-to-ne'al; pertaining to the peritoneum)

23. **Peristalsis** (P) _____ (R) _____

peristalsis (per"ĭ-stal'sis; around contraction; from [Gr. stalsis, contraction])

24. **Haustration** (R) _____ (S) _____

haustration (hos-tra'shun; pertaining to a haustra; from [L. hustor, drawer]; haustrations are small pouches or sacculations found in the colon and rectum)

25. **Antiemetic** (P) _____ (R) _____ (S) _____

antiemetic (an"tĭ-e-met'ik; pertaining to being against vomiting)

26. **Antidiarrheal** (P) _____ (R) _____ (S) _____

antidiarrheal (an"ti-di"ah-re'al; pertaining to being against diarrhea)

27. **Deglutition** (R) _____ (S) _____

deglutition (deg"loo-tish'un; the act of swallowing)

28. Defecation (R) _____ (S) _____

defecation (def"ĕ-ka'shun; the act of defecating [evacuation of the bowels])

29. Postprandial (P) _____ (R) _____ (S) _____

postprandial (post-pran'de-al; pertaining to after a meal)

30. Dysphagia (P) _____ (R) _____ (S) _____

dysphagia (dis-fa'je-ah; a state of difficult eating)

31. Stomatitis (R) _____ (S) _____

stomatitis (sto-mah-ti'tis; inflammation of the mouth)

32. Anorexia (P) _____ (R) _____ (S) _____

anorexia (an"o-rek'se-ah; a state without appetite)

33. Orogastric (R) _____ (CV) ___ (R) _____ (S) _____

orogastric (o"ro-gas'trik; pertaining to the mouth and stomach; clinically refers to the administration of food or medication by the passage of a tube from the mouth to the stomach)

34. Gastrectomy (R) _____ (S) _____

gastrectomy (gas"trek'to-me; cutting out [excision] of the stomach; clinically refers to a surgical procedure in which part or all of the stomach is removed)

35. Enterotomy (R) _____ (CV) ___ (S) _____

enterotomy (en"ter-ot'o-me; to cut the intestine; clinically refers to a surgical procedure in which the intestine is incised)

36. Enterostomy (R) _____ (CV) ___ (S) _____

enterostomy (en"ter-os'to-me; to create a mouth/opening in the intestine; clinically refers to the surgical creation of an artificial opening in the small intestine through the abdominal wall; usually for the placement of a feeding tube)

37. Intussusception (P) _____ (R) _____ (S) _____

intussusception (in"tus-sus-sep'shun; the act of receiving within; from [L. intus, within + suscipere, to receive]; clinically refers to telescoping of part of the intestine into an adjoining part)

38. Necrotic (R) _____ (CV) ___ (S) _____

necrotic (ne-krot'ik; pertaining to necrosis; from [Gr. nekros, dead])

12.2. Alimentary Anatomy and Physiology

12.2.1. ORAL CAVITY AND DENTITION

The oral cavity contains a muscular structure called the *tongue* (Fig. 12–1). The dorsal surface of the tongue is covered with numerous, small projections (*papillae*[1]). These projections contain taste receptors. In cats, the projections are pronounced and sharp, aiding with normal feline grooming practices. The base of the tongue is located in the ventral *oropharynx*. A *sublingual* band of connective tissue on the ventral midline of the tongue connects the remainder of the tongue to the floor of the oral cavity. This band of connective tissue is called the *frenulum*[2] (Fig. 12–2). The dorsal border of the oral cavity is formed by the *hard palate*. The hard palate provides a bony separation between the oral and nasal cavities. It is covered by connective tissues and mucous membranes, formed in ridges. Caudal to the hard palate, in the oropharynx, is the *soft palate*. The soft palate separates the nasopharynx from the oropharynx, providing protection for the nasal passages during *deglutition*.

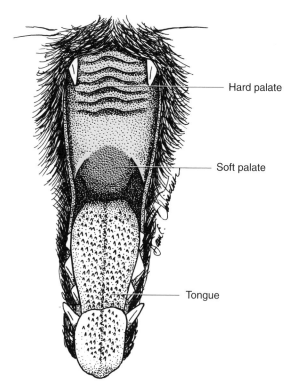

Hard palate

Soft palate

Tongue

FIGURE 12–1. Oral cavity (frontal view).

---

[1]Papillae (*pah-pil'e*); plural of papilla (*pah-pil'ah*); from [L. *papilla*, a small, nipple-shaped projection].
[2]Frenulum (*fren'u-lum*); from [L. dim. of *fraenum*, a small bridle].

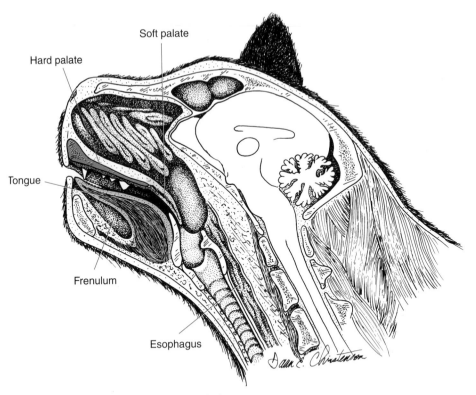

FIGURE 12–2. Oral cavity (midsagittal section).

The *gingiva* is the *periodontal* mucous membrane that covers the bone of the upper and lower jaws. The *gingival sulcus* is the tiny groove formed between the *neck* of the *tooth* and the free edge of the gingiva (Fig. 12–3). The *neck* of the *tooth* is found at the gingival margin, where the *crown* and the *root* meet. The crown of each tooth is covered in *enamel*, the hardest substance found in the body. Each root is covered in a mineralized substance called *cementum*. Directly beneath the enamel and cementum is a porous, bony substance called *dentin*; dentin makes up the bulk of each tooth. At the center of the dentin of each tooth is a canal, filled with soft tissue, blood vessels, and nerves. This is the *pulp cavity*. Nerves and vessels enter and exit the pulp cavity through the *apical delta*,[3] found at the apex of the root. The tooth is held in the bone of the jaw by the *periodontal ligament*.

Some dental surfaces are designated as either *labial, buccal, palatal* or *lingual*, by virtue of the mucosal tissue with which the tooth surface comes in contact/adjoins. The *occlusal* (*o-kloo'zal*) surface of a tooth is that which comes in contact with

[3]Apical delta; apical, pertaining to an apex; delta, as in a delta found at the mouth of a river, with numerous small divisions leading to the destination.

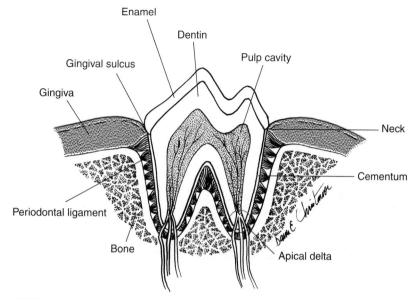

FIGURE 12–3. Tooth anatomy.

another tooth. Individual teeth are named according to right or left, *maxillary* (upper) or *mandibular* (lower), and the sequence number within the tooth type. A sequence number does not apply to the canine teeth because there is only a right and a left canine on each jaw. When citing dental abnormalities, it is important to name the specific tooth/teeth involved. Failure to do so may result in corrective actions being taken with the wrong tooth. Dental formulas provide veterinary professionals with a guide as to the types and numbers of teeth that should be found in an animal's mouth (Figs. 12–4 and 12–5 on pp. 210 and 211). The following are the dental formulas for adult dogs and cats:

Adult Canine Dental Formula ($\times$ 2):

$$\text{I}\ \frac{3}{3}\ \text{C}\ \frac{1}{1}\ \text{P}\ \frac{4}{4}\ \text{M}\ \frac{2}{3}$$

Adult Feline Dental Formula ($\times$ 2):

$$\text{I}\ \frac{3}{3}\ \text{C}\ \frac{1}{1}\ \text{P}\ \frac{3}{2}\ \text{M}\ \frac{1}{1}$$

Note that the numbers are shown in what appear to be fractions; the upper numbers reflect the maxillary teeth and the lower numbers reflect the mandibular teeth. All of the "fractions" shown are to be multiplied by two, because they represent the number of teeth found in only one half of the mouth. In the dental

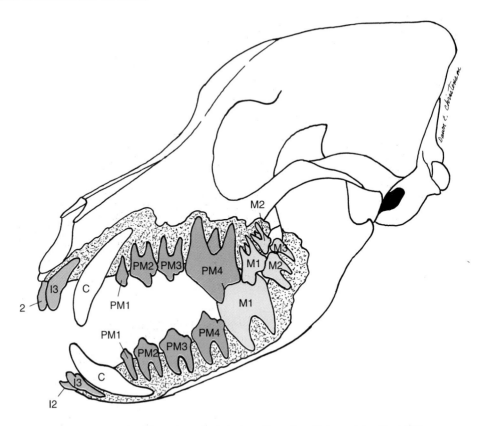

FIGURE 12–4. Canine dentition schematic. I, incisor; C, canine; PM, premolar; M, molar.

formulas, "I" indicates *incisors*, "C" indicates *canines*, "P" indicates *premolars*, and "M" indicates *molars*.

12.2.2. GASTROENTERIC ANATOMY

The *esophagus* is a muscular tube that serves as a passage from the *pharynx* to the *stomach* (Fig. 12–6 on p. 212). It lies dorsal to the trachea as it traverses the neck and thoracic cavity. The stomach is a pouch-like structure that lies in the left craniolateral quadrant of the *peritoneal cavity*. When empty, it lies very close to the diaphragm, liver, and spleen, partially protected by the caudal ribs. The *fundus* is the billowing, curved portion of the stomach near the *gastroesophageal* opening (Fig. 12–7 on p. 213). The *body* of the stomach is that portion which lies between the fundus and the pylorus. The *pylorus* is the narrow segment of the stomach, near the duodenum. The terminal portion of the stomach is marked by the *pyloric sphincter*.[4]

---

[4]Sphincter (*sfingk'ter*); from [Gr. *sphingkter*, that which binds tight]; a sphincter is a ring-like band of muscle fibers that constricts a natural opening.

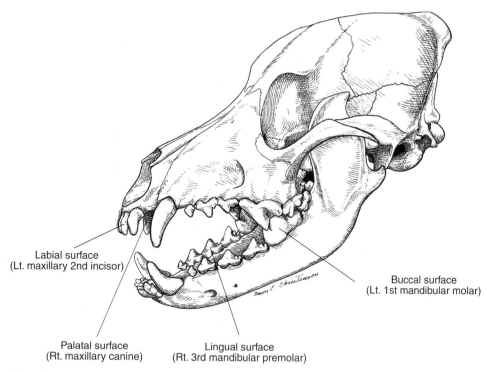

Labial surface
(Lt. maxillary 2nd incisor)

Buccal surface
(Lt. 1st mandibular molar)

Palatal surface
(Rt. maxillary canine)

Lingual surface
(Rt. 3rd mandibular premolar)

FIGURE 12–5. Canine dentition.

This sphincter is generally tightly closed, except during active gastric emptying. Only small volumes of liquid, like water, can trickle through the pyloric sphincter when it is closed. The wall of the stomach is muscular and has numerous folds. These folds provide tremendous expansive ability for the stomach and help to pulverize food. The gastric mucosa is covered with a thick layer of protective mucus.

The *small intestine* is composed of the *duodenum, jejunum,* and *ileum.* The duodenum is the proximal portion of the small intestine (see Fig. 12–7). It lies in the right lateral peritoneal cavity, from the pyloric sphincter to the jejunum. Its Latin origin, [*duodeni,* twelve at a time], was derived because, in humans, it is approximately 12 fingerbreadths long (ca. 12 inches). Obviously, with the size variances in domestic animals, the name cannot be used to estimate the length of this section of bowel. The *jejunum* is the middle portion of the small intestine, which actually comprises the longest segment of bowel (Fig. 12–8 on p. 214). It occupies the greater portion of the peritoneal cavity. The distal portion of the small intestine is the *ileum,* which lies between the jejunum and the cecum (Fig. 12–9 on p. 215).

The entire small intestine is simply a tube-like structure. The wall of the small intestine is muscular, with the muscle fibers oriented both in a longitudinal and a circular fashion. Coordinated muscular contractions create the worm-like, propulsive action called *peristalsis.* The enteric mucosa is composed of billions of

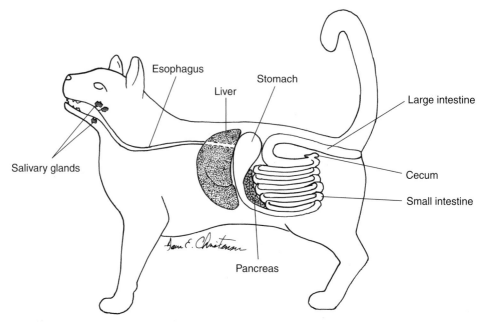

FIGURE 12–6. Schematic of the feline gastrointestinal tract.

finger-like projections called *villi*[5] (Fig. 12–10 on p. 216). The villi increase the surface area of the small intestine for maximal absorption of nutrients. Each *villus* is covered by simple columnar epithelium. Even the epithelial cells have their own finger-like projections, called *microvilli*, which increase the absorptive surface area even further. Near the bases of the villi are small crypts, also lined with simple columnar epithelium. The epithelium of the crypts produces protective mucus that coats the surface of the enteric lumen. In the center of each villus are a lymphatic vessel and blood vessels. The lymphatic vessel found at the center of each villus is called a *lacteal* (lak'te-al).

The *cecum* is a vestigial structure in dogs and cats that marks the end of the small intestine and the beginning of the *large intestine*, or colon (see Fig. 12–9). It is a small, blind sac, through which very little intestinal contents flow.

The large intestine is composed of several parts (see Fig. 12–9). The *ascending colon* lies along the right side of the peritoneal cavity. It traverses cranially from the cecum to the transverse colon. The *transverse colon* traverses the peritoneal cavity from right to left, between the ascending and descending portions of the colon. The *descending colon* lies on the left side of the peritoneal cavity and traverses the abdominal cavity caudally, between the transverse colon and the rec-

---

[5]Villi (*vil'i*), plural of villus (*vil'us*); from [L. *villus*, a tuft of hair].

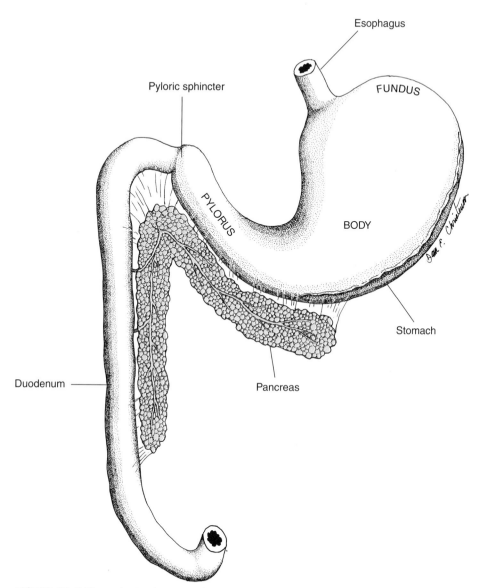

FIGURE 12–7. Stomach, duodenum, and pancreas.

tum. The *rectum* is the terminal portion of the colon, associated with the anal opening. An internal and an external *anal sphincter* are found at the anus.

The entire colon contains numerous, large *haustrations*. Longitudinal muscle fibers are not found throughout the wall of the colon. Instead, the longitudinal fibers are arranged in distinct bands. It is the tension created by these bands of muscle that actually creates the haustrations. The mucosal surface of the colon also differs from that of the small intestine, in that it does not have villi.

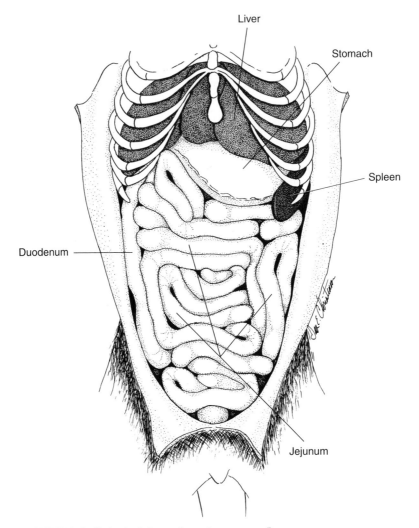

FIGURE 12–8. Abdominal viscera (omentum removed).

12.2.3. ACCESSORY ORGANS AND TISSUES

12.2.3.1. Liver and Biliary Tree

The *liver* occupies approximately the cranial third of the peritoneal cavity (see Fig. 12–8). It lies immediately caudal to the diaphragm and is well protected by the caudal ribs. The liver is composed of several large lobes, each of which is highly vascular and is constructed with numerous sinuses, channels, and canals lined with simple cuboidal epithelium (Fig. 12–11 on p. 217). The hepatic cells lining these *biliary canals* secrete bile and bile salts. Cholesterol is one of the precursor elements used by the *hepatocytes* to produce bile and bile salts. Yellow bile

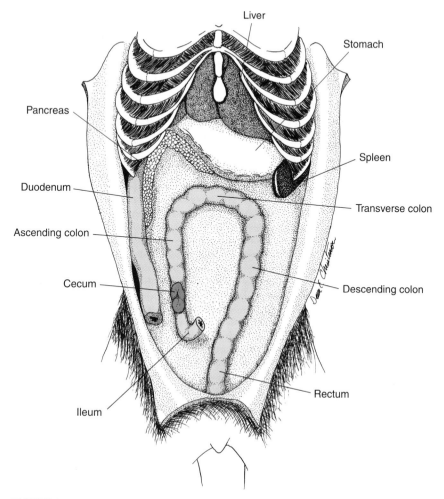

FIGURE 12–9. Ileum, cecum, and colon.

pigments come from bilirubin, which is a byproduct of hemoglobin[6] degradation. Back-up of these pigments into the blood due to hepatic disease may result in *icteric*-appearing mucous membranes and skin. All of the many biliary canals converge into larger *bile ducts*. The *common bile duct* connects all of the hepatic bile ducts with the duodenum (Fig. 12–12 on p. 218). The *gallbladder* is also connected to the common bile duct. It merely serves as a storage area for bile, which the gallbladder concentrates as it is stored there. Smooth muscle in the walls of the

---

[6]Hemoglobin (*he″mo-glo′bin*); *hem*(o)- , blood + *globin*; hemoglobin is the blood protein found in red blood cells responsible for the transport of oxygen.

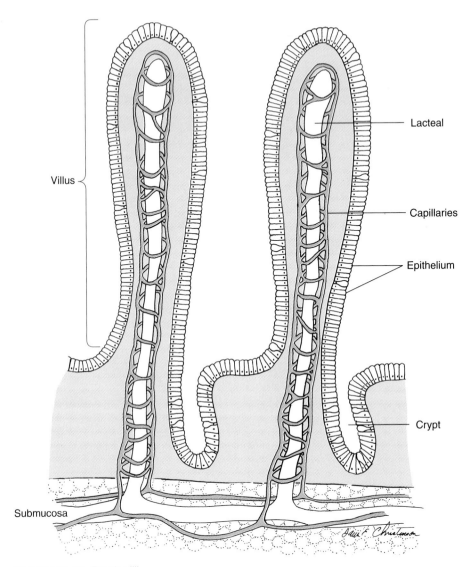

Lacteal

Capillaries

Epithelium

Crypt

Villus

Submucosa

FIGURE 12–10. Enteric villi.

gallbladder contracts during a meal to express bile into the common bile duct. This is especially important when meals high in fat are consumed.

The liver has many other functions, in addition to bile and bile salt production. All of the blood from the mesentery (*mes"en-ter'e*) must pass through the liver before entering general circulation. This is discussed along with the digestive process, in a later section. In addition, the liver is responsible for producing most of the plasma (blood) proteins, particularly many of the clotting factors. The liver can metabolize or, if necessary, it can store many nutrients in its tissues, like

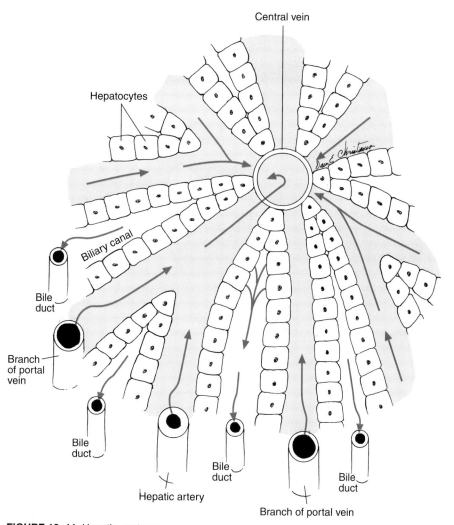

Central vein

Hepatocytes

Biliary canal

Bile
duct

Branch
of portal
vein

Bile
duct

Bile
duct

Hepatic artery

Bile
duct

Branch of portal vein

FIGURE 12–11. Hepatic anatomy.

lipid-soluble vitamins as well as sources of energy. It can also create, from "scratch," simple sugars to be used for energy (*gluconeogenesis*[7]). The liver is important for metabolism and biotransformation of many of the drugs administered to animals. The list of hepatic functions goes on and on; animals cannot survive without the liver. Fortunately, the liver is not easily destroyed and has a tremendous ability to repair and regenerate its tissues when damaged.

---

[7]Gluconeogenesis (*gloo″ko-ne″o-jen′ĕ-sis*); *gluc(o)-* , sugar + *ne(o)-* , new + *gen-* , produce + *-sis* the process of.

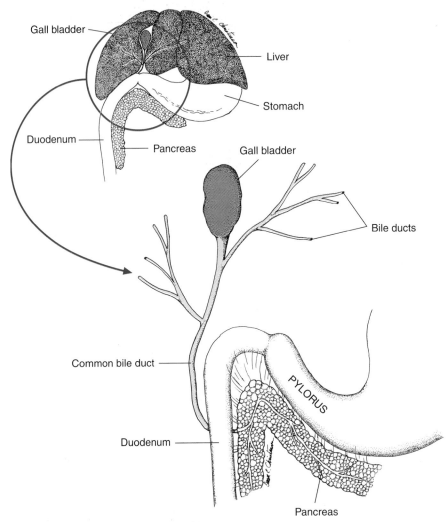

FIGURE 12–12. Biliary tree and gallbladder.

12.2.3.2. Pancreas

The *pancreas* is a glandular organ that lies in the right lateral peritoneal cavity, closely attached to the duodenum and pylorus (see Fig. 12–7). Ducts from the pancreas enter the duodenum, providing passage for pancreatic enzymes. The pancreas is a complex organ with both exocrine (digestive) functions as well as endocrine functions. Endocrine functions of the pancreas are discussed in Chapter 15.

12.2.3.3. Peritoneum, Omentum, and Mesentery

The *peritoneum* is the tissue that lines the walls of the abdominal cavity and covers the abdominal viscera. *Parietal peritoneum*[8] is that which lines the walls of the abdominal cavity, and *visceral peritoneum* is that which covers the organs. The parietal and visceral peritoneum are, for all practical purposes, continuous with one another. The large portion of peritoneal tissue that connects visceral and parietal portions is the *mesentery* (Fig. 12–13 on p. 220). The main attachment for the mesentery is found along the dorsum of the abdominal cavity. From there it forms a fan-like membrane that supports the mesenteric blood vessels, mesenteric lymph nodes and vessels, and nerves that supply the intestines and other abdominal organs. The mesentery provides the supportive attachments for most of the intestinal tract. The *omentum*[9] is a much more delicate tissue, made of loose connective tissue and adipose (Fig. 12–14 on p. 221). Attachments for the omentum are found from the fundus to the pylorus of the stomach. The rest of the omentum lies freely on the floor of the ventral abdomen. It helps to hold the intestines, stomach, and spleen in place. The truly unique characteristic of the omentum is that it will try to seal off or wall off damaged areas along the intestinal tract.

12.2.4. DIGESTIVE PHYSIOLOGY

The digestive process actually begins *preprandially*. Pavlov proved this by training a group of dogs to respond to the sound of a bell in anticipation of a meal. Once trained, the dogs would exhibit *hypersialosis* whenever the bell was rung. Not only is *saliva* produced excessively, in anticipation of a meal, but gastric and other digestive juices begin to prepare for the oncoming food, as well.

The tongue plays an important role in the *prehension*[10] of liquids for companion animals. Most domestic animals use suction to take water and other liquids into the mouth. Dogs and cats, however, use their tongues. They actually form sort of a ladle, by curling the end of the tongue backward. By repeatedly dipping the "ladle" into a body of water and drawing it up into the mouth, a dog or a cat is able to consume the liquid.

Prehension of food varies among domestic animals, depending on the structure of the mouth. Because dogs and cats are carnivorous, their teeth are designed for shearing and tearing of meat from a carcass. In the wild, pieces of meat are torn from the carcass and swallowed. Very little, if any, *mastication* (chewing) takes place. Domestication has provided dogs and cats with preformed kibbles and other such forms of food. Although not necessary, the instinctive prehensile activity may still be exhibited, in the gulping and shaking of food taken into the

---

[8]Parietal (*pah-ri'ĕ-tal*, [L. *parietalis*]) refers to the walls of a cavity.

[9]Omentum (*o-men'tum*); from [L. *omentum*, fat skin].

[10]Prehension (*pre-hen'shun*); from [L. *prehensio*]; the act of seizing or grasping; clinically refers to the act of taking food into the mouth.

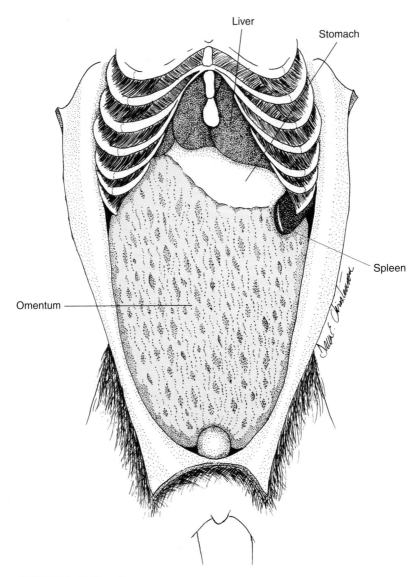

FIGURE 12–13. Omentum.

mouth. In addition, because many of today's foods are dry, many dogs and cats masticate the food. Mastication serves to mix the food with the saliva, making a moist, slippery food bolus to slide through the esophagus. That is the principal role of saliva, to moisten the food and to stick the particles together so that the food may be formed into a manageable bolus for *deglutition*. Unlike human saliva, the saliva of domestic animals has very little, if any, enzymes to initiate digestion.

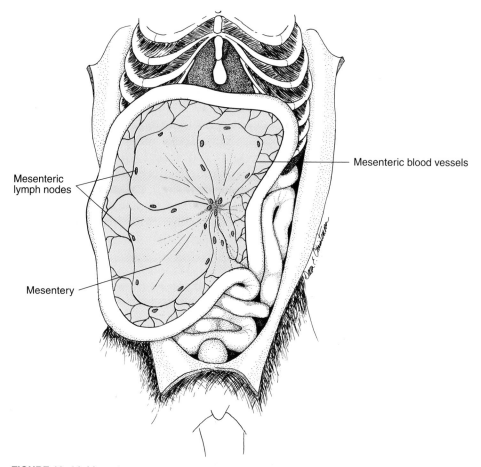

Mesenteric blood vessels

Mesenteric
lymph nodes

Mesentery

FIGURE 12–14. Mesentery.

Domestic animal saliva has two components, an aqueous (watery) part for moistening the food and a viscous part to aid in the formation of the food bolus.

After deglutition, peristaltic activity of the esophagus transports the food bolus to the stomach. When the food enters the stomach, it is tossed and turned by gastric contractions. The gastric motions pulverize the food further and mix it thoroughly with gastric secretions. *Hydrochloric acid* (HCl) and *pepsin* are the two principal secretions in the stomach. The hydrochloric acid is necessary to convert *pepsinogen*, the inactive form of the enzyme pepsin, into active pepsin. Pepsin is stored in an inactive form in the stomach to prevent *autodigestion*[11] of the stomach. Pepsin is a proteolytic[12] enzyme, for the initiation of protein digestion. Actu-

[11]Autodigestion; *auto-* , a prefix meaning "self."
[12]Proteolytic (*pro"te-o-lit'ik*); *prote(o)-* , protein + *-lytic,* pertaining to destruction.

ally, very little digestion takes place in the stomach. The stomach serves more as a holding or storage tank, until the rest of the digestive tract can handle the food that has been consumed. Little by little, the stomach contracts and squirts small volumes of its liquefied contents through the pyloric sphincter into the duodenum.

The duodenum is where digestion really gains momentum. Bile from the liver is secreted into the duodenum. The *bile* and bile salts are important for the emulsification of fats. When fats are emulsified, more lipid surface area is created on which pancreatic enzymes may work. Bile salts are also important for aiding in the absorption of fatty acids and some lipid-soluble vitamins. The pancreas also secretes its digestive juices into the duodenum. Three of the primary *pancreatic enzymes* are *lipase*[13] (for fat digestion), *amylase*[14] (for starch digestion), and *trypsin* (*trip'sin*; for protein digestion). As the ingesta is mixed by segmentation and peristalsis of the intestinal tract, the enzymes break down substances into usable nutrients.

Peristalsis carries the ingesta through the duodenum and the jejunum. Throughout these sections of the small intestine, the enzymes continue to work. Nutrients released by the digestive process are absorbed by the duodenum and jejunum. Most nutrients are absorbed by *active transport*. Most of the water contained in the ingesta at this point remains in the lumen of the intestine. The ileum is most important for reabsorption of bile and bile salts. Recycling may be popular in today's society, but the ileum has been recycling bile and bile salts for millennia.

Peristaltic activity continues to carry the remaining liquid material past the cecum and into the ascending colon. The cecum, in dogs and cats, is a vestigial structure that contributes little, if anything, to the digestive process. (It is much more important in herbivores, like horses and rabbits. In those animals, microbial fermentation of roughages takes place in the cecum.) Once the ingesta is in the colon, it passes slowly through the ascending, transverse, and descending portions of the colon. *Segmentation*, rather than peristalsis, is the predominant muscular activity of the colon. The haustrations, combined with segmentation, slowly mix and turn the bowel contents, much like spading the earth. This exposes a tremendous amount of surface area, to permit absorption of water and electrolytes from the ingesta. By the time the bowel contents have been slowly propelled to the descending colon and rectum, the fecal material has been *desiccated* (dried) into firm masses of waste material. The fecal material is stored and further desiccated in the rectum, until the animal voluntarily defecates.

Actually, *defecation* is partly an involuntary act and partly a voluntary act. Pressure of feces in the rectum stimulates involuntary relaxation of the internal anal sphincter. This causes the external anal sphincter to constrict. The external anal sphincter is relaxed only when the animal chooses to do so for defecation. At this time, most of the haustrations in the colon and rectum disappear, making it

---

[13]Lipase (*li'pās*); from *lip(o)-* , fat + *-ase*, a suffix indicating an enzyme.

[14]Amylase (*am'ĭ-lās*); from *amyl(o)-* , starch + *-ase*.

easier for peristaltic actions to evacuate the bowel. It should be noted that very young animals have not yet developed the voluntary control mechanisms involved with the external anal sphincter. Particularly when training a puppy in its elimination habits, the owner should be aware that the puppy experiences a *gastrocolic* reflex for defecation approximately 15 to 30 minutes *postprandial*. Because the puppy may not have full anal sphincter control, it would be wise for the owner to take him outside to eliminate within the previously stated time period.

Most of the nutrients absorbed throughout the intestinal tract, except lipids, eventually make their way into the *mesenteric blood vessels* (veins). These blood vessels carry the blood to the liver. While it percolates through the liver, hepatic macrophages remove bacteria and other organisms from the blood. The liver also detoxifies the blood, metabolizes (burns) some of the nutrients, and stores others. Eventually, the blood leaves the liver by way of the hepatic vein and flows back to the heart. In the normal animal, any blood returning to the heart from the peritoneal viscera must pass through the liver first.

Lipids are absorbed and transported to the bloodstream by a different route. Lipids must be digested into smaller-sized molecules called *fatty acids*. Fatty acids can readily diffuse across the cell membranes of the enteric epithelium. This is because cell membranes are composed largely of lipids. As a fatty acid passes through the endoplasmic reticula and Golgi apparatus of the *enterocyte*, it is packaged with protein. This new fatty acid–protein compound is called a *chylomicron*.[15] Chylomicrons are then absorbed by the lacteals. Once in the lacteals, the chylomicrons flow with the rest of the lymphatic fluids. They finally make their way to the bloodstream by passing through a structure called the *thoracic duct*. The thoracic duct provides a portal between the lymphatic system and the circulating blood. Eventually, the liver and body tissues remove the chylomicrons from the blood and use or store their components. Fatty acids provide a tremendous energy source for the body. Because most commercial diets for pets contain at least small amounts of fat, *postprandial lipemia*[16] is normal.

12.2.5. NUTRIENTS

The basic classifications of *nutrients* are (1) water, (2) carbohydrates, (3) lipids, (4) proteins, (5) vitamins, and (6) minerals. Those nutrients that provide sources of energy are the carbohydrates, lipids, and proteins.

Water is a very important nutrient. Approximately 70% of the body weight is from water. Animals and people may be able to live for periods of time without food, but without sufficient volumes of water, an animal dehydrates and eventually dies.

Carbohydrates provide the most easily digested nutrients for energy. They are basically compounds made of simple and complex sugar molecules. When di-

---

[15]Chylomicron (*ki"lo-mi'kron*); *chyl(o)-* , juice + [Gr. *micron*, a small thing]; *chyle* is the milky white fluid absorbed by the lacteals [*lact(o)-*, milky].

[16]Lipemia (*li-pe'me-ah*); *lip(o)-* , fat + *hem-* , blood + *-ia* a condition of; lipemic blood samples usually have cloudy, white plasma to some degree.

gested, it is the simple sugar molecule that is readily absorbed and used by the body. Carbohydrates in the diet usually come from various grains, like wheat.

Lipids provide the most concentrated form of energy. Lipids are packed with calories. Comparing lipids to carbohydrates, in terms of energy, is like comparing premium, high-octane gasoline to regular no-lead. They both provide usable fuel to burn, but performance is much better with the high-octane. For those animals who are under excessive physical demands, like herding or tracking dogs, additional fats in the diet help meet their energy needs without their having to consume excessively large volumes of food.

Proteins can also be used for energy. The digestive process needed to achieve usable energy from protein is complex. More important than providing an energy source, proteins are necessary in the diet to provide building blocks (amino acids) for ongoing tissue growth and repair. Protein in the diet must be of good quality to supply the needs of the body. Old boot leather or rawhide does not contain high-quality protein and essential amino acids for domestic animals. High-quality protein must come from good meats, dairy products, or some plants (particularly legumes, like soy). Cats are unique in that they require the essential amino acid taurine in their diets. In addition, cats require higher amounts of protein in their diets than do dogs. This is because cats are true carnivores and are designed to derive large amounts of energy from meat protein.

Vitamins are organic compounds found naturally in many different sources of food. They are required for many of the normal metabolic processes of the body. Vitamins are classified as either water soluble or lipid soluble. Water-soluble vitamins include vitamin C and the B complex vitamins. *Vitamin C* is found naturally in many fruits and other plants. Unlike people, most domestic animals do not require dietary supplementation of vitamin C because their bodies synthesize the compound. One common pet that does require vitamin C supplementation is the guinea pig. Vitamin C is an unstable vitamin that is easily destroyed by oxidation or by exposure to heat or light. Consequently, fresh sources of vitamin C must be provided for guinea pigs. These sources include citrus fruits, cabbage, tomatoes, potatoes, and leafy green vegetables. Vitamin C is important for numerous metabolic processes and particularly for the production of connective tissues. *B complex* vitamins are found in numerous meats, fruits, vegetables, and grains. B vitamins are important for normal cellular metabolism. Lipid-soluble vitamins include vitamins A, D, E, and K. Each of the lipid-soluble vitamins can be stored in large amounts by the liver, except vitamin K; only limited amounts of vitamin K may be stored there. Because the body can store lipid-soluble vitamins, oversupplementation with them could result in toxic side effects. *Vitamin A* is readily found in eggs, fish, liver, dairy foods, and vegetable sources. Many animals, including humans, can synthesize vitamin A from beta carotene (found in yellowish fruits and vegetables). Cats lack this ability, however, and must be provided with vitamin A directly from their food. Vitamin A is important for healthy eyes. Vitamin D also is synthesized by the body on exposure to sunlight. *Vitamin D* is important for the growth and maintenance of healthy bones. Dietary vitamin D is found in milk, eggs, and fish. *Vitamin E* helps maintain healthy hematopoietic and reproductive systems. It is found in eggs, liver, and many grains. It is considered to be an antioxidant because it tends to bind readily to oxygen, preventing oxidation of other compounds, like vitamins A and C. *Vitamin K* is important for the production of clotting factors for the blood and is found in eggs as well as many green, leafy plants, like spinach.

Minerals are inorganic elements and compounds, like iron, phosphorus, calcium, and so on. Iron is critical for the oxygen-carrying ability of the blood. Calcium and phosphorus are important for bone homeostasis. Calcium is poorly absorbed from the digestive tract, whereas phosphorus is readily absorbed. Inappropriate amounts or an inappropriate Ca–P ratio have a deleterious impact on bone growth and maintenance.

Fortunately for pet owners, dietary formulation has been simplified. Pet food companies formulate and package foods to meet the nutritional needs of domestic dogs and cats. Each prepackaged diet is completely balanced, including just the right amounts of carbohydrates, lipids, proteins, vitamins, and minerals to meet the pet's needs. Different formulations have been developed for young, middle-aged, active, and geriatric animals. Still other formulations have been developed specifically to help manage particular companion animal diseases. Provided an owner selects a name-brand diet appropriate for the age, activity level, and species of his or her pet, the commercial food should meet the nutritional needs of the pet. Supplementation usually is not required and in many situations is not advisable. The notion that dogs and cats need dietary variety is untrue. In fact, abrupt dietary changes usually result in gastroenteric upset and diarrhea. Owners should avoid abrupt dietary changes, as well as feeding "table food" to their pets. Not only is gastroenteritis a possibility from such practices, but obesity may be a problem. Unfortunately, most pet owners are compelled to give treats to their pets. If they do, they should be as "heart-smart" for their pets as they are for themselves, avoiding fats and salt. Healthy "people-food" treats may include fresh fruits and vegetables. Many pet owners enjoy giving milk and ice cream to their pets. Unfortunately, many dogs and cats do not have appropriate digestive enzymes for these types of foods. Therefore, feeding these types of dairy products to the pets is much like feeding them to a lactose-intolerant person: *gastroenteritis* and diarrhea usually result. There are dairy-like products on the market today, designed and marketed just for dogs and cats, that should be given to pets in lieu of milk and ice cream. Regardless of why or what the pet owner elects to feed as treats, they should always be given in moderation.

12.2.6. PATHOPHYSIOLOGY

12.2.6.1. Periodontal Disease

Periodontal disease is a progressive disorder of the mouth. It begins with the development of *plaque* (*plak*), which is a bacteria-laden film that coats the teeth and mucous membranes. The bacteria in plaque, if left unchecked, etch away the enamel and inflame and destroy periodontal tissues. Plaque is easily removed by brushing or by abrasives in the diet. If it is left to build up, it begins to thicken into a more solid substance called *tartar*. Tartar build-up along the gingival margin and in the gingival sulcus begins to force the gingiva away from the neck of the tooth. Bacteria continue their vandalism under the protective covering of the tartar. Excessive tartar build-up may begin to calcify, forming the hard substance called *calculus* (*kal'ku-lus*). The tartar and calculus continue to be deposited, in a snowball effect, over the crown and the root of the tooth. *Gingivitis* worsens because of the pressure of the tartar and the bacterial activity. All of these factors progressively begin to destroy the periodontal ligament attachments for the tooth, and gingival recession ensues. Eventually, the greater portion of the root is exposed, potentiating tooth loss as well as bacterial infection around and within the tooth. Advanced periodontal disease results in actual loss of dental bone, as well as mandibular and maxillary bone. Periodontal disease can affect other body systems and organs, diminishing the overall health of the animal. This is particularly true if the pet develops *dysphagia* and *anorexia* because of the *stomatitis*.

Periodontal disease can be prevented through appropriate oral hygiene. In general, on an annual basis, it is recommended that dogs and cats receive *dental prophylaxis* (*pro"fǐ-lak'sis*) provided by veterinary professionals. Some pets may require more frequent visits. The prophylaxis includes scaling (scraping) off the tartar build-up. Then the crowns of the teeth are polished with an abrasive paste. The polishing is important to remove pits and grooves in the enamel created by bacteria. This gives future plaque and tartar less of a foothold. Finally, all of the teeth are carefully inspected for looseness and *dental caries* (cavities), and the gingival sulci are measured to determine the condition of the periodontal ligaments. Oral care does not end here.

Owners must play an active role in the prevention of periodontal disease. Special brushes, veterinary toothpastes, and oral rinses have been developed for pet care at home. The veterinary toothpastes are flavored to be palatable for dogs and cats and they do not foam the way traditional toothpastes do. Toothpaste foam can be very disagreeable for many pets. Brushing just 2 to 3 times per week can make a marked difference in the health of a pet's mouth. Pet-safe, antiplaque chew toys, along with dry foods and biscuits, can also help minimize plaque and tartar build-up. In fact, some pet foods on the market today are designed specifically to minimize tartar accumulations. To use an old phrase, "an ounce of prevention is worth a pound of cure." Prevention of periodontal disease is the key to maintaining healthy teeth and mouths for pets.

12.2.6.2. Gastroenteric Disorders

There are numerous gastroenteric disorders of dogs and cats. Some disorders, infectious and noninfectious alike, can be life threatening. Many of the infectious diseases, including Canine Parvoviral Enteritis, Canine Infectious Hepatitis, Feline Panleukopenia, Canine Distemper, and Canine Coronaviral Gastroenteritis, can be prevented through routine immunization. Each of the aforementioned diseases can be fatal, especially in very young or old animals. For those animals who are unfortunate enough to acquire an infectious form of viral gastroenteritis, only supportive care with fluid therapy, *antiemetics*, and *antidiarrheals* can be provided. In puppies and kittens, vaccination protocols for these diseases usually begin around 8 weeks of age and continue at 3- to 4-week intervals until about 12 to 16 weeks of age. The final vaccination of puppies against Canine Parvovirus should be given after 18 to 20 weeks of age to provide optimal protection against the disease. Previously immunized adult animals should receive annual revaccination against these diseases to maintain immunity (i.e., resistance to disease).

Two of the most common noninfectious gastroenteric disorders are *gastric dilatation volvulus*[17] (GDV) and enteric obstruction. GDV is common in, but not exclusively seen in large, deep-chested breeds of dogs (e.g., Doberman Pinschers, Great Danes, German Shepherds). The most frequent scenario leading to GDV in these animals is consumption of large volumes of food or water, followed by play. The weight of the gastric contents makes the stomach more pendulous. Because of the large structure of the caudal chest and cranial abdomen, the pendulous stomach has room to move and may flip over on its own axis (volvulus). Obviously, the twisting action prohibits passage of anything through the gastroesophageal opening and the pylorus. Blood flow for the stomach and spleen is also impaired. Gas and toxins accumulate in the stomach, causing it to bloat. The stomach continues to expand until it is so stretched it sounds like a basketball when tapped (i.e., a "ping"). GDV is an emergency situation. Unless the stomach is quickly decompressed by passage of an orogastric tube, puncture with a trocar, or surgery, the animal will die. Death due to GDV occurs *rapidly*; therefore, prompt intervention by veterinary professionals is essential for patient survival. Surgery is also required to untwist the stomach. If a portion of the stomach wall has died because of lack of blood supply, *gastrectomy* of the *necrotic* area is performed. After a partial gastrectomy, the dog is not able to consume food *per os* (by mouth) until the stomach has had ample time to heal. To maintain the nutritional needs of the patient, an *enterostomy* tube may be temporarily placed. Small, frequent liquid meals can then be provided through the enterostomy. When no longer needed, the tube is removed and the openings in the intestine and abdominal cavity are closed. Dogs who have experienced GDV once are more likely to experience it again. Even if the stomach or the omentum are sutured to the abdominal wall, it is still possible for the dog to break those attachments and torse the stomach again. The pet owner of a former GDV patient should try to minimize potential for recurrence of the disorder by feeding smaller, more frequent meals (ca. 2–3/day), prohibiting consumption/gulping of large volumes of water at one time, and avoiding exercise and play for 1 to 2 hours postprandial.

Enteric obstructions are usually caused by some type of foreign body, like small rubber balls, rocks, or any other such objects that a precocious dog or cat might consume. The obstruction prevents passage of ingesta through the intestinal tract. The peristaltic activity can become so strong in the attempt to remove the insulting object, that an *intussusception* develops at or near the obstruction. *Necrosis* of the bowel at that site quickly ensues. An *enterotomy* is required to remove the foreign body and an enterectomy is performed to remove the necrotic

---

[17]Volvulus (*vol'vu-lus*); from [L. *volvere*, to twist around]; gastric dilatation volvulus is a twisting of the stomach, accompanied by excessive dilation with gas.

portion of the bowel. An *anastomosis*[18] joins the two healthy ends of the intestine together. The longer the obstruction has existed, the greater the risk of *peritonitis* developing, before or after surgery. Most obstructions like this are preventable by owners "pet-proofing" their homes and yards. Doing so could save the life of the pet and could also save the owner a costly hospital bill.

12.3. Self-Test

Using the previous information in this chapter, respond to each of the following questions using the most appropriate medical term(s). Do not use abbreviations.

1. The medical term that pertains to the time after a meal is _____.

2. Lipase, amylase, and trypsin are enzymes produced by the _pancreas_.

3. _gastroenteritis_ is the medical term meaning inflammation of the stomach and the intestines.

4. The _pyloric_ sphincter is a specialized band of muscle tissue that controls the passage of ingesta from the stomach to the duodenum.

5. The act of swallowing is medically termed _____.

6. Inappetence is medically termed _anorexia_.

7. A(n) _orogastric_ tube is a tube placed from the mouth to the stomach, often for the administration of medication or food.

8. The surgical connection of two ends of bowel is called a(n) _____.

9. _peridontal_ disease is a progressive disease of the tissues surrounding the teeth that can be prevented through proper oral hygiene.

10. The rhythmic, worm-like contractions of the digestive tract that propel ingesta through that tract are called _peristalsis_.

11. The surface of a tooth that naturally comes in contact with the cheek mucosa is called the _____ surface.

12. A(n) _____ is a drug used to deter vomiting.

13. Inflammation of the peritoneum is medically termed _peritonitis_.

14. The _liver_ is a large digestive organ that occupies approximately the cranial third of the abdominal cavity, and is responsible for the production of bile and bile salts.

---

[18]Anastomosis (*ah-nas"to-mo'sis*); from [Gr. *anastomosis*, opening, outlet].

15. The ___jejunum___ is the longest portion of the small intestine and occupies a large part of the abdominal cavity space.

16. The lacy tissue made of loose connective tissue and adipose that is attached to the greater curvature of the stomach, lies along the ventral abdomen, and helps to hold abdominal contents in place is the _____.

17. Excessive salivation is medically termed _____.

18. The medical term pertaining to the liver is ___hepatic___.

19. A(n) ___enterostomy___ is a surgical procedure in which an opening is created into the intestine, often for the placement of a postoperative feeding tube.

20. Surgical removal of all or part of the stomach is medically termed a(n) ___gastrectomy___.

21. ___glossal___ and ___lingual___ are both medical terms pertaining to the tongue.

22. ___GDV___, commonly called "bloat," is a life-threatening disorder in which the stomach twists on its own axis and becomes distended with gas.

23. The _____ is that region where the mouth and throat communicate.

24. _____ is the medical term used for the seizing or grasping of food for consumption.

25. The colon is formed with numerous, pouch-like structures called _____ that with segmentation activity help to mix and turn bowel contents for optimal desiccation.

26. The telescoping of a portion of the intestine onto an adjacent part is medically termed a(n) _____.

27. The _____ is the peritoneal tissue that supports the blood vessels, lymph nodes and vessels, and nerves that supply the intestinal tract. Its supportive attachments for the intestines are located along the dorsum of the abdominal cavity.

28. The _____ junction is the region of the bowel where the distal portion of the small intestine meets the cecum, marking the end of the small intestine and the beginning of the colon.

29. Inflammation of the pancreas would be medically termed ___pancreatitis___.

30. The porous, bony substance beneath the enamel and cementum of a tooth is called _____.

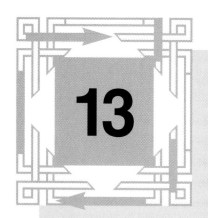

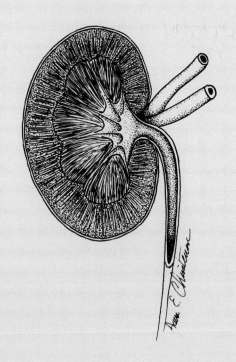

The Urinary System

GOALS AND OBJECTIVES

By the conclusion of this chapter, the student will be able to:

1. Recognize common root words, prefixes, and suffixes related to the urinary system.

2. Divide simple and compound words into their respective parts.

3. Recognize, correctly pronounce, and appropriately use common medical terms related to the urinary system.

4. Demonstrate an understanding of urinary anatomy.

5. Demonstrate an understanding of renal physiology, with regard to urine production, water homeostasis, waste excretion, and electrolyte homeostasis.

13.1. Introduction to Related Terms

Divide each of the following terms into its respective parts ("R" root, "P" prefix, "S" suffix, "CV" combining vowel).

1. **Renal**   (R) _____ (S) _____

   renal (re'nal; pertaining to the kidney)

2. **Prerenal**   (P) _____ (R) _____ (S) _____

   prerenal (pre-re'nal; pertaining to before the kidney)

3. **Postrenal**   (P) _____ (R) _____ (S) _____

   postrenal (post-re'nal; pertaining to after the kidney)

4. **Retroperitoneal**   (P) _____ (CV) ___ (R) _____ (S) _____

   retroperitoneal (re"tro-per"ĭ-to-ne'al, ret"ro-per"ĭ-to-ne'al; pertaining to behind the peritoneum)

5. **Nephritis**   (R) _____ (S) _____

   nephritis (ně-fri'tis; inflammation of the kidney)

6. **Pyelonephritis**   (R) _____ (CV) ___ (R) _____ (S) _____

   pyelonephritis (pi"ě-lo-ně-fri'tis; inflammation of the kidney and its pelvis)

7. **Pyelogram**   (R) _____ (CV) ___ (S) _____

   pyelogram (pi'ě-lo-gram"; to record the pelvis; clinically refers to a radiographic procedure in which radiopaque dye is used to visualize the renal pelvis and other structures)

8. **Cystogram**   (R) _____ (CV) ___ (S) _____

   cystogram (sis'to-gram; to record the bladder; clinically refers to a radiographic procedure used to visualize the urinary bladder)

9. **Cystocentesis**   (R) _____ (CV) ___ (R) _____

   cystocentesis (sis"to-sen-te'sis; puncture of the bladder; refers to the clinical procedure in which urine is withdrawn from the bladder using a syringe and needle, by puncture through the abdominal wall)

10. **Urethritis**   (R) _____ (S) _____

    urethritis (u"re-thri'tis; inflammation of the urethra)

11. **Urolithiasis**   (R) _____ (CV) ___ (R) _____ (CV) ___ (S) _____

    urolithiasis (u"ro-lĭ-thi'ah-sis; a condition of urinary stones)

12. **Hematuria**   (R) _____   (R) _____   (S) _____

hematuria (hem"ah-tu're-ah, he"mah-tu're-ah; a condition of bloody urine)

13. **Cystotomy**   (R) _____   (CV) _____   (S) _____

cystotomy (sis-tot'o-me; to cut the bladder; clinically refers to a surgical procedure in which the bladder is incised)

14. **Polyuria**   (P) _____   (R) _____   (S) _____

polyuria (pol"e-u're-ah; a condition of much urine; clinically refers to passage of large volumes of urine in a given period of time)

15. **Oliguria**   (P) _____   (R) _____   (S) _____

oliguria (ol"ĭ-gu're-ah; a condition of small urination; clinically refers to a small volume of urine in relation to fluid intake)

16. **Pollakiuria**   (R) _____   (CV) _____   (R) _____   (S) _____

pollakiuria (pol"ah-ke-u're-ah, pol"ak-ĭ-u're-ah; a condition of frequent urination)

17. **Dysuria**   (P) _____   (R) _____   (S) _____

dysuria (dis-u're-ah; a condition of difficult urination)

18. **Anuria**   (P) _____   (R) _____   (S) _____

anuria (ah-nu're-ah, an-u're-ah; a condition without urination)

19. **Nephrotoxic**   (R) _____   (CV) _____   (R) _____   (S) _____

nephrotoxic (nef"ro-tok'sik; pertaining to a kidney toxin [poison])

20. **Uremia**   (R) _____   (R) _____   (S) _____

uremia (u-re'me-ah; a condition of urine in blood; clinically refers to retention of wastes in the blood that should be excreted by the kidneys and the toxic condition produced)

21. **Azotemia**   (R) _____   (R) _____   (S) _____

azotemia (az"o-te'me-ah, a-zo-te'me-ah; a condition of nitrogen in the blood; clinically refers to excess urea and other nitrogenous compounds in the blood)

22. **Proteinuria**   (R) _____   (R) _____   (S) _____

proteinuria (pro"te-in-u're-ah; a condition of protein in the urine)

23. **Glycosuria**   (R) _____   (R) _____   (S) _____

glycosuria (gli"ko-su're-ah; a condition of glucose in the urine)

24. **Uropoiesis**   (R) _____ (CV) ___ (R) _____ (S) _____

   uropoiesis (u"ro-poi-e'sis; the process of producing urine)

25. **Urethrostomy**   (R) _____ (CV) ___ (S) _____

   urethrostomy (u"re-thros'to-me; to create a "mouth" in the urethra; clinically refers to a surgical procedure in which a permanent opening is made in the urethra to facilitate urination)

26. **Glomerular**   (R) _____ (S) _____

   glomerular (glo-mer'u-lar; pertaining to a glomerulus; [L. glomerulus, dim. of glomus, ball])

27. **Peritubular**   (P) _____ (R) _____ (S) _____

   peritubular (per"ĭ-tu'bu-lar; pertaining to around a tubule)

13.2. Urinary Anatomy and Physiology

13.2.1. URINARY SYSTEM ANATOMY

The *kidneys* lie *retroperitoneal*, near the dorsocranial abdominal cavity (Fig. 13–1). The right kidney tends to be on the right dorsolateral abdomen, slightly caudal to the last rib. It is typically attached fairly tightly along the dorsum. The left kidney is usually found on the left dorsolateral abdomen, slightly more caudal than the right kidney. It also tends to be attached slightly looser than the right kidney, making it easier to palpate. An easy phrase to help keep the positioning of each kidney straight is "righty tighty, lefty loosy and last."

   Attached to each kidney is a *ureter*. These fine, small tubes carry urine to the *urinary bladder* (see Fig. 13–1). The urinary bladder is found in the caudal abdominal cavity, closely associated with the pelvis. When the bladder is empty, it is found in the pubic area. As the bladder becomes full, it becomes more pendulous and progressively falls in a cranioventral direction in the peritoneal cavity. The bladder itself is composed of smooth muscle and its interior is lined with stratified squamous epithelium. At the neck of the bladder is a sphincter, used to control evacuation of urine.

   The *urethra* is a tube connecting the urinary bladder with the external environment (Figs. 13–2 on p. 236 and 13–3 on p. 237). As the urethra leaves the bladder it passes dorsal to the pelvis before progressing to its distal point, the urethral orifice. In male dogs, the urethra must pass through a bony structure in the penis (i.e., the *os penis*[1]). In addition, the prostate gland (a part of the male reproductive tract) surrounds the neck of the bladder. This area, as well as the os penis and the curvature over the pelvis, create natural areas for potential stricture, especially in animals prone to *urolithiasis*.

---

[1]Os penis (*os pe'nis*); from [L. *os*, bone + penis].

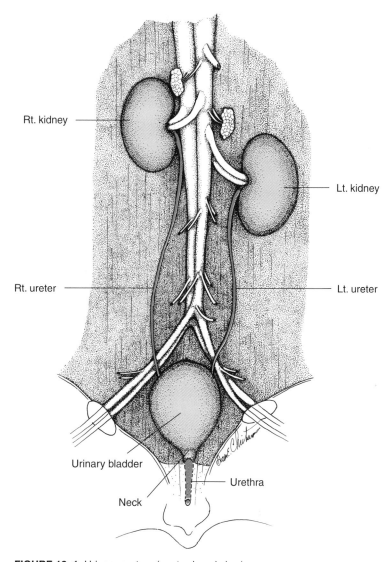

FIGURE 13–1. Urinary system (ventrodorsal view).

13.2.2. RENAL ANATOMY

The kidney is encased in a *renal capsule,* composed of tough, fibrous connective tissue (Fig. 13–4 on p. 238). The *renal cortex,*[2] which is closest to the renal capsule, is the outermost functional portion of the kidney. The renal cortex contains bil-

---

[2]Renal cortex (*re'nal kor'teks*); cortex from [L. *cortex,* shell].

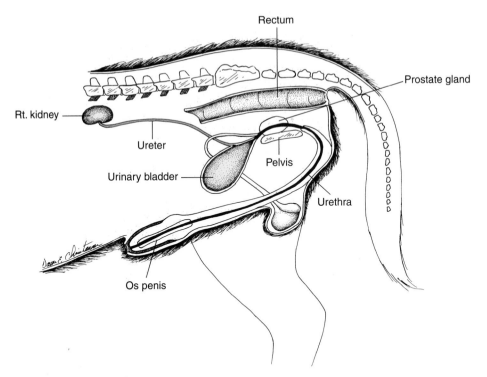

FIGURE 13–2. Canine male urinary tract.

lions of *nephrons*, the functional units of the kidney. The *renal medulla*[3] is surrounded by the renal cortex. The medulla is composed of numerous tubules that communicate with the other portions of the nephrons in the cortex and the collecting ducts, which lead to the *renal pelvis*. The renal pelvis merely serves as a large "funnel" to collect all of the urine from the numerous tubules and ducts to be passed onto the ureter.

13.2.3. NEPHRON

As stated earlier, the nephron is an individual functional unit of the kidney (Fig. 13–5 on p. 239). Each nephron is structured as a series of tubes that serve to keep essential elements for the body and excrete potentially toxic wastes. Fresh, oxygenated blood arrives at the kidney and is pumped through billions of glomeruli. A *glomerulus* is simply a twisted bundle of capillaries, surrounded by a spheroid structure called *Bowman's capsule*. Leading from Bowman's capsule is a progression of tubes. The proximal tubular structure is called the *proximal convoluted*[4]

---

[3]Renal medulla (*re'nal mĕ-dul'ah*); from [L. *medulla*, inmost part].

[4]Convoluted (*kon'vo-lūt-ed*); from [L. *convolutus*, coiled].

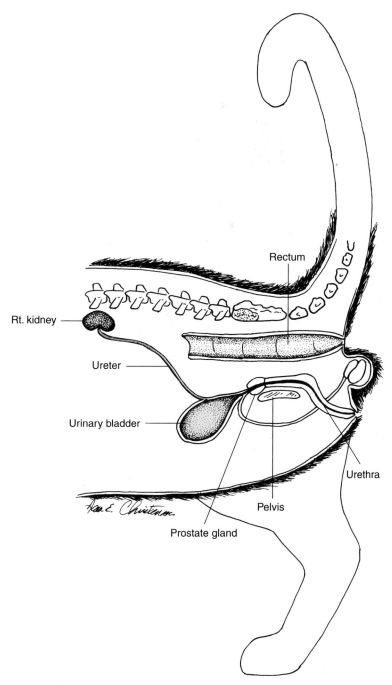

FIGURE 13–3. Feline male urinary tract.

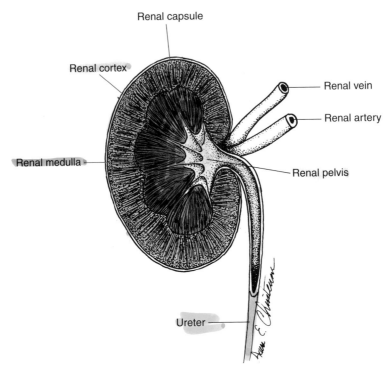

Renal capsule

Renal cortex

Renal vein

Renal artery

Renal medulla

Renal pelvis

Ureter

FIGURE 13–4. Sagittal kidney.

tubule. This leads to a structure that looks much like the elbow of a drain pipe under a sink. This "elbow" is referred to as the *loop of Henle*, named after Fredrich Gustav Jakob Henle, a German anatomist. The loop of Henle leads to the *distal convoluted tubule*. All of the distal convoluted tubules converge at collecting ducts, which lead to the renal pelvis. All of the tubules of the nephron are surrounded by numerous *peritubular* capillaries. The importance of the capillary-tubule relationship is discussed in the section on *uropoiesis*. The renal tubules are lined with simple cuboidal epithelium. This epithelial tissue is active in reabsorption of various nutrients for the body.

13.2.4. UROPOIESIS

Urine production is highly dependent on adequate blood pressure. Without sufficient blood pressure, water and wastes cannot be forced through the glomeruli for filtration. An opposing force of blood plasma osmotic pressure also affects filtration by the glomerulus. As blood enters the glomerulus, hydrostatic pressure[5]

---

[5]Hydrostatic pressure (*hi"dro-stat'ik*); [*hydr(o)-* , water + Gr. *statikos*, standing]; hydrostatic pressure is the force exerted by a liquid to maintain a state of equilibrium.

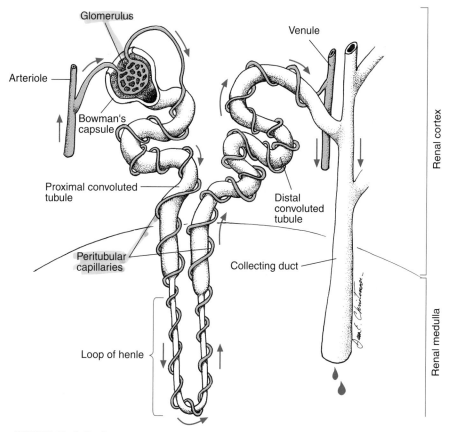

FIGURE 13–5. Nephron.

forces water and dissolved particles from the capillaries into Bowman's capsule. This glomerular filtrate passes through all of the renal tubules. Along the way, various portions of the tubules either reabsorb components for use by the body or excrete unnecessary components.

Most nutrients are reabsorbed in the proximal convoluted tubules by active transport and delivered to the peritubular capillaries. Some of the nutrients reabsorbed by the proximal convoluted tubules are glucose, various amino acids, proteins, and electrolytes (PO_4^-, SO_4^-, Ca^+, K^+, and Na^+). Water is reabsorbed by osmosis. As the filtrate continues and passes through the loop of Henle, additional water and sodium continue to be reabsorbed. The distal convoluted tubule is relatively impermeable to water; however, electrolytes like Na^+ continue to be reabsorbed there. In addition, the epithelium of the distal convoluted tubule excretes various substances to be eliminated in the urine (e.g., H^+, K^+, NH_4^-, and various drugs like penicillin). Finally, as the filtrate passes through the collecting ducts, water and Na^+ may continue to be absorbed. By the time the fluid passes from the collecting ducts into the renal pelvis and subsequently the ureter, the urine has been well concentrated. Nearly all of the sodium that was in the original filtrate has been reabsorbed. Most of the other nutrients, including water, that are needed by the body also have been reabsorbed. Excesses of nutrients and toxic wastes have been filtered out and excreted. One of the most important wastes to be eliminated by the kidneys is *urea*. Urea is a nitrogenous by-product of protein metabolism that can be very harmful to the body. Failure to remove urea from the blood results in serious disease manifestations.

13.2.5. PATHOPHYSIOLOGY

Renal function is critical to maintenance of homeostasis. Evaluation of the urine can reveal much about renal function, as well as the health of the individual. *Glycosuria* is often encountered in patients with diabetes mellitus. The glucose is passed in the urine because the kidneys can only handle reabsorption of so much glucose. Once the renal tubules have reached their threshold for glucose reabsorption, the remaining excess passes with the urine. *Proteinuria*, on the other hand, is more indicative of insufficient kidney function due to renal disease. Complete urinalysis, involving tests of specific gravity, chemical properties, and microscopic examination of the urine sediment, can be very useful diagnostically. For example, *polyuria* is a clinical manifestation of both *diabetes mellitus* and *diabetes insipidus*. Urinalysis alone may help the clinician distinguish between these two very different diseases. Polyuria due to diabetes mellitus is a secondary effect of the body's inability to regulate blood glucose concentrations. Diabetes insipidus, however, is a primary renal disorder in which the kidneys are unable to reabsorb water and therefore cannot concentrate the urine. Of course, one must not forget to collect a very thorough patient history, because many medications (e.g., prednisolone[6]) can also cause polyuria. Various cell types and casts seen in the urine sediment may provide evidence of *cystitis* versus *nephritis*. Other diagnostic tools, such as *cystograms* and *pyelograms*, help the veterinarian visualize areas of disease, particularly changes related to *uroliths* and obstructions.

There are many ways in which disease processes can affect renal function. For example, the most common cause of *prerenal azotemia* is low blood pressure. Low blood pressure could be caused by many things, such as low blood volume due to blood loss or dehydration, or cardiac disease. With insufficient blood pressure, the glomeruli cannot produce the filtrate for the removal of toxic compounds like urea and ammonia. Unless the primary cause of the low blood pressure is corrected, the kidneys progressively begin to fail. The resulting renal damage may be irreversible. Examples of renal and postrenal azotemia are demonstrated in the following discussions of ethylene glycol toxicity and *urolithiasis*.

---

[6]Prednisolone is a corticosteroid, anti-inflammatory medication.

13.2.5.1. Urolithiasis

Urolithiasis is a disorder that may plague dogs and cats alike. Male cats, however, are probably the most frequently seen patients with urolithiasis. Urethral obstruction due to urolith formation is common in male cats. Triple phosphate or struvite (*stroo'vīt*) crystals are the most common crystal involved with this syndrome in cats. For those cats prone to struvite crystal formation, the *postprandial alkaline tide*[7] can be a large contributing factor to the problem. In essence, the postprandial alkaline tide is a normal sequela to eating a meal. Hydrogen ions are drawn from the blood by the stomach for the formation of large amounts of hydrochloric acid for digestion. This results in alkaline circulating blood. In turn, the kidneys produce highly alkaline urine, which provides the perfect environment for struvite crystal and urolith formation. Male cats, with their very small urethral lumen, become easily obstructed by accumulations of struvite crystals and uroliths.

Male cats with urethral obstruction usually are presented on an emergency basis. Typically, the urinary bladder is extremely distended and must be quickly relieved by the passage of a urethral catheter, or *cystocentesis*. Unfortunately, the signs leading up to this traumatic, life-threatening event were probably unnoticed or misinterpreted by the owners. The obstruction develops progressively. Over time, crystals begin to accumulate in the bladder and the urethra. Soon cystitis and *urethritis* ensue. Between the inflammation and the urolith formation, urination becomes increasingly difficult for the cat. Many cat owners misinterpret the crying and *dysuria* in the litterbox for constipation. They typically do not see signs of the *hematuria* because the cat is so efficient at covering up the evidence with the litter. By the time many of these cats arrive at the hospital, they have severe *postrenal azotemia*. In fact, the cats are brought in most often not because of the urethral problem, but because of the vomiting, depression, and disorientation caused by *uremia*. Intense supportive medical care is usually required for these patients. Once the obstruction is removed and the toxic effects of uremia resolved, many of these patients can be managed dietarily. Specially formulated foods are available that help to create a more acidic urine. Thereby, struvite crystal formation can be minimized, if not eliminated. For chronic obstructive cases, the damage and scarring caused by each incident often requires the reconstructive surgery of a *urethrostomy*. Numerous large uroliths in the bladder may warrant a *cystotomy*, as well. For some cats, even a urethrostomy may not be enough to preclude urethral obstruction. The owners of such a cat must be well aware of the early signs of cystitis and urethritis, such as *oliguria*, *pollakiuria*, dysuria, and hematuria. If recognized early, complete obstruction may be avoided with rigorous medical intervention.

---

[7]Postprandial alkaline tide (*post-pran'de-al*); from [*post-* , after + *prandi(o)-* , meal + *-al* pertaining to]; the transient alkalinity of the body after a meal.

13.2.5.2. Ethylene Glycol Toxicity

Ethylene glycol (antifreeze) is a deadly proposition for dogs, cats, and other unsuspecting animals. Every year, countless animals die needlessly from the *nephrotoxic* effects of ethylene glycol. The incidents usually occur in the spring and particularly in the fall, when people are flushing and refilling their automobile radiators in preparation for oncoming harsh weather. Even the smallest pool of sweet-smelling antifreeze is very attractive to most dogs and cats; a small amount (less than 1 tsp.) can be lethal.

An animal who has consumed antifreeze rapidly sustains complete renal failure. *Renal azotemia*, uremia, and *anuria* quickly ensue, as a result of glomerular damage. Even with rigorous emergency medical care, many of these patients die. If an owner merely suspects that his or her pet may have consumed some antifreeze, that pet should be taken to the veterinarian for immediate medical services. The longer the time from ingestion to medical intervention, the smaller the chances of salvaging enough renal function to prolong life. Survival of ethylene glycol toxicity is the exception rather than the rule.

Pet owners must be made aware of the hazards of ethylene glycol for their pets, children, and wildlife. They must ensure safe storage and disposal of the agent. Today, they could avoid use of ethylene glycol completely, with the advent of nontoxic antifreeze compounds. Death due to renal failure caused by ethylene glycol toxicity is completely preventable. The burden of prevention falls to everyone who uses antifreeze or coolants containing ethylene glycol.

13.3. Self-Test

Using the previous information in this chapter, respond to each of the following questions using the most appropriate medical term(s).

1. The kidneys lie _____ in relation to the abdominal cavity.

2. The ___*glomerulus*___ is that portion of the nephron that is composed of a bundle of capillaries and is responsible for filtering wastes and other components from the blood.

3. Blood in the urine is medically termed ___*hematuria*___.

4. Urethral obstruction is a common cause of postrenal _____, which is an accumulation of nitrogenous substances in the blood.

5. Ethylene glycol is a _____ chemical that, when consumed by an animal, results in death due to damage to the kidneys.

6. _____ is a disease syndrome of the urinary system in which urinary stones are formed.

7. The procedure in which urine is withdrawn via puncture of the bladder using a syringe and needle through the abdominal wall is medically termed ___Cystocentesis___.

8. Glucose in the urine is medically termed _____.

9. Frequent urination is medically termed _____.

10. A(n) _____ is a radiographic procedure in which contrast media are used to evaluate the bladder.

11. ___nephritis___ is inflammation of the kidney(s).

12. _____ is a condition in which excessive amounts of urine are produced.

13. Difficulty urinating is medically termed ___dysuria___.

14. A(n) _____ is a surgical procedure in which the urethra is incised, creating a permanent opening.

15. Inflammation of the kidney and its pelvis is medically termed

_____.

16. A(n) _____ is a surgical procedure in which the bladder is incised, often for the removal of urinary stones.

17. The ___ureter___ is a small tube that carries urine from the kidney to the bladder.

18. _____ is the medical term meaning "urine production."

19. The proximal _____ is the portion of the nephron through which most nutrients and water are reabsorbed.

20. Production of small amounts of urine is medically termed

_____.

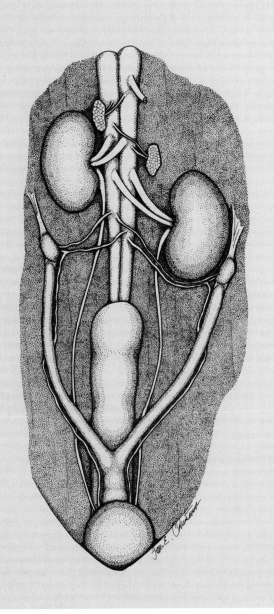

The Reproductive System

GOALS AND OBJECTIVES

By the conclusion of this chapter, the student will be able to:

1. Recognize common root words, prefixes, and suffixes related to the reproductive system.
2. Divide simple and compound words into their respective parts.
3. Recognize, correctly pronounce, and appropriately use common medical terms related to the reproductive system.
4. Demonstrate an understanding of reproductive anatomy (male and female).
5. Demonstrate an understanding of reproductive physiology as it relates to estrus, gestation, parturition, lactation, and, in the male, spermatogenesis.

14.1. Introduction to Related Terms

Divide each of the following terms into its respective parts ("R" root, "P" prefix, "S" suffix, "CV" combining vowel).

1. **Cryptorchid**   (R) _____   (R) _____

   cryptorchid (krip-tor'kid; hidden testicles; clinically refers to an animal whose testes have not yet dropped into the scrotum)

2. **Monorchid**   (R) _____   (R) _____

   monorchid (mon-or'kid; one testicle; clinically refers to an animal who has only one testicle in the scrotum)

3. **Orchiectomy**   (R) _____   (S) _____

   orchiectomy (or"ke-ek'to-me; excision of the testes; i.e. castration; cf. orchidectomy)

4. **Spermatogenesis**   (R) _____   (CV) ___   (R) _____   (CV) ___   (S) _____

   spermatogenesis (sper"mah-to-jen'ĕ-sis; the process of sperm production)

5. **Ovariohysterectomy**   (R) _____   (CV) ___   (R) _____   (S) _____

   ovariohysterectomy (o-va"re-o-his"ter-ek'to-me; excision of the ovaries and the uterus; cf. spay)

6. **Pyometra**   (R) _____   (CV) ___   (R) _____

   pyometra (pi"o-me'trah; pus in the uterus)

7. **Mastitis**   (R) _____   (S) _____

   mastitis (mas-ti'tis; inflammation of the breasts/mammary tissue)

8. **Gestation**   (R) _____   (S) _____

   gestation (jes-ta'shun; the state of bearing; clinically refers to the stage of the reproductive cycle in which the female is carrying young in utero)

9. **Parturition**   (R) _____   (S) _____

   parturition (par"tu-ri'shun; the state of birthing)

10. **Lactation**   (R) _____   (S) _____

    lactation (lak-ta'shun; the state of milking)

11. **Postparturient**   (P) _____   (R) _____   (S) _____

    postparturient (post-par"tūr're-ent; pertaining to after birthing; cf. postpartum)

12. **Dystocia**   (P) _____   (R) _____   (S) _____

    dystocia (dis-to'se-ah; the process of difficult birth)

13. **Neonatal**   (P) _____   (R) _____   (S) _____

   neonatal (ne"o-na'tal; pertaining to newly born)

14. **Mutagenic**   (R) _____   (R) _____   (S) _____

   mutagenic (mu"tah-jen'ik; pertaining to change producing; clinically refers to anything that alters the DNA to create genetic abnormalities)

15. **Teratogenic**   (R) _____   (CV) ___   (R) _____   (S) _____

   teratogenic (ter"ah-to-jen'ik; pertaining to monster producing; clinically refers to anything that causes physical defects in the developing embryo/fetus)

16. **Proestrus**   (P) _____   (R) _____

   proestrus (pro-es'trus; before estrus; clinically refers to the period of the reproductive cycle before sexual receptivity)

17. **Metestrus**   (P) _____   (R) _____

   metestrus (met-es'trus; beyond/after estrus; clinically refers to the period of the reproductive cycle after sexual receptivity)

18. **Anestrus**   (P) _____   (R) _____

   anestrus (an-es'trus; absence of estrus; clinically refers to the period of the reproductive cycle in which the female animal is in sexual quiescence)

19. **Monestrous**   (P) _____   (R) _____   (S) _____

   monestrous (mon-es'trus; pertaining to one estrus; clinically refers to those animals who experience one estrous cycle in a sexual season)

20. **Polyestrous**   (P) _____   (R) _____   (S) _____

   polyestrous (pol"e-es'trus; pertaining to much [many] estrus; clinically refers to those animals who experience numerous estrous cycles during a sexual season)

21. **Pseudocyesis**   (R) _____   (CV) ___   (R) _____

   pseudocyesis (su"do-si-e'sis; false pregnancy)

22. **Metritis**   (R) _____   (S) _____

   metritis (me-tri'tis; inflammation of the uterus [womb])

14.2. Reproductive Anatomy and Physiology

14.2.1. FEMALE REPRODUCTIVE ANATOMY

Female animals have a pair of *ovaries,* located near the dorsum of the abdominal cavity (Figs. 14–1 and 14–2). They are firmly attached to the body wall with fibrous connective tissue. In the mature female, the ovaries contain *oocytes*[1] at vari-

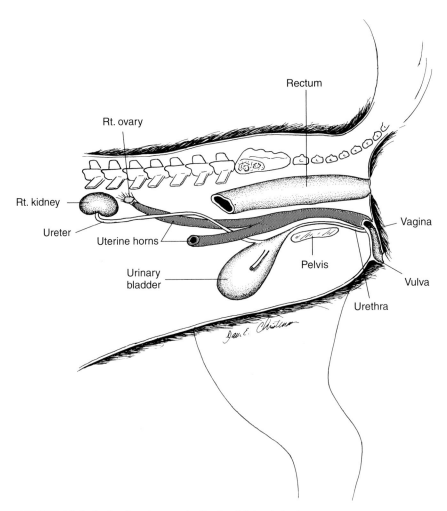

FIGURE 14–1. Canine female reproductive tract (lateral view).

---

[1]Oocyte (*o'o-sīt*); from [Gr. *oon,* egg + *-cyte*].

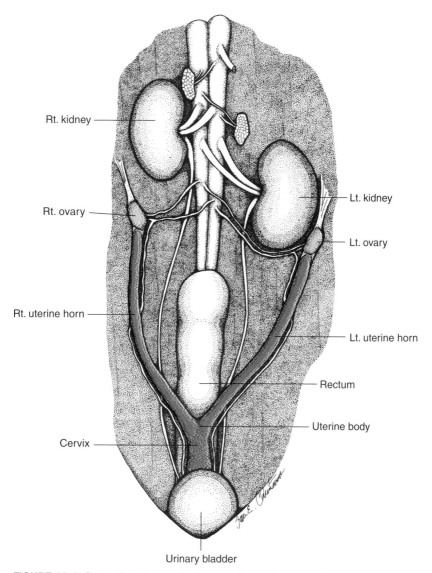

FIGURE 14–2. Canine female reproductive tract (ventrodorsal view).

ous stages of development. Oocytes are created by *meiosis*[2] from primary ovarian cells. Each oocyte contains half of the genetic information found in the parent cell (half that required to produce offspring). Some chemicals and other agents can

---

[2]Meiosis (*mi-o′sis*); a special method of cell division of sex cells, in which daughter cells receive only half the chromosomes of the parent cell.

have *mutagenic* effects on the primary ovarian cells. Oocytes produced from these altered cells produce genetically abnormal offspring.

The ovaries are closely associated with the *uterine horns.* At *ovulation,*[3] oocytes are deposited into the *infundibulum*[4] of each uterine horn. Unlike humans, animals tend to produce multiple offspring from a single pregnancy. Therefore, the uterus is subdivided into two horns, facilitating carriage of multiple fetuses during *gestation.* The uterine horns converge caudally at the *uterine body.* The *cervix* (*ser'viks*), a strong sphincter, demarcates the uterus from the vagina. The *vagina* (*vah-ji'nah*) serves as a passageway not only for the reproductive tract, but for the urinary tract as well. The urethral orifice is found along the ventral floor of the vagina, in the caudal third of the passage. The uterus and the vagina are lined with stratified squamous epithelium. Cytologic analysis of these epithelial linings can be helpful in determining where the animal is with regard to the estrous cycle. The *labia* (*la'be-ah*) of the *vulva* (*vul'vah*) provide some protection for the vaginal opening and tissue.

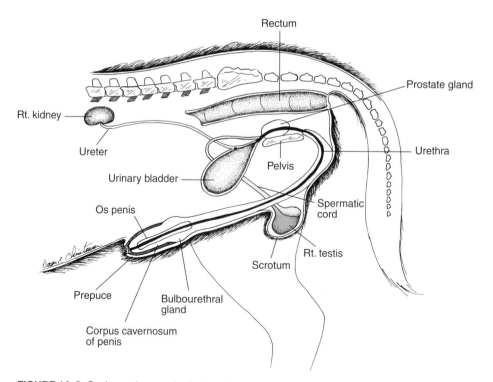

FIGURE 14–3. Canine male reproductive tract.

---

[3]Ovulation (*o"vu-la'shun*); the release of an oocyte from the ovary.

[4]Infundibulum (*in"fun-dib'u-lum*); from [L. *infundibula,* funnel]; the infundibulum of the uterine horn is a funnel-shaped structure designed to "catch" the oocyte on ovulation.

14.2.2. MALE REPRODUCTIVE ANATOMY

The *testes* of mature male animals are suspended by the *spermatic cord* in the *scrotum*[5] (Fig. 14–3). The spermatic cord and testes are covered by a fibrous connective tissue sheath. Within the sheath of the spermatic cord are the *vas deferens*[6] and the testicular artery and vein. The spermatic cord passes through the inguinal rings into the abdominal cavity. The vas deferens ultimately terminate at the proximal urethra, near the prostate gland. The *prostate (pros'tāt) gland* encircles the neck of the bladder, and is a reproductive structure responsible for contributing a transparent fluid to semen. The *urethra* in males serves a dual purpose: (1) as a passage for urine from the bladder during urination, and (2) as a passage for semen during *copulation*.[7] The urethra is centrally located in the *penis*. Among domestic animals, the male dog is unique in that he has a bony structure called the *os penis*, through which the urethra passes. In most male animals, the penis is composed of highly vascular, sponge-like tissue called the *corpus cavernosum (kor-pus' kav"er-no'sum)*. During copulation, the penile tissue becomes engorged with blood, creating a somewhat rigid structure. The *bulbus glandis*, located at the proximal end of the penis, is of particular importance in male dogs. During copulation, the bulbus glandis enlarges tremendously and is responsible for the "tie."[8] The penis itself is covered by a moist mucous membrane and protected by the *prepuce (pre'pūs)*. The male cat is unique in that his penis is not positioned along the ventral midline of the abdomen. The penis of the male cat is directed caudally (Fig. 14–4 on p. 252). In addition, it is covered with numerous barb-like projections.

The testes originate in the abdominal cavity. As the male animal matures, the testes progressively migrate caudally. Ultimately, they should pass through the inguinal rings into the scrotal sac. Some males, however, may retain one or both testes in the abdominal cavity. Clinically, these occurrences are referred to as *monorchidism* and *cryptorchidism*, respectively.

14.2.3. SPERMATOGENESIS

The testes are structured for continuous production of sperm (Fig. 14–5 on p. 253). Spermatogenic cells throughout the testes continually develop new sperm. As the sperm develop, they collect in the *seminiferous tubules*,[9] which are

---

[5]Scrotum (*skro'tum*); from [L. *scrotum*, bag]; the scrotum is a pouch of skin that contains the testes.

[6]Vas deferens (*vas def'er-enz*); from [L. *vas*, vessel] and [L. *deferens*, different]; the vas deferens are vessels that transport sperm from the testes to the urethra.

[7]Copulation (*kop"u-la'shun*); sexual union between a male and a female animal.

[8]The "tie" is the period of copulation between a male and female dog during which the two animals are physically locked together. The male cannot completely dismount until the bulbourethral gland reduces in size.

[9]Seminiferous tubules (*se"mĭ-nif'er-us, sĕ"mi-nif'er-us*); from [L. *semen*, seed + *ferre*, to bear + *-ous*, pertaining to]; the seminiferous tubules are tiny channels throughout the testes in which spermatozoa develop and through which they leave the glandular tissue.

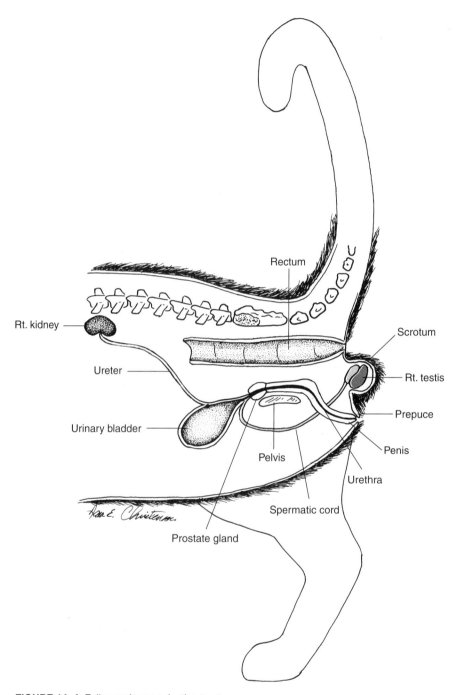

FIGURE 14–4. Feline male reproductive tract.

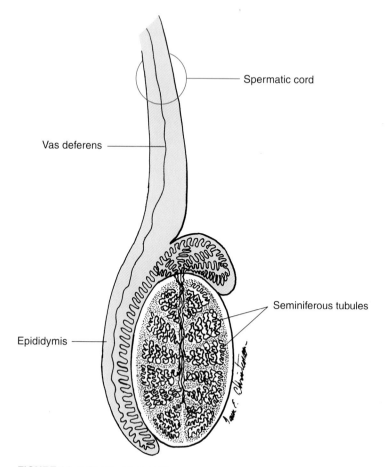

FIGURE 14–5. Testis cross-section.

coiled throughout the testes. Eventually, they pass into the vas deferens of the *epididymis*[10] for a period of maturation. Ultimately, mature sperm cells make their way through the vas deferens of the spermatic cord and through the urethra for insemination of the female.

Spermatozoa contain only half of the genetic information required to create a new animal of that species. Their basic structure facilitates active mobility (Fig. 14–6). Each sperm has a *head* that is partially covered by a small cap called the *acrosome* (ak'ro-sōm). The head is the actual nucleus of the sperm cell, containing the chromosomes. The acrosome contains lysosomal enzymes to facilitate penetration and fertilization of the oocyte. Only one sperm cell is permitted entry into

---

[10]Epididymis (ep"ĭ-did'ĭ-mis); from *epi-*, upon + [Gr. *didymos*, testis].

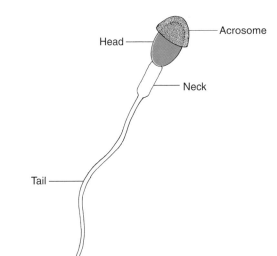

FIGURE 14–6. Spermatozoon.

any one oocyte. Adjacent to the head is the *neck* or body, which contains numerous mitochondria. The *tail* of the sperm cell is a long, slender structure that contains a temporary energy store for the cell. This energy is required for the whipping movement of the tail that propels the sperm. On fertilization of the ovum, the sperm cell loses its neck and tail.

14.2.4. ESTROUS CYCLE

Female domestic animals differ widely with regard to the length and frequency of their estrous cycles. Some are *monestrous* whereas others are *polyestrous.* Regardless of the frequency or length of the *estrous cycle,* each animal progresses through the same stages of *estrus. Proestrus* is the stage in which the female animal prepares for conception. Ovarian follicles form with ready oocytes and the uterine wall begins to engorge with blood in preparation for embryonic/fetal development. *Estrus* is that stage of the cycle in which the female is receptive to the male and can conceive. *Metestrus* is the period following estrus. If conception has not taken place, the ovarian follicles regress and the uterine wall returns to a more normal state. *Anestrus* is the period of sexual quiescence in the female. Behavioral changes during each of these stages of the estrous cycle are variable among each of the domestic species. The single most consistent behavior exhibited by domestic animals in estrus is acceptance of the male. Estrus is the only time during which the female accepts the advances of a male and is able to conceive.

14.2.5. CONCEPTION AND GESTATION

On copulation of a female in estrus, millions of sperm "swim" through the female's reproductive tract in search of oocytes. (Many female domestic animals release multiple oocytes with each estrous cycle. This facilitates the production of multiple offspring from a single breeding. Dogs and cats are most inclined to produce "litters" of young. Sheep frequently produce twins. Horses and cattle usually produce single offspring.) Each oocyte encountered along the reproductive tract is surrounded by sperm. Each sperm begins to attempt penetration of the oocyte by using proteolytic enzymes found in the acrosome. Vigorous tail lashing propels the sperm. Only one sperm is permitted entry. As soon as one sperm penetrates the ovum, the cell wall of the ovum becomes impermeable to any other sperm. The combined DNA of the sperm cell and the oocyte provide complete information for the creation of a new being. The fertilized *ovum* undergoes mitosis and implants in the uterine wall. The *placenta* develops, providing a highly vascular, stable attachment for the developing embryo. Hormones produced by the ovarian follicle and the placenta maintain the pregnancy. All blood and nutrients pass from the mother through the placenta to the developing embryo/fetus, whereas all wastes from the offspring are transported back to the mother for elimination. Because of this shared arrangement, it is important to avoid administration of potentially *teratogenic* agents to the mother during the pregnancy. Even the administration of some immunizations during gestation could have teratogenic effects. Before anything is given to a pregnant female, a veterinarian should be consulted.

The gestation period varies from species to species. Refer to Table 14–1 for average gestation periods for each of the domestic species.

TABLE 14–1. Average Gestation Periods

SPECIES	GESTATION PERIOD (DAYS)	AVERAGE NO. OF YOUNG
Bovine	280–290	1
Canine	60–65	8–10
Equine	330–340	1
Feline	60–65	8–10
Ovine	140–150	1–2

14.2.6. PARTURITION

Parturition is the actual birthing process. Hormonal changes signal the onset of parturition. Most domestic animals exhibit behavioral changes before the onset of actual labor. Most females appear anxious and restless, and engage in "nesting" behaviors. Once the cervix has sufficiently dilated and uterine contractions intensify, the fetus is forced from the uterine horn through the uterine body and into the birth canal (vagina). Continued contractions force the fetus from the body of the female. The most common presentation of young is with the fetus positioned in sternal recumbency with the forefeet and head caudal in the mother. Malpositioning of the fetus or excessively large fetuses often result in *dystocia*. As soon as the neonate is born, the mother begins to remove the fetal membranes from it. She severs the *umbilical cord*, usually by chewing through it. Shortly after giving birth to the *neonate*, placental attachments break down, and uterine contractions expel the placenta. This is often referred to as the "afterbirth." Many female animals consume the afterbirth. This is a protective mechanism, so that predators are not attracted to her and her young. In animals who produce multiple offspring, it is important to account for a placenta for each neonate. A retained placenta could result in *postparturient* complications, such as *metritis*.

14.2.7. LACTATION

Hormones usually stimulate *lactation* a number of hours or even days before parturition. The mammary glands become laden with milk and may even leak small amounts from the teats/nipples before parturition. The first milk produced by the female is called *colostrum* (ko-los'trum). It contains large quantities of maternal antibodies, that provide the neonate(s) with temporary immunity. It is extremely important for neonates to suckle as soon as possible postpartum. The colostrum is contained only in the first milk produced, and the neonates can readily absorb the antibodies only during the first hours of life. In most domestic animals, absorption of colostral antibodies drops significantly after 12 hours postpartum. Milk produced after the initial colostrum is much richer in milk fats, providing a better energy source for the young. The female continues to lactate, provided she is stimulated through natural suckling or mechanical milking. In those species that tend to produce multiple offspring, each neonate tends to select a specific teat from which it will nurse. Subsequent feedings are likely to be from the same teat as the first. The time of weaning varies from species to species and female to female. On the average, however, most young are weaned between three to six weeks of age. If *mastitis* develops, the young must be weaned earlier or bottle fed with a milk replacer until an appropriate weaning time can be achieved. Of course, dairy calves are fed milk replacers in lieu of milk from the cow, so that the milk can be marketed. Careful milking practices and husbandry of dairy cattle is important to prevent mastitis. Mastitis in dairy cattle can have a profound economic impact on the dairy operation and the industry.

14.2.8. PSEUDOCYESIS

Pseudocyesis occurs most commonly in dogs. Hormonal and physical changes in the female's body follow with a typical gestation period. She may develop mammary enlargement and may even lactate briefly. Psychologically, the female is inclined to behave with maternal instincts. In the absence of offspring, she may nurture stuffed toys or other such objects. The incidence of metritis and *pyometra* is much greater in cases of pseudocyesis, and these animals therefore should be watched closely for signs of disease.

14.2.9. POPULATION CONTROL

Overpopulation of dogs and cats in the United States is a serious problem. Millions of unwanted dogs and cats are put to death every year by animal control agencies and humane societies. This ugly circumstance could be avoided if people would exercise responsible pet ownership by having their pets spayed or neutered. The idea that every female should have one litter before she is spayed is a myth. In actuality, the earlier a female is spayed the less likely she is to develop mammary cancer. Even older females can have their risk of mammary cancer reduced through an *ovariohysterectomy.* The optimal time to perform an ovariohysterectomy for prevention of mammary cancer and birth control is before the female's first estrous cycle (i.e., between 4 to 10 months, depending on the breed of dog or cat). *Orchiectomy* of a male reduces his inclination to roam and reduces some tendencies toward aggression. Annoying behaviors such as "mounting" inanimate objects or people are curbed. Prostate disorders are also significantly reduced by orchiectomy. It is recommended that males be neutered before 6 months of age. The myth that spaying or neutering pets causes them to gain weight has no basis; overfeeding and lack of exercise result in overweight pets.

14.3. Self-Test

Using the previous information in this chapter, respond to each of the following questions using the most appropriate medical term(s).

1. The inflammation of mammary tissue is medically termed

    _____ .

2. A(n) _____ is a newborn animal.

3. _____ is a specialized process of cellular division of sexual cells, in which only half of the original chromosomes of the parent cell are found in the daughter cells.

4. Any type of agent that can alter the DNA of sexual cells, resulting in genetic defects in off-spring, is called a(n) _____ agent.

5. _____ is the process of difficult birth.

6. The _____ is a strong muscular sphincter that separates the uterus from the vagina.

7. Animals who experience numerous estrous cycles during a sexual season are termed _____.

8. The _____ gland, which surrounds the neck of the urinary bladder in the male, is responsible for secreting a fluid component found in semen.

9. A(n) _____ is a surgical procedure in which the ovaries and uterus are removed from the female. It is commonly referred to as a spay operation.

10. The production of sperm is medically termed _____.

11. A male animal in which neither of the testes descends into the scrotal sac is referred to as a(n) _____.

12. The period in which a female animal is in sexual quiescence is termed _____.

13. A condition in which pus accumulates in the uterus is medically termed a(n) _____.

14. _____ is literally a false pregnancy.

15. A(n) _____ or castration is a surgical operation in which the testes are removed from the male.

16. A(n) _____ agent is anything that alters fetal development in utero, resulting in birth defects.

17. The period of female receptivity, during which a female animal accepts the advances of a male to permit breeding, is termed _____.

18. The _____ period is the period of time after the birth of young.

19. A male animal in which only one testis descends into the scrotal sac is referred to as a(n)

_____.

20. A(n) _____ female is any female animal who experiences only one estrous cycle during a sexual season.

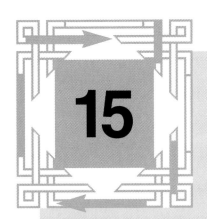

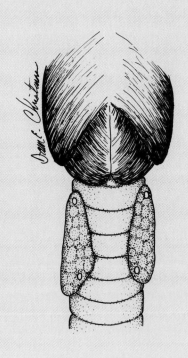

The Endocrine System*

GOALS AND OBJECTIVES

By the conclusion of this chapter, the student will be able to:

1. Recognize common root words, prefixes, and suffixes related to the endocrine system.
2. Divide simple and compound words into their respective parts.
3. Recognize, correctly pronounce, and appropriately use common medical terms related to the endocrine system.
4. Demonstrate an understanding of endocrine anatomy.
5. Demonstrate an understanding of endocrine physiology with regard to hormones and negative feedback.
6. Demonstrate an understanding of endocrine physiology with regard to principal functions and effects of each of the major endocrine organs.

---

*Author's note: It is advisable that this chapter be attempted only after Chapters 1 through 14 have been successfully completed. Assumptions of anatomic and physiologic knowledge of previous body systems are made throughout this chapter.

15.1. Introduction to Related Terms

Divide each of the following terms into its respective parts ("R" root, "P" prefix, "S" suffix, "CV" combining vowel).

1. Adrenal   (P) _____ (R) _____ (S) _____

adrenal (ah-dre'nal; pertaining to near the kidney; clinically refers to the adrenal glands, which are located close to the kidneys)

2. Adrenergic   (R) _____ (R) _____ (S) _____

adrenergic (ad"ren-er'jik; pertaining to adrenal working; clinically refers to activity stimulated by adrenaline [epinephrine])

3. Adrenocorticotropic
(R) _____ (CV) ___ (R) _____ (CV) ___ (R) _____ (S) _____

adrenocorticotropic (ad-re"no-kor"tĭ-ko-tro'pik; pertaining to adrenal cortex stimulating/influencing; cf. adrenocorticotrophic)

4. Adenohypophysis
(R) _____(CV) ___ (P) _____ (CV) ___ (S) _____

adenohypophysis (ad"ĕ-no-hi-pof'ĭ-sis; growth of a gland below; clinically refers to the glandular, anterior portion of the pituitary gland)

5. Neurohypophysis
(R) _____(CV) ___ (P) _____ (CV) ___ (S) _____

neurohypophysis (nu"ro-hi-pof'ĭ-sis; growth of nerves below; clinically refers to the neural, posterior portion of the pituitary gland)

6. Parathyroid   (P) _____ (R) _____

parathyroid (par"ah-thi'roid; beside the thyroid)

7. Hypothyroidism   (P) _____ (CV) ___ (R) _____ (S) _____

hypothyroidism (hi"po-thi'roid-izm; a state of low thyroid; clinically refers to below-normal levels of hormones produced by the thyroid gland)

8. Antidiuretic   (P) _____ (R) _____ (S) _____

antidiuretic (an"tĭ-di"u-ret'ik; pertaining to being against urination)

9. Hypoglycemia
(P) _____ (CV) ___ (R) _____(R) _____ (S) _____

hypoglycemia (hi"po-gli-se'me-ah; a state of low glucose in the blood)

10. Hyperglycemia   (P) _____ (R) _____(R) _____ (S) _____

hyperglycemia (hi"per-gli-se'me-ah; a state of excessive glucose in the blood)

11. **Gluconeogenesis**

(R) _____   (CV) ___   (R) _____ (R) _____   (CV) ___   (S) _____

gluconeogenesis (gloo"ko-ne"o-jen'ĕ-sis; the process of new glucose production; physiologically it is the production of glucose from noncarbohydrate molecules; cf. glyconeogenesis)

15.2. Endocrine Anatomy and Physiology

The endocrine system is composed of numerous glands and other tissues that produce *hormones*. Hormones are chemicals that stimulate reactions in various organs and tissues of the body. Most hormones are organ specific or tissue specific. The endocrine system is a silent partner among all of the body systems, and plays a large role in the maintenance of homeostasis. Unlike all the other body systems, we cannot physically see the endocrine organs working. Evaluation of the endocrine system must be made through observing the activity of other body tissues and organs in response to secretion of the various hormones. Because endocrine organs are highly vascular and use the blood to transport their secretions throughout the body, hormones can be measured in the laboratory using special hematologic testing procedures.

15.2.1. ENDOCRINE ORGANS

15.2.1.1. Pituitary Gland (Hypophysis)

The *hypophysis* is located on the ventral midline of the cerebral hemispheres and midbrain (Fig. 15–1). A small depression in the floor of the cranial vault cradles the pituitary gland. The gland itself is subdivided into two distinct lobes: the *anterior pituitary* or the *adenohypophysis,* and the *posterior pituitary* or the *neurohypophysis.* The pituitary gland may appear to be a small, insignificant structure, but it exerts tremendous control over most of the body. It produces approximately eight different hormones, only some of which are discussed here. *Antidiuretic hormone* (ADH) is produced by the neurohypophysis and targets the renal tubules for control of water retention or loss by the kidney. In the presence of ADH, the renal tubules become more permeable to water, allowing for reabsorption of water for the body. The resultant effect of ADH is reduced urine output. The adenohypophysis produces *growth hormone* (GH). As its name implies, GH regulates growth of the body. Even in the adult animal, GH is necessary for such things as facilitation of wound repair. At the cellular level, GH controls ribosomal protein synthesis, transcription of DNA into RNA by the nucleoli, and mobilization of cellular energy stores. Consequently, mitotic activity could not take place without

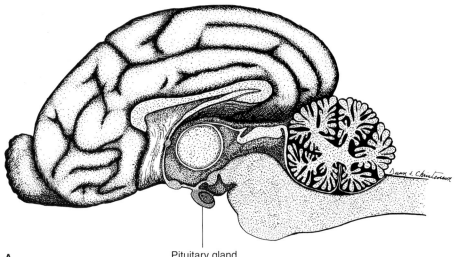

A

Pituitary gland

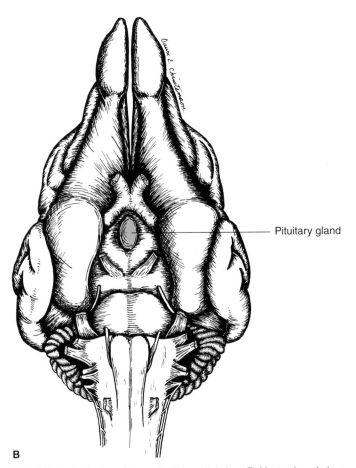

B

FIGURE 15–1. Pituitary Gland. **A**, Midsagittal view; **B**, Ventrodorsal view.

GH. *Thyroid-stimulating hormone* (TSH), produced by the adenohypophysis, stimulates the thyroid gland to produce its hormones.

15.2.1.2. Thyroid Gland

The *thyroid gland* is located on the ventrolateral aspect of the trachea, slightly caudal to the larynx (Fig. 15–2). In most of the domestic animals, the thyroid is found as two lateral lobes of glandular tissue that, depending on the species, may or may not be connected by an isthmus. Activity of the thyroid gland is stimulated by the adenohypophysis. As a result of stimulation, one of the hormones produced by the thyroid gland is *thyroxine* (thi-rok′sin; T₄). Thyroxine controls the body's metabolic rate. In the presence of thyroxine, cellular activity and, consequently, metabolism increase. In cases of *hypothyroidism*, the thyroid gland fails to respond adequately to TSH. *Calcitonin* (kal″sĭ-to′nin), also produced by the thyroid gland, helps control concentrations of calcium and phosphorus ions. In the presence of calcitonin, blood levels of calcium and phosphorus are lowered. This is accomplished by stimulating increased deposition of these ions in bone, as well as increased excretion of calcium and phosphorus by the kidney.

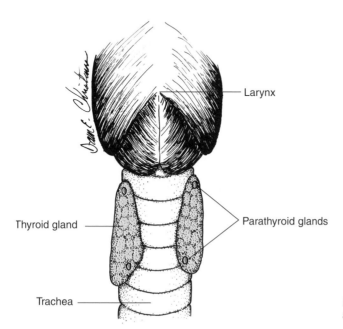

Larynx

Thyroid gland

Parathyroid glands

Trachea

FIGURE 15–2. Canine thyroid and parathyroid glands.

15.2.1.3. Parathyroid Glands

The *parathyroid glands* are found in pairs on the surface of each of the lobes of the thyroid gland (see Fig. 15–2). The four parathyroid glands are small in comparison to the thyroid. *Parathyroid hormone* (PTH, also called *parathormone*) is produced by the parathyroid glands. It is responsible for increasing blood calcium concentrations and decreasing blood phosphorus concentrations. PTH targets various organs to affect blood concentrations of these ions. It regulates the absorption of calcium from the digestive tract, the excretion of phosphorus and the absorption of calcium by the kidneys, and the release of calcium from bone.

15.2.1.4. Adrenal Glands

The *adrenal glands* were so named because they lie near to the kidneys (Fig. 15–3). These two small glands are structured similarly to the kidneys, in that they have an adrenal cortex and an adrenal medulla. Each of these areas secretes different hormones. The adrenal medulla secretes *epinephrine* (*ep"ĭ-nef'rin*; adrenaline) and *norepinephrine*. Both of these hormones are sympathomimetic in their effects. Epinephrine is constantly secreted. During times of need (i.e., epinephrine stress response, "fight or flight"), the adrenal medulla increases its rate of secretion. When the crisis is over, secretion of epinephrine returns to normal levels. The *adrenergic* or sympathomimetic effects of epinephrine include increased cardiac output, bronchodilation, peripheral vasoconstriction, and vasodilation in vital organs and muscles. It is by virtue of epinephrine that people and animals are sometimes capable of extraordinary feats of strength in crisis situations.

On stimulation of the adrenal cortex by *adrenocorticotropic hormone* (ACTH) from the adenohypophysis, cortisol[1] is secreted. Probably the most familiar and popular effect of cortisol is its anti-inflammatory activity. In the presence of chronic disease or stress, secretion of cortisol is stimulated. This *glucocorticosteroid stress response*[2] is a protective mechanism intended to promote rapid mobilization of amino acids and fatty acids from energy stores in the body, and to stimulate *gluconeogenesis* by the liver. In so doing, blood glucose levels are maintained in a normal range between meals and during times of anorexia. Hydrocortisone also inhibits the permeability of vessels to macrophages and other blood constituents,

---

[1]Cortisol (*kor'tĭ-sol*); a corticosteroid produced by the adrenal cortex; also called hydrocortisone.

[2]Glucocorticosteroid stress response (*glu"ko-kor"tĭ-ko-ster'oid*); a process in which cortisol is secreted in large amounts to reduce inflammation and provide energy, in the form of glucose, for the body. This response is usually associated with chronic disease or injury.

providing anti-inflammatory action. However, with neutrophils and monocytes unable to escape from the bloodstream into the tissues, tissue defense against pathogenic microorganisms is impaired. Animals suffering from chronic disease/stress or who are medicated with systemic corticosteroids are more susceptible to infectious diseases.

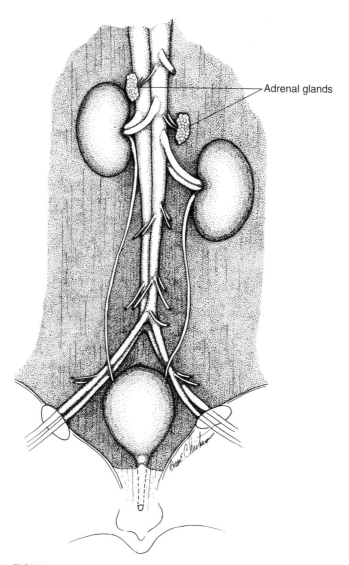

Adrenal glands

FIGURE 15–3. Adrenal glands.

15.2.1.5. Pancreas

The exocrine activity of the pancreas is discussed in Chapter 12. The endocrine function of the pancreas is critical to the maintenance of homeostasis with regard to glucose. *Insulin* (*in'su-lin*) is a pancreatic hormone responsible for lowering blood glucose concentrations. In the presence of insulin, active transport of glucose into cells is promoted. By facilitating active transport and utilization or storage of glucose, blood glucose concentrations are lowered. In opposition to the effect of insulin, the pancreatic hormone *glucagon* (*gloo'kah-gon*) increases blood glucose concentrations. Glucagon stimulates the liver to convert glycogen into glucose and to undergo *gluconeogenesis*. In so doing, glucagon facilitates increased blood glucose levels.

15.2.1.6. Ovaries and Testes

Numerous ovarian hormones are produced in the female. Secretion of most ovarian hormones is ultimately controlled by the pituitary gland. *Estrogen* (*es'tro-jen*) is the ovarian hormone responsible for the development of feminine characteristics. *Progesterone*,[3] on the other hand, is produced largely by follicles associated with ovulation. Such follicles remain and continue to secrete progesterone throughout gestation, to maintain the pregnancy. The most abundant male hormone secreted by the testes is *testosterone* (*tes-tos'tě-rōn*). It is responsible for the development of masculine characteristics seen in animals and humans.

The preceding information covers only a small portion of the many hormones produced in the body. Hormones are not secreted exclusively by the glands and organs outlined earlier. Numerous other hormones are secreted by many different tissues. For example, gastric and enteric cells secrete the hormone *gastrin*, which in turn stimulates production of various digestive juices. The kidney secretes *erythropoietin*, which stimulates the bone marrow to produce erythrocytes. It is through the carefully regulated, harmonious secretion of the body's many hormones that homeostasis is maintained.

15.2.2. NEGATIVE FEEDBACK SYSTEM

The negative feedback system is simply a mechanism through which hormonal secretions are controlled. It is a delicate system of checks and balances that pre-

---

[3]Progesterone (*pro-jes'tě-rōn*); a hormone produced by the corpus luteum of the ovary, as well as the adrenal cortex and the placenta

vents oversecretion of hormones. Without such a system, body tissues and organs would become exhausted and eventually fail. The principle behind negative feedback is quite simple. An endocrine organ secretes a hormone. That hormone causes a specific tissue to perform a function. When the function is carried out sufficient to the body's needs, a message such as, "Whoa! Stop! I can't take it anymore!!" is sent back to the endocrine organ to stop secreting the hormone.

To clarify this further, it is helpful to review Antidiuretic Hormone (ADH) production by the neurohypophysis. The body, through various sensory receptors, senses when tissues are becoming dehydrated. To prevent further dehydration, the neurohypophysis begins to secrete ADH. ADH travels to the renal tubules, causing them to become permeable to water. The tubules continue to reabsorb water as long as ADH is present. The resultant urine is very concentrated and produced in small volume. When the body senses that the tissues are adequately hydrated, the neurohypophysis is told to "stop!" secreting ADH. Through this continuous "give-and-take" mechanism, water homeostasis is maintained. In cases of *diabetes insipidus* (di"ah-be'tēz in-sip'ĭ-dus), the neurohypophysis fails to secrete enough ADH. As a result, excessive water is lost from the body because the renal tubules cannot reabsorb water in the absence of ADH.

The pancreatic hormone, insulin, provides another example of negative feedback at work. In a normal animal, insulin is secreted by the pancreas in response to elevated blood glucose levels. As the insulin is secreted, blood glucose concentrations are lowered to a normal, acceptable range. As normal blood glucose concentrations are achieved, the pancreas is told to stop secreting insulin. If, however, blood glucose concentrations continue to fall into a *hypoglycemic* state, the pancreas is stimulated to secrete glucagon. Glucagon stimulates the conversion of glycogen to glucose, and, if needed, initiates gluconeogenesis in the liver. As a result, blood glucose concentrations are raised and again maintained in a normal, acceptable range. Failure to maintain appropriate blood glucose concentrations results in severe pathology. Both *hyperglycemia* and hypoglycemia can result in encephalopathies. In patients with diabetes mellitus, insufficient insulin is produced. Without sufficient insulin, the patient becomes hyperglycemic. As the renal threshold is reached, some of the excess glucose spills over into the urine, resulting in *glycosuria*. If blood glucose concentrations continue to rise, the patient may fall into a coma and eventually die. Patients afflicted with *diabetes mellitus* (di"ah-be'tēz mel'ĭ-tus) must be maintained on a strict regimen, including insulin administration and dietary management. Administration of insulin to diabetic patients must be carefully coordinated with meals so that the patient does not become hypoglycemic and succumb to insulin shock. Although hormones like insulin can be administered to patients, nothing can truly replace the natural regulatory mechanisms of the negative feedback system.

15.3. Self-Test

Using the previous information in this chapter, respond to each of the following questions using the most appropriate medical term(s). Do not use abbreviations.

1. The ___parathyroid___ gland secretes parathyroid hormone.

2. ___ADH___ hormone is produced by the posterior pituitary gland and targets the renal tubules to promote reabsorption of water.

3. The ___adrenal___ glands are located close to the kidneys and produce hormones, some of which stimulate sympathomimetic activity.

4. Growth hormone is produced by the ___adenohypophysis___ or the anterior pituitary gland.

5. ___hyperglycemia___ or high blood glucose levels occur in patients with diabetes mellitus due to insufficient secretion of insulin.

6. The ___thyroid___ gland is located on the ventrolateral trachea, caudal to the larynx.

7. The ___pituitary___ gland is located on the ventral midline of the cerebral hemispheres and midbrain and is responsible for regulating many other endocrine glands of the body.

8. _____ hormone, produced by the adenohypophysis, stimulates the adrenal cortex to secrete cortisol.

9. The posterior pituitary gland is also called the _____.

10. _____ is a condition in which the thyroid gland produces insufficient amounts of its hormones.

11. Insulin is a hormone secreted by the ___pancreas___ and is responsible for lowering blood glucose levels.

12. ___thyroxine___ is a hormone secreted by the thyroid gland that is largely responsible for controlling the metabolic rate of the body.

13. ___calciton___ is another hormone secreted by the thyroid gland that is in part responsible for controlling blood calcium and phosphorus concentrations.

14. _____ is a pancreatic hormone that increases blood glucose concentrations.

15. A state in which a patient suffers from below-normal blood glucose concentrations is medically termed _____.

16

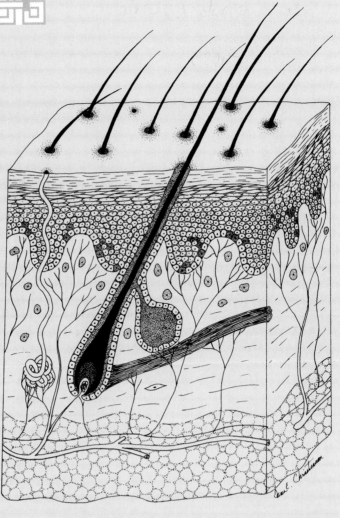

The Integumentary System

GOALS AND OBJECTIVES

By the conclusion of this chapter, the student will be able to:

1. Recognize common root words, prefixes, and suffixes related to the integumentary system.
2. Divide simple and compound words into their respective parts.
3. Recognize, correctly pronounce, and appropriately use common medical terms related to the integumentary system.
4. Demonstrate an understanding of integumentary anatomy.
5. Demonstrate a basic understanding of integumentary physiology and pathophysiology with regard to functions including hair growth, wound healing, and allergic dermatitis.

16.1. Introduction to Related Terms

Divide each of the following terms into its respective parts ("R" root, "P" prefix, "S" suffix, "CV" combining vowel).

1. **Dermatitis**   (R) _dermal_ (S) _itis_

   dermatitis (der"mah-ti'tis; inflammation of the skin)

2. **Epidermal**   (P) _epi_   (R) _derm_ (S) _al_

   epidermal (ep"ĭ-der'mal; pertaining to upon the dermis)

3. **Intradermal**   (P) _intra_ (R) _derm_ (S) _al_

   intradermal (in"trah-der'mal; pertaining to within the dermis)

4. **Subcutis**   (P) _sub_   (R) _cutis_

   subcutis (sub-ku'tis; beneath the skin)

5. **Erythematous**   (R) _erythema_(S) _ous_

   erythematous (er"ĭ-them'ah-tus; pertaining to erythema [Gr. erythema, flush upon the skin]; clinically, an erythematous lesion would appear reddened)

6. **Pruritus**   (R) _prurit_ (S) _us_

   pruritus (proo-ri'tus; the state of itching)

7. **Melanocyte**   (R) _melan_ (CV) _o_ (S) _cyte_

   melanocyte (mel'ah-no-sīt, me-lan'o-sīt; a black cell)

8. **Piloerection**   (R) _pil_   (CV) _o_ (R) _erection_

   piloerection (pi"lo-ĕ-rek'shun; hair erection)

9. **Fibroplasia**   (R) _fibr_   (CV) _o_ (R) _plas_ (S) _ia_

   fibroplasia (fi"bro-pla'se-ah; the process of fiber forming)

10. **Circumoral**   (P) _circum_ (R) _or_   (S) _al_

    circumoral (ser"kum-o'ral; pertaining to around the mouth)

11. **Interdigital**   (P) _inter_ (R) _digit_ (S) _al_

    interdigital (in"ter-dij'ĭ-tal; pertaining to between toes)

12. **Perianal**   (P) _peri_ (R) _an_ (S) _al_

    perianal (per"e-a'nal; pertaining to around the anus)

13. **Allergen**   (R) _allerg_ (R) _gen_

    allergen (al'er-jen; allergy producing)

14. **Carcinoma**   (R) _carcin_ (S) _cma_

carcinoma (kar"sĭ-no'mah; a cancerous tumor; clinically, carcinoma refers to a type of malignant growth that originates from epithelial cells)

16.2. Integumentary Anatomy and Physiology

The skin is the largest organ of the body. It serves many important functions, such as protecting underlying tissues and structures, that help maintain homeostasis. This protective covering prevents entry into the body by many harmful agents, including microorganisms and some chemicals. The skin also helps maintain water homeostasis by preventing dehydration of underlying tissues. The skin also plays an integral role in regulating body temperature. Through vasoconstriction, *piloerection*, vasodilation, and sweating, the skin can facilitate conservation or loss of body heat as needed. Tactile sensory perception is possible through sensory nerve endings found in the skin. Even vitamin D is synthesized by the skin. Each of the layers of the skin contributes to the overall function of the integument.

16.2.1. EPIDERMIS

The *epidermis* is the most superficial of the skin layers (Fig. 16–1 on p. 276). It is composed of stratified squamous epithelium. It is the keratinized cells of the epidermis, in conjunction with oily secretions from glands found in the dermis, that provide protection against entry of microorganisms and prevent absorption of some chemicals. Also found in the epidermis are *melanocytes*. The dark cytoplasmic granules of the melanocytes impart pigmentation to the skin. Such pigmentation provides protection of deeper tissues from the harmful effects of ultraviolet radiation. The melanic granules of the cells absorb light energy, rather than permitting it passage through the epidermis. Animals with little or no pigmentation are more susceptible to the harmful effects of ultraviolet light and are more likely to develop diseases such as squamous cell *carcinoma*.

16.2.2. DERMIS

The *dermis* is composed of fibroelastic connective tissue, making the skin a very tough yet elastic structure (see Fig. 16–1). The dermis is the thickest of the two skin layers, connected to the epidermis with finger-like projections called *papillae*.[1] These papillae interlock with the folds and ridges of the epidermis, forming a relatively strong bond between the two skin layers. Within the dermis are many other important structures, such as vessels and nerves. The nerves are

---

[1]Papillae (*pah-pil'e*); plural of papilla (*pah-pil'ah*); a small, nipple-shaped projection.

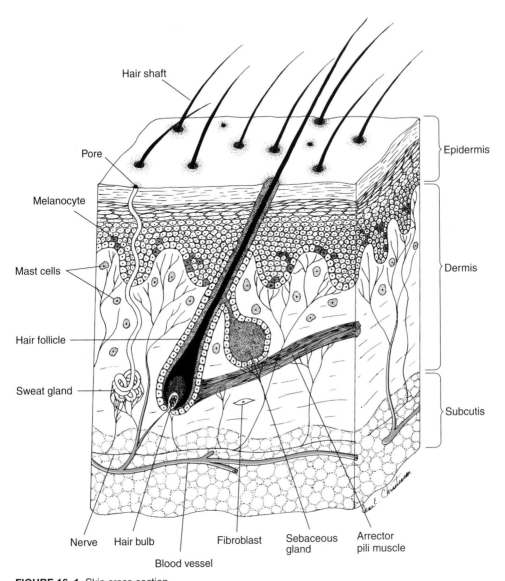

Hair shaft

Pore

Melanocyte

Mast cells

Hair follicle

Sweat gland

Epidermis

Dermis

Subcutis

Nerve   Hair bulb   Fibroblast   Sebaceous   Arrector
                                        gland   pili muscle

Blood vessel

FIGURE 16–1. Skin cross-section.

predominantly sensory, many of which terminate at the epidermal–dermal interface. The *intradermal* capillary network provides nourishment for the dermis and
the avascular epidermis; it also provides an efficient mechanism through which
body heat may be lost. Vasodilation of these intradermal capillaries facilitates the
loss of excess body heat and is clinically apparent as *erythema*. *Erythematous* lesions may also appear in areas of localized inflammation.

Allergic dermatitis is a frequent cause of erythema, pruritus, and urticaria[2] in companion animals. Domestic animals have large numbers of mast cells in the dermis. Mast cells are the facilitators of many allergic reactions. When presented with a recognizable allergen, a mast cell releases its histamine-containing granules. A cascade of events unfolds, resulting ultimately in inflammation.

16.2.3. SUBCUTIS

The subcutis is composed of adipose and loose connective tissues, loosely attaching the skin to underlying tissues and structures (see Fig. 16–1). The adipose tissue is important for providing insulation for the body. Because of the structural nature of the subcutaneous tissues, the subcutis is an excellent location for deposition of some medications. Vaccinations, medications, and fluids are frequently administered to domestic animals by subcutaneous injections.

16.2.4. ACCESSORY SKIN STRUCTURES

Numerous glands are found in the dermis. Sebaceous glands[3] produce sebum,[4] an oily substance that keeps the skin and fur relatively soft, pliable, and waterproof. Sebaceous glands are usually associated with hair follicles (see Fig. 16–1). Some sebaceous-type glands secrete scent markers called pheromones.[5] Pheromones are used by domestic animals for territorial marking and for attraction of mates. Circumoral glands in cats are used frequently to mark territory; that is why cats tend to rub their faces and chins on objects and people. Interdigital glands are often found in cloven-hoofed animals, such as sheep and goats. Interdigital glands provide an efficient means to mark trails as the animals walk along. Many horned animals, such as goats, also have pheromone-producing glands near the base of the horns. Hence, these animals are frequently observed head-butting and rubbing on objects. Perianal glands tend to mark territory when animals defecate. Dogs are frequently found greeting and identifying other dogs by sniffing in the region of the perianal glands. Sweat glands are found in abundance over the entire body of horses. In most other domestic animals, however, sweat glands are found in limited numbers. In dogs and cats, for instance, appreciable numbers of sweat glands are found only in the foot pads. With the exception of the horse, most domestic animals cannot use sweating as a means of reducing body temperature. Hence, these animals tend to succumb to intense heat more readily than do humans or horses. Note in Figure 16–1 that many sweat glands are not associated with hair follicles; rather, they secrete their products through pores in the skin.

---

[2]Urticaria (ur"tĭ-ka're-ah); from [L. urtica, "stinging nettle" + -ia] wheal formation on the skin; commonly referred to as "hives."

[3]Sebaceous (sĕ-ba'shus); from [L. sebaceus, pertaining to sebum].

[4]Sebum (se'bum); from [L. sebum, suet].

[5]Pheromone (fer'o-mōn); scent marker that elicits certain behaviors in others of the same species.

Toenails, hooves, and *horns* are all formed from specialized keratinized epithelial cells (Figs. 16–2 and 16–3). The growth regions for these structures are found at the proximal border. The growth area for the hoof is frequently referred to as the *coronet* or *coronary band.*[6] The specialized epithelial cells in the growth area produce new cells that rapidly keratinize. The keratinized layer of cells, making up the nail, hoof, or horn wall, is attached to the dermis with corrugated, laminar folds. The dermis found under the nail or hoof of animals is commonly referred to as the *"quick."*

Hair follicles originate in the dermis (see Fig. 16–1). They are lined with epithelium and traverse the epidermis to the surface of the skin. Each follicle has an *arrector pili muscle* (*ah-rek'tor pī'li*) associated with it. These muscles are responsible for piloerection, used to conserve body heat by creating a dead space of air next to the body. The *hair bulb,* which gives rise to the *hair shaft,* is found at the base of the follicle. Just as nails and hooves developed from specialized epithelial cells, so do hairs. During hair growth periods, the hair bulb is large and has a vigorous blood supply (Fig. 16–4). As the hair shaft grows in length, the hair follicle begins to extend deeper into the dermis. On entering the resting phase of hair growth, the hair bulb regresses. Eventually, the hair follicle shrinks in length, forcing the now poorly attached hair shaft out. This normal cycle of hair growth and loss occurs on a seasonal basis. It is truly seasonal, because hair growth and loss are closely correlated with the amount of daylight. That is why most domestic animals, even if housed indoors, begin to shed heavily during late winter and begin to acquire thicker, more luxurious coats during the fall. *Alopecia*[7] may be

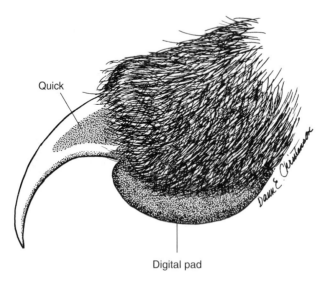

Quick

Digital pad

FIGURE 16–2. Feline claw.

[6]Coronary (*kor'o-na-re*); from [L. *corona,* pertaining to encircling].

[7]Alopecia (*al"o-pe'she-ah*); from [Gr. *alopekia,* a disease in which the hair falls out].

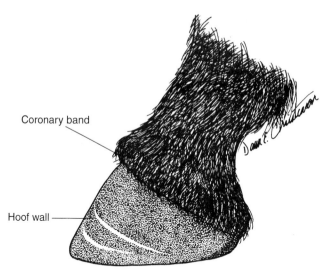

Coronary band

Hoof wall

FIGURE 16–3. Equine hoof.

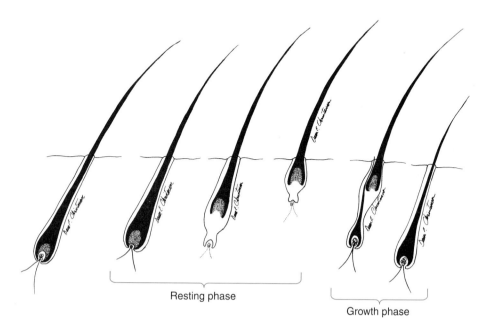

Resting phase

Growth phase

FIGURE 16–4. Hair growth.

observed resulting from primary dermatologic diseases or from systemic diseases. Some endocrine disorders, for example, commonly result in alopecia as well as other dermatologic symptoms.

16.2.5. WOUND HEALING

Wound healing is divided into four distinct stages: the inflammatory stage, the debridement stage, the repair stage, and the maturation stage. For the purpose of simplifying the healing process, a simple laceration is used to demonstrate each of the stages (Fig. 16–5 A–E).

Immediately after a skin laceration, the *inflammatory stage* of the healing process ensues. There is hemorrhage from all of the intradermal and subcutaneous vessels. Bleeding is important to help cleanse the wound and provide ready access to macrophages. Inflammation quickly ensues, characterized by pain, edema, erythema, heat, and some loss of function of the body part. Severed vessels vasoconstrict to minimize blood loss. Clotting factors and platelets aggregate and form a thrombus in the wound. This thrombus provides a weak matrix to hold the wound edges together for approximately the first four

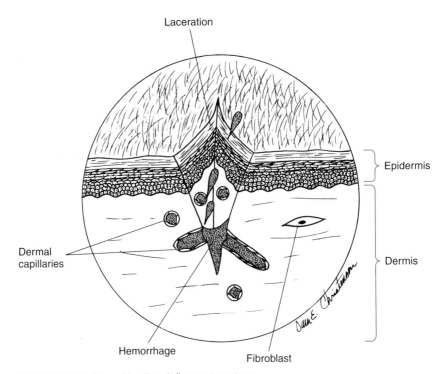

FIGURE 16–5A. Wound healing: Inflammatory stage.

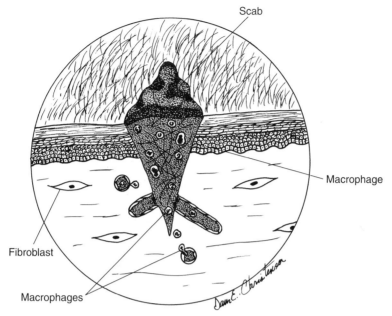

FIGURE 16–5B. Wound healing: Debridement stage.

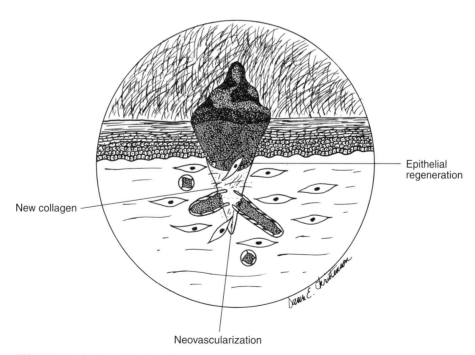

FIGURE 16–5C. Wound healing: Repair stage.

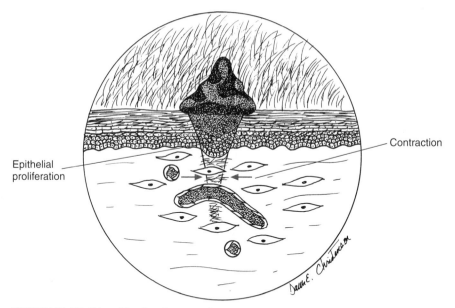

FIGURE 16–5D. Wound healing: Late repair stage.

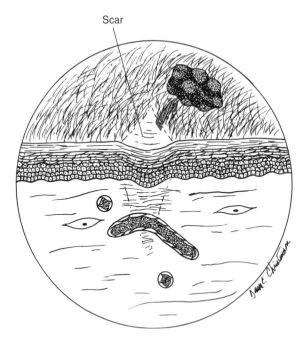

FIGURE 16–5E. Wound healing: Maturation stage.

days. Desiccation (drying) of the surface of the thrombus (i.e., "scab") prevents entry into the wound of additional microorganisms and debris.

During the *debridement stage* of wound healing, multitudes of macrophages infiltrate the wound. They debride the wound by phagocytizing microorganisms and cellular debris. At the height of the debridement stage, a *purulent exudate*[8] may be seen suppurating from the wound. In addition to and equally important to the actual debridement of the wound, is the stimulation of fibroblastic activity. Macrophages in the wound and other sentinels of inflammation stimulate the migration of fibroblasts to the wound site.

During the *repair stage,* two concurrent events take place: *fibroplasia* and *epithelial regeneration.* Although these events are discussed separately, it is important to note that they occur concurrently. Fibroplasia is the means by which the dermis is repaired. Fibroblasts that have been called to the wound begin to deposit collagen (the basic component of connective tissue). In the normal wound, fibroplasia is heavily underway and providing reasonable wound strength after day 5. Remodeling of the collagen results in wound contraction, drawing the edges of the wound closer together. Collagen continues to be deposited and remodeled, peaking in one to two weeks (hence the standard suture removal time of 7 to 10 days). By the third week postwounding, the numbers of fibroblasts present in the area and the amount of new collagen being deposited have significantly diminished.

On top of the fibroplastic healing of the dermis, epithelial regeneration is occurring in the epidermis. Cells in the basal cell layer undergo mitosis. Progressively, the newly formed epithelial cells migrate from the wound edges to the center of the wound. On covering the wound breadth, the epithelial cells proliferate to fill the epidermal void. Pruritus is frequently evident once the epithelial cells have covered the surface of the dermis. The sensory nerve endings associated with pruritus can function only if the epidermis is intact. As the epithelial cells proliferate in the wound, they progressively dissolve any attachments of the thrombus. It is at this stage that most "scabs" fall off. Premature removal of a scab frequently destroys portions of the epithelial cells that are regenerating.

During the *maturation stage* of wound healing, collagen fibers continue to be remodeled and contract. Average maturation of scar tissue may last for several weeks or nearly 1 year beyond the repair stage. The final scar tissue is nearly as strong as the surrounding normal tissue. Elasticity of the scar never equals that of normal skin.

16.2.6. ALLERGIC DERMATITIS

Mast cells in domestic animals are found predominantly throughout the dermis. Other tissues of domestic animals that have relatively high numbers of mast cells are in the digestive tract and the pulmonary airways. Regardless of location or

---

[8]Purulent exudate (*pu'roo-lent eks'u-dāt*); a purulent exudate contains pus; exudates are fluids that in general contain a high proportion of protein, cells, and cellular debris.

cause, the release of histamine by mast cells usually results in profound inflammation. Therefore, allergic dermatitis frequently results from contact, inhalant, as well as food allergens. Allergic reactions do not occur with the first exposure to an allergen. The first exposure serves to *sensitize* the animal. As in the case with most food allergies, multiple exposures to the allergen are required before the animal becomes *hypersensitive*[9] to the agent. Once the animal is hypersensitive, his or her body overreacts to subsequent exposures (*challenges*) to the insulting allergen(s).

To isolate specific allergens, *intradermal skin testing* is performed. A series of intradermal injections is administered to the patient. Each injection contains a specified volume and concentration of an individual allergen. A *positive control* site is injected with histamine and a *negative control* site is injected with sterile water. After the allergens have been administered, the injection sites are observed over a 15- to 20-minute period for *wheal*[10] formation. Wheals formed in response to allergens are measured and compared to the positive and negative control sites. Any wheals less than or equal to the size of the negative control are considered negative. All others are graded on a scale of 1 to 4, with 4 being equal to or greater than the size of the positive control. Determination of specific allergens helps the owner remove the insulting allergens from the pet's environment or diet. For those allergens that cannot be eliminated, the pet may be engaged in *desensitization therapy*. Desensitization therapy is a slow, progressive process. Allergens are injected subcutaneously, usually at weekly or biweekly intervals. Over time, the concentration of the allergens is progressively increased. The goal of desensitization therapy is to administer doses of allergens that are low enough so that a hypersensitivity reaction is not stimulated, yet high enough to stimulate a different, more appropriate immune response by the body. Ultimately, the animal no longer reacts adversely to challenge situations with those allergens.

Flea allergy dermatitis is the most common isolate from intradermal skin testing. Dogs and cats with flea allergy dermatitis are allergic to the flea's saliva. It takes only one flea bite in a severely allergic animal to send him or her into intense dermatitis. The dermatitis from the single flea bite may last up to 8 weeks. That is why it is so important for owners to follow through with and maintain an adequate flea control protocol. Effective flea control protocols must include treatment of *all* pets in the household, the house itself, and the outdoor environment. Pet owners should consult with veterinary professionals about currently available flea control products that may be suitable for their pets and home situations.

---

[9]Hypersensitive (*hi″per-ˌsen′sĭ-tiv*); *hyper-* , above normal + *sensitive;* an exaggerated response to something, in this context an allergen.

[10]Wheal (*wēl*); a smooth, raised, circumscribed, erythematous skin lesion.

16.3. Self-Test

Using the previous information in this chapter, respond to each of the following questions using the most appropriate medical term(s). Do not use abbreviations.

1. The sensation of itching is medically termed ___pruritus___ .

2. ___alopecia___ is abnormal hair loss in any amount.

3. The ___epidermis___ is the most superficial layer of the skin, composed of stratified squamous epithelium.

4. A(n) ___subcutaneous___ injection is an injection administered into the loose connective tissue beneath the skin.

5. A(n) ___melanocyte___ is a cell type that contains black granules, designed to absorb harmful light energy.

6. The repair stage of wound healing includes two concurrent events: epithelial regeneration and ___fibroplasia___ .

7. An injection administered directly into the dermis is medically termed a(n) ___intradermal___ injection.

8. ___circumoral___ glands are located around the mouths of cats. They secrete pheromones for territorial marking.

9. The positive control for allergic skin testing is ___histamine___ .

10. Any cancerous, malignant growth that involves epithelial tissue is referred to as ___carcinoma___ .

11. Inflammation of the skin is medically termed ___dermatitis___ .

12. Excessive redness of the skin, due to vasodilation of capillaries, is medically termed ___erythema___ .

13. A(n) ___allergen___ is any agent that stimulates a hypersensitive allergic reaction.

14. Red, raised, pruritic lesions, commonly called "hives," are medically referred to as ___urticaria___ .

15. ___piloerection___ occurs when the muscles attached to the hair follicles contract, causing the hairs to stand upright. In cold environments, this provides an insulating layer of air trapped in the animal's coat.

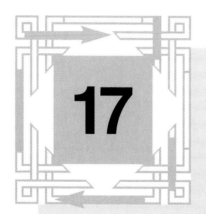

17

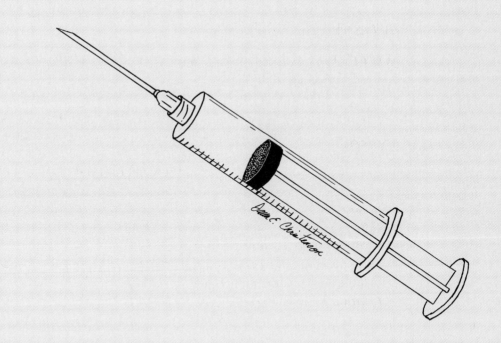

Pharmacology*

GOALS AND OBJECTIVES

By the conclusion of this chapter, the student will be able to:

1. Recognize common root words, prefixes, and suffixes related to pharmacology.

2. Divide simple and compound words into their respective parts.

3. Recognize, correctly pronounce, and appropriately use common medical terms related to pharmacology.

4. Demonstrate an understanding of the metric system with regard to weights, volumes, and conversions to apothecary and household measures.

5. Demonstrate an understanding of medication administration with regard to the five rights.

6. Demonstrate an understanding of medication administration with regard to relative rates of drug uptake per the different routes.

7. Demonstrate an understanding of prescription writing and transcription.

---

*Author's note: The purpose of this chapter is to familiarize the student with common terminology and abbreviations used in pharmacology. Dosage calculations, drug classifications, and pharmacokinetics are not covered because these topics stray from the original intent of this text. It is the author's hope that the tables and descriptions of weights and volumes will provide a valuable resource for students elsewhere in their studies. It is highly recommended that this chapter be attempted only after Chapters 1 through 16 have been successfully completed.

17.1. Introduction to Related Terms

Divide each of the following terms into its respective parts ("R" root, "P" prefix, "S" suffix, "CV" combining vowel).

1. **Pharmacology**   (R) _____   (CV) ____   (S) _____

   pharmacology (fahr"mah-kol'o-je; the study of medicine; clinically refers to the study of drug activity on the body)

2. **Iatrogenic**   (R) _____   (CV) ____   (R) _____   (S) _____

   iatrogenic (i"at-ro-jen'ik; pertaining to physician produced; clinically refers to any disorder in a patient that results from the actions of medical personnel)

3. **Parenteral**   (P) _____   (R) _____   (S) _____

   parenteral (pah-ren'ter-al; pertaining to around the intestines; clinically refers to various routes of medication administration that do not use the digestive tract)

4. **Kilogram**   (P) _____   (R) _____

   kilogram (kil'o-gram; one thousand grams)

5. **Hectogram**   (P) _____   (R) _____

   hectogram (hek'to-gram; one hundred grams)

6. **Decagram**   (P) _____   (R) _____

   decagram (dek'ah-gram; ten grams)

7. **Deciliter**   (P) _____   (R) _____

   deciliter (des'ĭ-le"ter; ten volumes; a unit of volume in the metric system that is one-tenth of a liter)

8. **Centimeter**   (P) _____   (R) _____

   centimeter (sen'tĭ-me"ter; a hundred measures; a unit of length in the metric system that is one one-hundredth of a meter)

9. **Milliliter**   (P) _____   (R) _____

   milliliter (mil'ĭ-le"ter; a thousand volumes; a unit of volume in the metric system that is one one-thousandth of a liter)

10. **Microgram**   (P) _____   (R) _____

    microgram (mi'kro-gram; a small weight; a unit of weight in the metric system that is one one-millionth of a gram or one one-thousandth of a milligram)

11. **Percent**   (P) _____   (R) _____

    percent (per-sent'; for each one hundred)

12. Anthelmintic   (P) _____   (R) _____   (S) _____

anthelmintic (ant"hel-min'tik; pertaining to against worms; anthelmintics are commonly referred to as "deworming" agents)

13. Antipyretic   (P) _____   (R) _____   (CV) ___   (S) _____

antipyretic (an"tĭ-pi-ret'ik; pertaining to against fever; an antipyretic agent is a drug that is used for fever reduction)

14. Antibiotic   (P) _____   (R) _____   (S) _____

antibiotic (an"tĭ-bi-ot'ik; pertaining to against life; clinically antibiotics are drugs that are used either to kill or inhibit growth of bacteria)

15. Contraindication   (P) _____   (R) _____   (S) _____

contraindication (kon"trah-in"dĭ-ka'shun; a state opposed to the indicated; clinically a contraindication is a situation in which an action/therapy is improper or undesirable because of the patient's condition)

16. Asepsis   (P) _____   (R) _____   (S) _____

asepsis (a-sep'sis; a state without decay; clinically refers to a state free from infection with microorganisms; cf. sterile)

17.2. Metric System

The metric system is a system of measure based on multiples of 10 and fractions of 10. There are three basic units of measure within the system. The meter is used for measurement of length (abbr. M or m). The liter is used for measurement of volume (abbr. L or l). Finally, the gram is used for measurement of weight (abbr. G, Gm, g, or gm). Standard prefixes are attached to each of the base units of measure to clearly indicate the multiple or fraction of 10 as appropriate (Table 17–1).

17.2.1. WEIGHT

Grams are a common unit of measure for weight in *pharmaceuticals*.[1] Dosages are frequently given as *milligrams* of drug per *kilogram* of body weight. Grams and milligrams are the most commonly used weights of pharmaceuticals. *Micrograms* are used less frequently. Table 7–2 shows the conversion equivalents for these commonly used weights.

---

[1]Pharmaceutical (fahr"mah-su'tĭ-kal); pertaining to a drug or pharmacy.

TABLE 17–1. Metric Prefixes

PREFIX	PHONETICS	ABBREVIATION	DECIMAL VALUE	SCIENTIFIC NOTATION	MEANING
tera	*ter'ah*	T	1,000,000,000,000	10^{12}	trillion
giga	*jĭ'gah*	G	1,000,000,000	10^{9}	billion
mega	*meg'ah*	M	1,000,000	10^{6}	million
kilo	*kil'o*	k	1,000	10^{3}	thousand
hecto	*hek'to*	h	100	10^{2}	hundred
deka	*dek'ah*	dk	10	10^{1}	ten
deci	*des'ĭ*	d	0.1	10^{-1}	one tenth
centi	*sen'tĭ*	c	0.01	10^{-2}	one-hundredth
milli	*mil'ĭ*	m	0.001	10^{-3}	one-thousandth
micro	*mi'kro*	μ or mc	0.000 001	10^{-6}	one-millionth
nano	*nan'o*	n	0.000 000 001	10^{-9}	one-billionth
pico	*pi'co*	p	0.000 000 000 001	10^{-12}	one-trillionth
femto	*fem'to*	f	0.000 000 000 000 001	10^{-15}	one-quadrillionth
atto	*at'to*	a	0.000 000 000 000 000 001	10^{-18}	one-quintillionth

17.2.2. VOLUME

Liters are a common unit of measure for volume in pharmaceuticals. Liquid drugs are frequently administered in milliliters. This is especially true when dealing with injections. Because a *cubic centimeter* is the equivalent volume of a *milliliter*, they may be used interchangeably. Table 17–3 shows the conversion equivalents for these commonly used volumes.

Concentration of liquid medications is expressed a number of ways. Many agents state a specific weight of the drug per volume (e.g., 10 mg/mL). Others express the concentration in *percent*. Because the strict definition of the term "percent" is "per one hundred," percent solutions are interpreted as weight in grams per 100 mL. For instance, a 5% solution of Lasix (furosemide; Hoechst-Roussel Pharmaceuticals, Somerville, NJ) contains 5 g of drug in every 100 mL of solution. Still others express concentration in ratios (e.g., 1:1000). In such a ratio, the number preceding the colon represents the drug weight in grams and the number following the colon represents the volume in milliliters. Therefore, a concentration of 1:1000 is interpreted as containing 1 g of drug in every 1000 mL of fluid.

TABLE 17–2. Metric Weights

WEIGHT	SYMBOL	EQUIVALENCY
1 kilogram	1 kg	1000 grams
1 gram	1 g	1 gram (1000 mg)
1 milligram	1 mg	0.001 gram; 1/1000 gram
1 microgram	1 mcg	0.000001 gram

TABLE 17–3. Metric Volumes

VOLUME	SYMBOL	EQUIVALENCY
1 liter	1 L	1 liter (1000 mL)
1 milliliter	1 mL	0.001 liter; 1/1000 liter
1 cubic centimeter	1 cc	0.001 liter; 1/1000 liter

17.2.3. CONVERSION TO APOTHECARY AND HOUSEHOLD SYSTEMS

The metric system is understood throughout the world. However, there are circumstances in which apothecary[2] or household measures are easier to use. This is often the case for pet owners because they are familiar with apothecary or household units of measure and have ready access to measuring implements for them. Most U.S. scales provide weight in pounds. However, many medications are dosed as milligrams per kilogram. In these circumstances, conversion of the patient's body weight in pounds to kilograms is required before any dosage calculation may be completed. Because it is often necessary to convert to and from metric, apothecary, and household units of measure, Table 17–4 has been provided.

TABLE 17–4. Metric, Apothecary, and Household Equivalencies

METRIC	APOTHECARY	HOUSEHOLD
	Weight	
1 kg	2.2 lb	2.2 lb
453.6 g	16 oz	1 lb
~ 30 g (31.1 g)	1 oz	
1 g	~ 15 gr (15.4 gr)	
~ 65 mg (64.8 mg)	1 gr	
~ 16 mg (16.2 mg)	¼ gr	
~ 0.5 mg (0.54 mg)	1/120 gr	
	Volume	
3.8 L	128 fl oz	1 gal (4 qt)
946.3 mL (cc)	32 fl oz	1 qt (2 pt)
473.2 mL	16 fl oz	1 pt
~ 240 mL (236.6 ml)	8 fl oz	1 c
~ 30 mL (29.6 ml)	1 fl oz	2 tbsp
~ 15 mL (14.8 ml)	0.5 fl oz (4 fl dr)	1 tbsp (3.7 tsp)
~ 4 mL (3.7 ml)	1 fl dr (60 ℥)	1 tsp
1 mL	~ 16 ℥ (16.7 ℥)	
0.06 mL	1 ℥	

Note that approximate (~) weights and volumes in the table above are commonly used for calculation purposes. Actual equivalencies follow each approximation in parentheses.

17.3. Medication Administration

17.3.1. FIVE RIGHTS OF MEDICATION ADMINISTRATION

Iatrogenic disorders and even fatalities are not uncommon in any of the medical professions. Veterinary medical professionals are not immune to the human error that can accompany medication administration. Iatrogenic problems in veterinary patients due to medication administration can be avoided, if the five rights of medication administration are reviewed before every drug is given. The "five rights" provide a simple checklist to ensure correct administration of medications. All one has to do is ask himself or herself the following questions: "Do I have the right patient? The right drug? The right dosage?" "Am I giving it via the right route?" and "Is this the correct time?"

Right patient? Veterinary patients who are hospitalized should be identified with labels on the cage as well as on each animal. Many small animal hospitals prefer to remove personal collars and harnesses to prevent injury. Without distinctive physical characteristics or other mechanisms for identifying patients, mistakes are more likely to occur. Think of the consequences in the case of an *antibiotic* to be administered to one of two black Labradors who look identical. Suppose that one of those two dogs (i.e., the one not intended to receive the drug) is severely allergic to the agent. Administration of the antibiotic to the wrong patient could result in death. Adequate identification of each Labrador would help prevent a fatal error in this situation. Veterinary practices may purchase any of a number of commercial patient identification devices that are safe and cost effective. Regardless of how patients are marked for identification, anyone administering medications should make every effort to ensure that the right patient is receiving the drug. Imagine a situation in which two patients named "Buffy" are hospitalized because of unexplained fever. A drug order has been given for one "Buffy" to receive an *antipyretic.* "Buffy" the dog can safely receive most of the common antipyretic agents, like aspirin or Tylenol (acetaminophen; McNeil Consumer Products, Fort Washington, PA). "Buffy" the cat, however, cannot. Tylenol, even in small doses, is highly toxic and can be lethal in cats. Even aspirin can have toxic effects in cats. Taking just a moment to clarify the drug order for a correct patient can avert an iatrogenic crisis.

Right drug? Several things must be checked to ensure that one has the right drug. Verify the veterinarian's drug order. Compare the drug order to the drug label. Evaluate the label for the drug name, concentration, and expiration date. Evaluate the contents of the container for spoilage or contamination. Last, check to see that the drug is in the correct form. Table 17–5 provides common prescription abbreviations for the various forms of medications.

---

[2]Apothecary (*ah-poth'ĕ-ka"re*); from [Gr. *apotheke*, storehouse]; refers to a pharmacy or pharmacist.

Right dosage? Verify the veterinarian's drug order. Is the order dosed per pounds body weight or per kilograms body weight? Whenever calculating drug dosages, always be certain to carry through with the appropriate units in the mathematical equation. Label the final answer of the calculation in the units that are to be administered. On obtaining the drug to be administered, compare the volume in-hand to the calculated volume once again. Table 17–6 gives common units by which drugs are administered.

Right route? Verify the veterinarian's drug order. How or where is the medication to be administered? Is the form of drug and the in-hand volume appropriate for the ordered route? If the in-hand volume seems to exceed that which may be reasonably given by the ordered route, double-check the calculations. If the calculations are found to be correct, perhaps the veterinarian who gave the order should be consulted. The veterinarian may deem the calculated volume within acceptable limits of the selected route, or he or she may choose an alternate route. Acceptable volumes to be administered by various routes are discussed in upcoming sections. Table 17–7 contains prescription abbreviations and their meanings for commonly used routes of medication administration.

Right time? Verify the veterinarian's drug order. How frequently is the medication to be administered? Should the medication be given before a meal for optimal absorption? Should the medication be given after meals to avoid gastric upset? The timing of medication administration is very important. Giving a drug too frequently could result in toxic side effects. Giving a drug beyond the prescribed period (i.e. late) could result in low blood levels of the agent, consequently making it ineffective. Most medication administration periods are based on the half-life of the drug. The time schedule for administration of medications

TABLE 17–5. Medication Form Abbreviations

Rx ABBREVIATION	MEANING
aq	Water [L. *aqua*]
cap	Capsule
elix	Elixir
emuls	Emulsion
ext	Extract
mixt	Mixture
supp	Suppository
susp	Suspension
syr	Syrup
tab	Tablet
tr, tinct	Tincture
ung	Ointment [L. *unguentum*]

TABLE 17–6. Medication Unit Abbreviations

ABBREVIATION	MEANING	ABBREVIATION	MEANING	ABBREVIATION	MEANING
cc	cubic centimeter	gtt	drop	℥, min, M	minim
dr	dram	kg	kilogram	oz	ounce
fl dr	fluid dram	L	liter	pt	pint
fl oz	fluid ounce	mcg, μg	microgram	qt	quart
gal	gallon	mEq	milliequivalent	tbsp, T	tablespoon
g, gm, G, Gm	gram	mg	milligram	tsp, t	teaspoon
gr	grain	ml, mL	milliliter	U	unit

should be strictly adhered to, as written in the prescription. Table 17–8 contains prescription abbreviations and their meanings for common times of medication administration.

17.3.2. PER OS

Per os administration is one of the most widely used routes of medication administration. Many would advocate, "if the gut works, use it." When the length of time for uptake of a drug is not critical, per os administration is useful. The per os route provides one of the slower routes for uptake of drugs. Giving per os medications to animals does present challenges at times, particularly if the agent is not palatable. *Anthelmintics* are probably one of the most frequently used per os

TABLE 17–7. Medication Administration Route Abbreviations

R_x ABBREVIATION	MEANING
A.D., ad	Right ear [L. *auris dextra*]
A.S., as	Left ear [L. *auris sinistra*]
A.U., au	Both ears [L. *auris uterque*]
ID	Intradermal
IM	Intramuscular
IP	Intraperitoneal
IV	Intravenous
O.D., od	Right eye [L. *oculus dexter*]
O.S., os	Left eye [L. *oculus sinister*]
O.U., ou	Both eyes [L. *oculus uterque*]
P.O., po	By mouth [L. *per os*]
SC, SQ	Subcutaneous

TABLE 17–8. Medication Administration Time Abbreviations

Rx ABBREVIATION	MEANING	Rx ABBREVIATION	MEANING
A.C., ac	Before meals [L. *ante cibum*]	qd	Every day
ad lib	As desired [L. *ad libitum*]	qh	Every hour [L. *quaque hora*]
B.i.d., Bid, bid	Twice daily [L. *bis in die*]	q2h	Every 2 hours
c̄	With	q4h, qqh	Every 4 hours [L. *quaque quarta hora*]
h	Hour	q6h	Every 6 hours
hs	At bedtime [L. *hora somni*]	q8h	Every 8 hours
noct	At night [L. *nocte*]	Q.i.d., Qid, qid	Four times daily [L. *quarta in die*]
NPO	Nothing by mouth	Qod, qod	Every other day
P.C., pc	After meals [L. *post cibum*]	s̄	Without
per	By	SOS	Once if needed [L. *si opus sit*]
PRN, prn	As needed [L. *pro re nata*]	STAT	Immediately [L. *statim*]
q	Every	T.i.d., Tid, tid	Three times daily [L. *ter in die*]
qAM	Every morning		

medications. Most of the paste and liquid anthelmintics are manufactured to be palatable, to facilitate easier administration. Antibiotics are also frequently administered per os.

Some antibiotics, as well as other drugs, have the tendency to cause gastritis. For such agents, manufacturers have produced enteric-coated tablets. The enteric coating protects the stomach from the drug because the coating is only fully removed from the tablet once it is in the intestinal tract, hence the name, "enteric coated." Enteric-coated tablets are not intended to be broken into smaller doses; to do so would defeat the purpose of the coating.

With regard to volumes of medication that can be administered per os, the only limiting features are the patient's stomach size and the correct dosage of the specific drug to be given. In general, most per os medications are administered in manageable, diminutive doses. Per os administration is one of the easiest routes to use, particularly for pet owners. Even if an owner cannot master "pilling" his or her pet, tablets and capsules can be easily hidden in tasty treats for the pets, provided that the food is not *contraindicated*.

17.3.3. PARENTERAL

Parenteral routes of medication administration include any of the injectable modalities. Each of the methods of injection is briefly discussed in the following.

17.3.3.1. Subcutaneous

Subcutaneous injections can be administered nearly anywhere that enough loose skin can be found on the animal. This route is frequently used for administration of immunizations, antibiotics, and (in small animals) subcutaneous fluids. The uptake of drug from subcutaneous sites is slower than from intramuscular and intravenous routes because of the lesser blood supply in the subcutis. Depending on the drug given, the subcutaneous route does provide a faster uptake than that of per os. Most subcutaneous injections are less than 5 to 10 cc in volume. If subcutaneous fluids are to be administered to a dog or a cat, the size and conformation of the animal must be considered. In general, 20 to 50 mL is an acceptable range per site for subcutaneous fluids in dogs and cats. Large volumes of fluids are rarely, if ever, administered to large animals subcutaneously.

17.3.3.2. Intramuscular

Intramuscular injections are administered into large muscle masses. Specific intramuscular injection sites are discussed in Chapter 6. The uptake of drug from intramuscular injection sites is far more rapid than from either the per os or subcutaneous routes. The excellent blood supply to skeletal muscle facilitates the rapid drug onset. There are greater volumetric limitations to intramuscular injections than in most of the other routes. Obviously, species, breed, size, and muscular condition of the animal play major roles in determining reasonable volumes that may be administered intramuscularly. Generally accepted per site volume ranges for intramuscular injections are 3 to 6 mL in dogs and cats and 10 to 20 mL in cattle and horses.

17.3.3.3. Intravenous

Intravenous administration of medications provides the fastest onset of any of the routes. Specific phlebotomy/intravenous injection sites are discussed in Chapter 7. For any agents in which a very rapid onset is indicated, or are potentially caustic to perivascular tissues, or require large fluid volumes to be given concurrently, the intravenous route is the administration method of choice. Usually, only sterile *solutions* are acceptable for intravenous administration. There are few exceptions to this rule. With the exceptions of total parenteral nutrition and propofol (an anesthetic agent), unless the solution is transparent (i.e., devoid of any particulate matter), intravenous administration is contraindicated. The intravenous route is the modality of choice for fluid therapy. Volumes of fluids for deficit replacement, as well as hydration maintenance, are based on the body weight of the individual patient. Any parenteral injection requires adherence to *aseptic* protocols, but because of the direct entry into the bloodstream, *asepsis* is most critical for intravenous injections.

17.3.3.4. Intradermal

Intradermal injections are used predominantly in veterinary medicine for allergy skin testing and tuberculosis testing. The latter is routinely performed in cattle and primates. Because of the minute tissue thickness of the dermis, volumes that may be injected are significantly restricted. In general, volumes less than 0.3 mL are acceptable for intradermal injection sites. Obviously, given the limited blood supply found in the dermis, uptake of agents injected intradermally is negligible. Most activity remains localized at the injection site.

17.3.3.5. Intraperitoneal

Intraperitoneal injections are used most frequently in small laboratory animals, such as mice. Uptake of medications by this route is comparable to that of intramuscular injections. Occasionally, intraperitoneal fluids are administered to large animals, such as sheep and goats. In dogs and cats, intraperitoneal dialysis may be performed in renal failure patients.

17.3.4. TOPICAL

Anything that is applied to the surface of the skin, eyes, or ears is considered a topical agent. Most ophthalmic and otic preparations are sterile. Therefore, care must be taken to avoid contamination of the applicator tip when the drug is administered. Ophthalmic and otic solutions are generally prescribed to be given by the drop. Ophthalmic solutions should always be applied before ophthalmic ointments. Ophthalmic ointments contain a petroleum base that prevents the absorption of aqueous solutions applied afterward. Dermatologic agents come in a variety of forms. For those that cannot or should not be applied directly from the original container, latex gloves or another suitable device should be used to apply the drug. This protects the patient's wounds from contamination by human skin; it also protects the person applying the medication from absorbing the agent. The issue of personnel safety is very important when topical pesticides[3] are being applied to patients.

---

[3]Pesticide (*pes'tĭ-sīd*); to kill pests; any of a number of chemical poisons used to destroy various pests, including insects, arachnids, and fungi.

17.4. Prescription Writing and Transcribing

Prescriptions are written in a fairly standardized format. Once the student has mastered the prescription abbreviations contained in previous tables, transcription to laymen's terms should be easy. Each written prescription begins with the superscription or heading symbol "R$_x$." The information that follows this "recipe" symbol contains information regarding the specific drug to be given. This information should include the name of the drug, its concentration, quantity, and any relevant compounding instructions. The signature (represented by the symbol "S." or "Sig.," meaning "mark" or "give") contains specific instructions for patient dosing that should be included on the receptacle. Of course, it goes without saying that pertinent patient information, the date, and veterinarian's signature should also be included on the written prescription. If the veterinarian issued the prescription verbally or by telephone, the notation "VO" (verbal order) or "TO" (telephone order) should accompany the order in the patient's medical record. Figure 17–1 provides an example of a written prescription.

It would be inappropriate to expect a pet owner to read and understand the instructions in the preceding prescription. The information must be transcribed into a form understood by the average person. All of the information found in the

---

Veterinary Medical Center, P.C.
3000 S. Fork Road
Anytown, MI 01234
(012) 345-6789
J. A. Smith, DVM

Patient: _"Sadie" Christenson_   I.D. # _642351_

R$_x$: _Prednisolone, 5 mg tabs, #30_

Sig: _1 tab PO bid pc × 5d, then 1 tab PO qd pc × 5d, then 1 tab PO qod pc until gone_

_0_ Refills

Dr. _J.A. Smith_   Date: _7-25-95_

FIGURE 17–1. Prescription example.

```
┌─────────────────────────────────────────────────────────────┐
│                 Veterinary Medical Center                     │
│             3000 S. Fork Rd., Anytown, MI 01234               │
│                      (012) 345-6789                           │
│   Dr. J. A. Smith                          Date: 07-25-95     │
│              Patient: Sadie Christenson #642351               │
│   Rₓ: Give 1 tablet orally twice daily after meals for 5 days,│
│   then give 1 tablet orally once daily after a meal for 5 days,│
│   then give 1 tablet orally every other day after a meal until│
│   gone.                                                       │
│   30 Prednisolone 5 mg tablets              0 Refills         │
│   Expiration date: 7-25-96                       dec          │
│                                                               │
└─────────────────────────────────────────────────────────────┘
```

FIGURE 17–2. Prescription label.

written prescription must be included on the receptacle label. In addition, the initials of the person filling the prescription, as well as the drug's expiration date, should be included. Figure 17–2 is representative of the label that should be placed on the bottle to be sold to the owner of the preceding patient.

17.5. Self-Test

Using the previous information in this chapter, respond to each of the following questions using the most appropriate medical term(s). Do not use abbreviations.

1. A(n) _____ disorder in a patient is one that was caused by the actions of medical personnel.

2. A drug, like aspirin, that is used to reduce fever is medically termed a(n) _____.

3. A(n) _____ is a drug that may commonly be referred to as a dewormer.

4. A(n) _____ is a metric unit of weight equal to one thousand grams.

5. The metric unit of volume equal to one one-thousandth of a liter or one cubic centimeter is the _____.

6. The parenteral medication administration route in which medication is injected beneath the skin is a(n) _____ injection.

7. Given the following excerpt from a prescription—Sig: 3 gtt od qid × 14d—by what route (i.e., where) should the medication be given? _____

8. The metric unit of weight that constitutes one one-thousandth of a gram is the

   _____.

9. A drug used to kill or inhibit growth of bacterial microorganisms is a(n)

   _____.

10. Given the following excerpt from a prescription—Sig: 250 mg po hs × 5d—what is the correct time of administration? _____

11. Given the following excerpt from a prescription—Sig: 20 mg IV STAT—by what route should the medication be given? _____

12. A patient's medical condition precluding the administration of a certain drug is termed a(n) _____.

13. The _____ system is one in which volumes are measured in fluid drams and ounces.

14. Given the following excerpt from a prescription—Sig: ½ tab po bid × 7d—how frequently should the drug be administered? _____

15. Given the following excerpt from a prescription—Sig: 2 gtt os q4h × 5d—what is the correct dosage of the medication to be administered? _____

16. Given the following excerpt from a prescription—Sig: 5 mg IM q6h × 2d—what is the correct route of medication administration? _____

17. The term _____ literally means "for every one hundred."

18. _____ should be strictly observed whenever parenteral medications, especially intravenous medications, are administered to prevent contamination with microorganisms.

19. Given the following excerpt from a prescription—Sig: 2 cap po tid ac × 10d—what is the correct time/frequency of medication administration? _____

20. What are the five rights of medication administration? _____

APPENDIX A

Chemical Symbol–Element Cross Reference

Atomic No.	Symbol	Name	Atomic No.	Symbol	Name	Atomic No.	Symbol	Name
1	H	hydrogen	37	Rb	rubidium	73	Ta	tantalum
2	He	helium	38	Sr	strontium	74	W	tungsten
3	Li	lithium	39	Y	yttrium	75	Re	rhenium
4	Be	beryllium	40	Zr	zirconium	76	Os	osmium
5	B	boron	41	Nb	niobium	77	Ir	iridium
6	C	carbon	42	Mo	molybdenum	78	Pt	platinum
7	N	nitrogen	43	Tc	technetium	79	Au	gold
8	O	oxygen	44	Ru	ruthenium	80	Hg	mercury
9	F	fluorine	45	Rh	rhodium	81	Tl	thallium
10	Ne	neon	46	Pd	palladium	82	Pb	lead
11	Na	sodium	47	Ag	silver	83	Bi	bismuth
12	Mg	magnesium	48	Cd	cadmium	84	Po	polonium
13	Al	aluminum	49	In	indium	85	At	astatine
14	Si	silicon	50	Sn	tin	86	Rn	radon
15	P	phosphorus	51	Sb	antimony	87	Fr	francium
16	S	sulfur	52	Te	tellurium	88	Ra	radium
17	Cl	chlorine	53	I	iodine	89	Ac	actinium
18	Ar	argon	54	Xe	xenon	90	Th	thorium
19	K	potassium	55	Cs	cesium	91	Pa	protactinium
20	Ca	calcium	56	Ba	barium	92	U	uranium
21	Sc	scandium	57	La	lanthanum	93	Np	neptunium
22	Ti	titanium	58	Ce	cerium	94	Pu	plutonium
23	V	vanadium	59	Pr	praseodymium	95	Am	americium
24	Cr	chromium	60	Nd	neodymium	96	Cm	curium
25	Mn	manganese	61	Pm	promethium	97	Bk	berkelium
26	Fe	iron	62	Sm	samarium	98	Cf	californium
27	Co	cobalt	63	Eu	europium	99	Es	einsteinium
28	Ni	nickel	64	Gd	gadolinium	100	Fm	fermium
29	Cu	copper	65	Tb	terbium	101	Md	mendelevium
30	Zn	zinc	66	Dy	dysprosium	102	No	nobelium
31	Ga	gallium	67	Ho	holmium	103	Lr	lawrencium
32	Ge	germanium	68	Er	erbium	104	Rf	rutherfordium
33	As	arsenic	69	Tm	thulium	105	Ha	hahnium
34	Se	selenium	70	Yb	ytterbium	106	*	*
35	Br	bromine	71	Lu	lutetium			
36	Kr	krypton	72	Hf	hafnium			

*Undetermined at time of publication.

APPENDIX B

Answer Keys for Introduction to Related Terms and Self-Test Exercises

Chapter 1 Answer Keys

SECTION 1.1.7. INTRODUCTION TO RELATED TERMS

1. (R) anter (CV) i (S) or
2. (R) caud (S) ad
3. (R) crani (S) al
4. (R) caud (CV) o (R) crani (S) al
5. (R) crani (CV) o (R) caud (S) al
6. (R) dors (S) al
7. (R) palm (S) ar
8. (R) dors (CV) o (R) palm (S) ar
9. (R) plant (S) ar
10. (R) dors (CV) o (R) plant (S) ar
11. (R) ventr (S) al
12. (R) dors (CV) o (R) ventr (S) al
13. (R) later (S) al
14. (R) medi (S) al
15. (R) medi (CV) o (R) later (S) al
16. (R) palmar (CV) o (R) dors (S) al
17. (R) plantar (CV) o (R) dors (S) al
18. (R) poster (CV) i (S) or
19. (R) rostr (S) al

SECTION 1.4. SELF-TEST

1. root
2. combining vowel
3. suffix
4. combining form
5. prefix
6. rostrad
7. ventrodorsal
8. sagittal
9. transverse
10. dorsopalmar
11. cranial
12. caudal
13. dorsal
14. medial
15. lateral
16. transverse
17. distal
18. proximal
19. oblique
20. median

Chapter 2 Answer Keys

SECTION 2.1. INTRODUCTION TO RELATED TERMS

1. (P) micr (CV) o (R) scop (S) ic
2. (R) cyt (CV) o (S) logy
3. (R) lys (CV) o (R) som (S) al
4. (P) intra (R) cellul (S) ar
5. (P) extra (R) cellul (S) ar
6. (R) nucle (S) ar
7. (R) chrom (CV) o (S) some
8. (R) nucle (S) olus
9. (P) endo (R) plasm (S) ic
10. (R) centr (CV) i (S) ole
11. (R) cyt (CV) o (R) plasm (S) ic
12. (R) vacu (S) ole
13. (R) chromat (S) ic
14. (R) phag (CV) o (R) cyt (CV) o (S) sis
15. (R) pin (CV) o (R) cyt (CV) o (S) sis
16. (P) ex (CV) o (R) cyt (CV) o (S) sis
17. (R) mit (CV) o (S) sis
18. (R) nucle (S) i
19. (P) inter (R) cellul (S) ar
20. (R) organ (S) elle
21. (R) physi (CV) o (S) logy
22. (R) reticul (S) ar
23. (R) rib (CV) o (R) som (S) al
24. (P) centr (CV) o (S) mere

SECTION 2.3. SELF-TEST

1. cytology
2. mitochondria
3. intracellular
4. intercellular
5. phagocytosis
6. cytoplasm
7. Golgi apparatus
8. exocytosis
9. ribosome
10. vacuole
11. nucleus
12. chromatin
13. extracellular
14. lysosome
15. rough endoplasmic reticulum
16. mitosis
17. chromosomes
18. active transport or facilitated diffusion
19. nucleolus
20. diffusion
21. anatomy
22. physiology
23. centrioles
24. Pinocytosis

Chapter 3 Answer Keys

SECTION 3.1. INTRODUCTION TO RELATED TERMS

1. (R) hemat (CV) o (R) poie (S) tic
2. (R) lymph (CV) a (S) tic
3. (R) muscul (CV) o (R) skelet (S) al
4. (R) cardi (CV) o (R) vascul (S) ar
5. (P) re (R) spirat (S) ory
6. (R) neur (CV) o (R) log (CV) i (S) cal
7. (R) aliment (S) ary
8. (R) urin (S) ary
9. (P) re (R) product (S) ive
10. (P) endo (R) crine
11. (R) integument (S) ary
12. (R) viscer (S) al
13. (R) crani (S) al
14. (R) thorac (S) ic
15. (R) abdomin (S) al
16. (R) epitheli (S) al
17. (R) endotheli (S) al
18. (R) cub (S) oidal

19. (R) squam (S) ous
20. (R) column (S) ar
21. (R) my (CV) o (S) cyte
22. (R) home (CV) o (S) stasis
23. (R) path (CV) o (S) logy
24. (P) syn (R) erg (S) ism
25. (P) sym (R) bio (S) sis
26. (R) bio (S) logy
27. (R) atom (S) ic
28. (R) molecul (S) ar

SECTION 3.3. SELF-TEST

1. molecule
2. Synergism
3. electron
4. protons

5. symbiotic
6. thoracic
7. hematopoietic
8. Homeostasis
9. epithelial
10. Amino acids
11. Pathology
12. integumentary
13. covalent
14. Water
15. Biology
16. inert
17. Electrolytes
18. endocrine
19. Pseudostratified
20. Adipose

Chapter 4 Answer Keys

SECTION 4.1. INTRODUCTION TO RELATED TERMS

1. (R) hemat (CV) o (S) logy
2. (R) morph (CV) o (S) logy
3. (P) erythr (CV) o (S) cyte
4. (R) reticul (CV) o (S) cyte
5. (P) poly (R) chrom (S) asia
6. (P) anis (CV) o (R) cyt (CV) o (S) sis
7. (P) poly (R) cyt (R) hem (S) ia
8. (P) an (R) em (S) ia
9. (P) pan (R) cyt (CV) o (S) penia
10. (P) leuk (CV) o (S) cyte
11. (P) leuk (CV) o (S) penia
12. (P) leuk (CV) o (R) cyt (CV) o (S) sis
13. (P) neutr (CV) o (S) penia
14. (P) bas (CV) o (R) phil (S) ic
15. (P) eosin (CV) o (R) phil (S) ia
16. (R) lymph (CV) o (R) cyt (CV) o (S) sis
17. (P) mono (R) cyt (CV) o (S) sis
18. (P) poly (R) morph (CV) o (R) nucle (S) ar

19. (R) thromb (CV) o (S) cyte
20. (R) hem (CV) o (S) stasis
21. (R) thromb (S) us
22. (R) phag (CV) o (S) cyte
23. (P) macr (CV) o (S) phage
24. (P) anti (R) coagul (S) ant
25. (R) hem (CV) o (S) lysis
26. (R) hem (CV) o (S) rrhage
27. (R) hemat (S) oma
28. (R) hemat (CV) o (S) crit
29. (P) mega (R) kary (CV) o (S) cyte
30. (R) poikil (CV) o (R) cyt (CV) o (S) sis

SECTION 4.3. SELF-TEST

1. Erythrocytes
2. Neutrophils
3. monocyte
4. hematoma
5. plasma
6. hemolysis
7. leukocytes
8. eosinophil

9. thrombocytes
10. Hemostasis
11. lymphocyte
12. leukocytosis
13. panleukopenia
14. basophilia
15. Hemoglobin
16. Erythrocytes
17. anticoagulant
18. Reticulocytes
19. thrombocytopenia
20. anisocytosis
21. serum
22. pancytopenia
23. anemia
24. hematocrit
25. poikilocytosis

Chapter 5 Answer Keys

SECTION 5.1. INTRODUCTION TO RELATED TERMS

1. (R) lymph (R) aden (CV) o (S) pathy
2. (R) splen (S) ic
3. (R) lymph (R) ang (S) itis
4. (R) lymph (CV) o (S) cyte
5. (R) splen (CV) o (S) megaly
6. (P) inter (R) stiti (S) al
7. (P) macr (CV) o (S) phage
8. (R) phag (CV) o (R) cyt (CV) o (S) sis
9. (R) path (CV) o (R) gen (S) ic
10. (R) tonsill (S) ectomy
11. (R) tonsill (S) itis
12. (R) lymph (S) oid

3. edema
4. macrophages
5. pathogens
6. thymus
7. prescapular
8. Lymphangitis
9. splenomegaly
10. tonsillitis
11. tonsillectomy
12. spleen
13. lymphadenopathy
14. axillary
15. superficial inguinal
16. splenectomy
17. Osmosis
18. Capillaries
19. Interstitial
20. immunity

SECTION 5.3. SELF-TEST

1. popliteal
2. Antibodies

Chapter 6 Answer Keys

SECTION 6.1.2. INTRODUCTION TO RELATED TERMS—WORD EXERCISES

1. (R) scapul (CV) o (R) humer (S) al
2. (R) humer (CV) o (R) radi (CV) o (R) uln (S) ar

3. (R) carp (S) al
4. (P) meta (R) carp (S) al
5. (P) meta (R) carp (CV) o (R) phalang (CV) e (S) al
6. (P) inter (R) phalang (CV) e (S) al
7. (R) cox (CV) o (R) femor (S) al

8. (R) femor (CV) o (R) tibi (S) al
9. (R) tars (S) al
10. (P) meta (R) tars (S) al
11. (P) meta (R) tars (CV) o (R) pha-lang (CV) e (S) al
12. (R) cervic (S) al
13. (P) inter (R) vertebr (S) al
14. (R) lumb (CV) o (R) sacr (S) al
15. (R) coccyg (CV) e (S) al
16. (P) ep (R) axi (S) al
17. (P) inter (R) cost (S) al
18. (R) cost (CV) o (R) chondr (S) al
19. (R) stern (S) al
20. (P) epi (R) physis
21. (P) meta (R) physis
22. (P) dia (R) physis
23. (P) peri (R) oste (S) al
24. (P) endo (R) oste (S) um
25. (P) syn (R) ovi (S) al
26. (R) arthr (S) itis
27. (R) myos (S) itis
28. (R) orth (CV) o (R) ped (S) ic
29. (R) flex (S) ion
30. (P) ex (R) ten (S) sion
31. (P) ab (R) duc (S) tion
32. (P) ad (R) duc (S) tion
33. (P) circum (R) duc (S) tion
34. (P) intra (R) muscul (S) ar

SECTION 6.3. SELF-TEST

1. coxofemoral
2. cervical
3. intercostal
4. Abduction
5. arthritis
6. periosteum
7. flexor
8. ligament
9. myositis
10. Coccygeal
11. femorotibial
12. intramuscular
13. humeroradioulnar
14. interphalangeal

15. metatarsus
16. thoracic
17. adduction
18. Synovial
19. Orthopedic
20. extensor
21. epiphysis
22. endosteum
23. comminuted
24. Intervertebral
25. tendons
26. costochondral
27. epiphyseal plate
28. scapulohumeral
29. diaphysis
30. gluteal

CANINE ANATOMY CHALLENGE (FIG. 6-15)

1. skull
2. maxilla
3. mandible
4. cervical vertebrae
5. scapula
6. scapulohumeral joint
7. humerus
8. humeroradioulnar joint
9. radius
10. ulna
11. carpus
12. accessory carpal bone
13. metacarpus
14. phalanges
15. proximal sesamoid bones
16. distal sesamoid bones
17. thoracic vertebrae
18. ribs
19. sternum
20. lumbar vertebrae
21. sacrum
22. ilium
23. coxofemoral joint
24. femur
25. femorotibial joint

26. patella
27. tibia
28. fibula
29. tarsus
30. calcaneus
31. metatarsus
32. phalanges
33. proximal sesamoid bones
34. distal sesamoid bones
35. coccygeal vertebrae

EQUINE ANATOMY CHALLENGE (FIG. 6-16)

1. skull
2. maxilla
3. mandible
4. cervical vertebrae
5. scapula
6. scapulohumeral joint
7. humerus
8. humeroradioulnar joint
9. radius
10. ulna
11. carpus
12. accessory carpal bone
13. third metacarpal bone
14. metacarpophalangeal joint
15. proximal sesamoid bones
16. proximal (first) phalanx
17. proximal interphalangeal joint
18. middle (second) phalanx
19. distal interphalangeal joint
20. distal (third) phalanx
21. distal sesamoid bone
22. thoracic vertebrae
23. ribs
24. sternum
25. lumbar vertebrae
26. sacrum
27. ilium
28. coxofemoral joint
29. femur
30. femorotibial joint
31. patella
32. tibia
33. fibula
34. tarsus
35. calcaneus
36. third metatarsal bone
37. metatarsophalangeal joint
38. proximal sesamoid bones
39. proximal (first) phalanx
40. proximal interphalangeal joint
41. middle (second) phalanx
42. distal interphalangeal joint
43. distal (third) phalanx
44. distal sesamoid bone
45. coccygeal vertebrae

Chapter 7 Answer Keys

SECTION 7.1. INTRODUCTION TO RELATED TERMS

1. (R) cardi (S) ac
2. (R) cardi (CV) o (R) log (S) ist
3. (P) peri (R) cardi (S) al
4. (P) epi (R) cardi (S) um
5. (R) my (CV) o (R) cardi (S) al
6. (P) endo (R) cardi (S) um
7. (R) atri (S) al
8. (R) ventricul (S) ar
9. (R) atri (CV) o (R) ventricul (S) ar
10. (R) aort (S) ic
11. (R) pulmon (S) ic
12. (R) arter (CV) i (S) al
13. (R) arter (CV) i (S) ole
14. (R) ven (S) ous
15. (R) ven (S) ule
16. (R) phleb (CV) o (S) tomy
17. (R) phleb (S) itis
18. (R) cardi (CV) o (R) my (CV) o (S) pathy

19. (R) electr (CV) o (R) cardi (CV) o (S) gram
20. (R) echo (R) cardi (CV) o (S) gram
21. (R) angi (CV) o (S) gram
22. (P) intra (R) ven (S) ous
23. (P) peri (R) vascul (S) ar
24. (P) brady (R) cardi (S) ia
25. (P) tachy (R) card (S) ia
26. (R) systol (S) ic
27. (R) diastol (S) ic
28. (P) a (R) systole
29. (R) sten (CV) o (S) sis
30. (R) cardi (CV) o (S) megaly
31. (P) hyper (R) trophy
32. (P) inter (R) atri (S) al
33. (P) inter (R) ventricul (S) ar
34. (P) a (R) rrhythm (S) ia
35. (R) vas (CV) o (R) constric (S) tion
36. (R) vas (CV) o (R) dila (S) tion
37. (R) sphygm (CV) o (R) man (CV) o (S) meter

SECTION 7.3. SELF-TEST

1. Systole
2. left atrioventricular valve
3. pericardial
4. myocardium
5. left atrium
6. aorta
7. Phlebitis

8. bradycardia
9. electrocardiogram
10. pulmonic
11. phlebotomist
12. angiogram
13. arteriole
14. cardiologist
15. asystole
16. diastole
17. Cardiomegaly
18. stenosis
19. P wave
20. interatrial septum
21. pulmonic and aortic
22. tachycardia
23. capillary
24. systemic circulation
    vena cavae
    right atrium
    right atrioventricular valve
    right ventricle
    pulmonic valve
    pulmonary arteries
    lungs
    pulmonary veins
    left atrium
    left atrioventricular valve
    left ventricle
    aortic valve
    aorta
    systemic circulation

Chapter 8 Answer Keys

SECTION 8.1. INTRODUCTION TO RELATED TERMS

1. (R) pleur (S) al
2. (R) pneumon (S) ia
3. (R) trache (CV) o (R) bronch (S) itis
4. (P) endo (R) trache (S) al
5. (R) trache (CV) o (S) tomy
6. (R) trache (CV) o (S) stomy

7. (R) laryng (S) itis
8. (R) rhin (S) itis
9. (R) rhin (CV) o (R) pneumon (S) itis
10. (R) pneum (CV) o (R) thorax
11. (R) hem (CV) o (R) thorax
12. (P) py (CV) o (R) thorax
13. (R) atel (S) ectasis
14. (P) tachy (R) pnea

15. (P) brady (R) pnea
16. (P) hyper (R) pnea
17. (P) dys (R) pnea
18. (P) a (R) pnea
19. (P) hyper (R) capn (S) ia
20. (P) hyp (R) ox (S) ia
21. (R) alveol (S) ar
22. (R) sinus (S) itis
23. (P) inter (R) cost (S) al
24. (R) bronch (CV) i (S) ole
25. (P) in (R) spira (S) tion
26. (P) ex (R) pira (S) tion
27. (P) a (R) spira (S) tion
28. (R) cyan (CV) o (S) sis
29. (R) hem (CV) o (S) ptysis
30. (P) anti (R) tuss (S) ive
31. (P) epi (R) glottis
32. (P) intra (R) nas (S) al
33. (P) a (R) chondr (S) al
34. (R) nas (CV) o (R) pharynx
35. (R) nas (CV) o (R) gastr (S) ic

SECTION 8.3. SELF-TEST

1. dyspnea
2. tracheobronchitis
3. Atelectasis
4. Cyanosis
5. Rhinitis
6. nasal turbinates
7. vital capacity
8. hemoptysis
9. antitussive
10. alveoli
11. epiglottis
12. tachypnea
13. apnea
14. tidal
15. tracheotomy
16. epistaxis
17. Bronchioles
18. pleuritis
19. pyothorax
20. intercostal

Chapter 9 Answer Keys

SECTION 9.1. INTRODUCTION TO RELATED TERMS

1. (R) neur (S) itis
2. (R) cerebr (S) al
3. (R) cerebell (S) ar
4. (P) af (R) ferrent
5. (P) ef (R) ferrent
6. (R) sympathet (S) ic
7. (P) para (R) sympathet (S) ic
8. (P) aut (CV) o (R) nom (S) ic
9. (R) cholin (R) erg (S) ic
10. (R) sympath (CV) o (R) mimet (S) ic
11. (R) synapt (S) ic
12. (R) neur (CV) o (S) glial
13. (R) astr (CV) o (S) cyte
14. (P) olig (CV) o (R) dendr (CV) o (S) cyte
15. (R) ependym (S) al

16. (P) micr (CV) o (S) glial
17. (P) bi (R) pol (S) ar
18. (P) uni (R) pol (S) ar
19. (P) multi (R) pol (S) ar
20. (R) axon (S) al
21. (R) mening (S) itis
22. (R) cerebr (CV) o (R) spin (S) al
23. (P) hemi (R) sphere
24. (R) brachi (S) al
25. (R) lumb (CV) o (R) sacr (S) al
26. (P) inter (R) vertebr (S) al
27. (R) electr (CV) o (R) encephal (CV) o (S) gram
28. (P) an (R) alges (S) ia
29. (P) an (R) esthes (S) ia
30. (P) para (R) ly (S) sis
31. (P) para (S) plegia
32. (P) tetra (S) plegia
33. (P) quadri (S) plegia

34. (P) hemi (S) plegia
35. (P) mono (S) plegia
36. (P) hemi (R) paresis
37. (P) a (R) tax (S) ia
38. (R) olfact (S) ory
39. (R) myel (CV) o (S) gram
40. (R) zoo (R) nos (S) is

SECTION 9.4. SELF-TEST

1. cerebrum
2. afferent
3. blood–brain barrier
4. cerebellum
5. intervertebral
6. sympathomimetic
7. Cerebrospinal
8. Analgesia
9. gray
10. pia mater
11. efferent
12. myelogram
13. zoonotic
14. Tetraplegia, quadriplegia
15. cholinergic
16. Oligodendrocytes
17. encephalomyelitis
18. brachial plexus
19. action potential
20. nodes of Ranvier
21. white
22. dura mater
23. Anesthesia
24. Hemiplegia
25. ataxia
26. electroencephalogram
27. parasympathetic
28. Paraplegia
29. sympathetic
30. sciatic
31. monoparesis

Chapter 10 Answer Keys

SECTION 10.1. INTRODUCTION TO RELATED TERMS

1. (R) ophthalm (CV) o (S) logy
2. (P) intra (R) ocul (S) ar
3. (P) peri (R) ocul (S) ar
4. (P) extra (R) ocul (S) ar
5. (R) opt (S) ic
6. (R) palpebr (S) al
7. (R) conjunctiv (S) al
8. (R) corne (S) al
9. (R) kerat (CV) o (R) conjunctiv (S) itis
10. (R) irid (CV) o (R) corne (S) al
11. (R) scler (S) al
12. (R) mi (CV) o (S) sis
13. (R) mydria (S) tic
14. (P) anis (CV) o (R) cor (S) ia
15. (R) nas (CV) o (R) lacrim (S) al
16. (R) phot (CV) o (R) phob (S) ia
17. (R) uve (S) itis
18. (R) blephar (CV) o (S) spasm
19. (R) distichi (CV) a (S) sis
20. (P) ec (R) trop (CV) i (S) on
21. (P) en (R) trop (CV) i (S) on
22. (R) retin (CV) o (S) pathy
23. (R) ophthalm (CV) o (R) log (S) ist
24. (P) contra (R) later (S) al
25. (P) uni (R) later (S) al
26. (R) bu (R) phthalmos

SECTION 10.3. SELF-TEST

1. ophthalmologist
2. Mydriasis
3. optic
4. ectropion
5. Glaucoma
6. conjunctiva
7. retina

8. nasolacrimal
9. uvea
10. distichiasis
11. cornea
12. synechia
13. sclera
14. iridocorneal
15. posterior chamber
16. miosis
17. keratoconjunctivitis
18. photophobia
19. Anisocoria
20. optic disc
21. nictitating membrane
22. epiphora
23. Blepharospasm
24. vitreous humor or vitreous body
25. buphthalmos

Chapter 11 Answer Keys

SECTION 11.1. INTRODUCTION TO RELATED TERMS

1. (R) ot (S) ic
2. (R) ot (S) itis
3. (R) acoust (S) ic
4. (R) audi (CV) o (S) logy
5. (R) vestibul (S) ar
6. (P) semi (R) circul (S) ar
7. (R) cochle (S) ar
8. (R) tympan (S) ic
9. (R) aur (S) al
10. (R) ot (CV) o (S) scope
11. (R) ot (CV) o (R) tox (S) ic
12. (R) cerumin (S) al
13. (R) retr (CV) o (S) grade
14. (R) ot (CV) o (R) lith
15. (R) dynam (S) ic

SECTION 11.3. SELF-TEST

1. otic
2. acoustic meatus
3. Otitis interna
4. otoscope
5. cochlea
6. eustachian
7. aural
8. *Otodectes cynotis*
9. tympanic membrane
10. otoliths
11. malleus, incus, stapes
12. semicircular canals
13. retrograde
14. Audiology
15. round window

Chapter 12 Answer Keys

SECTION 12.1. INTRODUCTION TO RELATED TERMS

1. (R) gloss (S) al
2. (R) lingu (S) al
3. (R) bucc (S) al
4. (R) labi (S) al
5. (P) peri (CV) o (R) dont (S) al
6. (R) gingiv (S) al
7. (R) or (CV) o (R) pharynx
8. (P) hyper (R) sial (CV) o (S) sis
9. (R) esophag (CV) e (S) al
10. (R) gastr (S) ic
11. (R) pylor (S) ic
12. (R) enter (S) ic
13. (R) duoden (S) al
14. (R) jejun (S) al
15. (R) ile (CV) o (R) cec (S) al
16. (R) hepat (S) ic

17. (R) bili (S) ary
18. (R) icter (S) ic
19. (R) pancreat (S) ic
20. (R) gastr (CV) o (R) enter (S) itis
21. (R) col (S) itis
22. (R) peritone (S) al
23. (P) peri (R) stalsis
24. (R) haustra (S) tion
25. (P) anti (R) emet (S) ic
26. (P) anti (R) diarrhe (S) al
27. (R) degluti (S) tion
28. (R) defeca (S) tion
29. (P) post (R) prandi (S) al
30. (P) dys (R) phag (S) ia
31. (R) stomat (S) itis
32. (P) an (R) orex (S) ia
33. (R) or (CV) o (R) gastr (S) ic
34. (R) gastr (S) ectomy
35. (R) enter (CV) o (S) tomy
36. (R) enter (CV) o (S) stomy
37. (P) intus (R) suscep (S) tion
38. (R) necr (CV) o (S) tic

SECTION 12.3. SELF-TEST

1. postprandial
2. pancreas
3. Gastroenteritis
4. pyloric
5. deglutition
6. anorexia
7. orogastric
8. anastomosis
9. Periodontal
10. peristalsis
11. buccal
12. antiemetic
13. peritonitis
14. liver
15. jejunum
16. omentum
17. hypersialosis
18. hepatic
19. enterostomy
20. gastrectomy
21. Glossal, lingual
22. Gastric dilatation volvulus
23. oropharynx
24. Prehension
25. haustrations
26. intussusception
27. mesentery
28. ileocecal
29. pancreatitis
30. dentin

Chapter 13 Answer Keys

SECTION 13.1. INTRODUCTION TO RELATED TERMS

1. (R) ren (S) al
2. (P) pre (R) ren (S) al
3. (P) post (R) ren (S) al
4. (P) retr (CV) o (R) peritone (S) al
5. (R) nephr (S) itis
6. (R) pyel (CV) o (R) nephr (S) itis
7. (R) pyel (CV) o (S) gram
8. (R) cyst (CV) o (S) gram
9. (R) cyst (CV) o (R) centesis
10. (R) urethr (S) itis
11. (R) ur (CV) o (R) lith (CV) i (S) asis
12. (R) hemat (R) ur (S) ia
13. (R) cyst (CV) o (S) tomy
14. (P) poly (R) ur (S) ia
15. (P) olig (R) ur (S) ia
16. (R) pollak (CV) i (R) ur (S) ia
17. (P) dys (R) ur (S) ia
18. (P) an (R) ur (S) ia
19. (R) nephr (CV) o (R) tox (S) ic
20. (R) ur (R) em (S) ia
21. (R) azot (R) em (S) ia
22. (R) protein (R) ur (S) ia
23. (R) glycos (R) ur (S) ia
24. (R) ur (CV) o (R) poie (S) sis

25. (R) urethr (CV) o (S) stomy
26. (R) glomerul (S) ar
27. (P) peri (R) tubul (S) ar

SECTION 13.3. SELF-TEST

1. retroperitoneal
2. glomerulus
3. hematuria
4. azotemia
5. nephrotoxic
6. Urolithiasis
7. cystocentesis
8. glycosuria
9. pollakiuria
10. cystogram
11. Nephritis
12. Polyuria
13. dysuria
14. urethrostomy
15. pyelonephritis
16. cystotomy
17. ureter
18. Uropoiesis
19. convoluted tubule
20. oliguria

Chapter 14 Answer Keys

SECTION 14.1. INTRODUCTION TO RELATED TERMS

1. (R) crypt (R) orchid
2. (P) mon (R) orchid
3. (R) orchi (S) ectomy
4. (R) spermat (CV) o (R) gen (CV) e (S) sis
5. (R) ovari (CV) o (R) hyster (S) ectomy
6. (R) py (CV) o (R) metra
7. (R) mast (S) itis
8. (R) gesta (S) tion
9. (R) parturi (S) tion
10. (R) lacta (S) tion
11. (P) post (R) parturi (S) ent
12. (P) dys (R) toc (S) ia
13. (P) neo (R) nat (S) al
14. (R) muta (R) gen (S) ic
15. (R) terat (CV) o (R) gen (S) ic
16. (P) pro (R) estrus
17. (P) met (R) estrus
18. (P) an (R) estrus
19. (P) mon (R) estr (S) ous
20. (P) poly (R) estr (S) ous
21. (R) pseud (CV) o (R) cyesis
22. (R) metr (S) itis

SECTION 14.3. SELF-TEST

1. mastitis
2. neonate
3. Meiosis
4. mutagenic
5. Dystocia
6. cervix
7. polyestrous
8. prostate
9. ovariohysterectomy
10. spermatogenesis
11. cryptorchid
12. anestrus
13. pyometra
14. Pseudocyesis
15. orchiectomy, orchidectomy
16. teratogenic
17. estrus
18. postparturient
19. monorchid
20. monestrous

Chapter 15 Answer Keys

SECTION 15.1. INTRODUCTION TO RELATED TERMS

1. (P) ad (R) ren (S) al
2. (R) adren (R) erg (S) ic
3. (R) adren (CV) o (R) cortic (CV) o (R) trop (S) ic
4. (R) aden (CV) o (P) hyp (CV) o (S) physis
5. (R) neur (CV) o (P) hyp (CV) o (S) physis
6. (P) para (R) thyroid
7. (P) hyp (CV) o (R) thyroid (S) ism
8. (P) anti (R) diure (S) tic
9. (P) hyp (CV) o (R) glyc (R) em (S) ia
10. (P) hyper (R) glyc (R) em (S) ia
11. (R) gluc (CV) o (R) neo (R) gen (CV) e (S) sis

SECTION 15.3. SELF-TEST

1. parathyroid
2. Antidiuretic
3. adrenal
4. adenohypophysis
5. Hyperglycemia
6. thyroid
7. pituitary
8. Adrenocorticotropic
9. neurohypophysis
10. Hypothyroidism
11. pancreas
12. Thyroxine
13. Calcitonin
14. Glucagon
15. hypoglycemia

Chapter 16 Answer Keys

SECTION 16.1. INTRODUCTION TO RELATED TERMS

1. (R) dermat (S) itis
2. (P) epi (R) derm (S) al
3. (P) intra (R) derm (S) al
4. (P) sub (R) cutis
5. (R) erythemat (S) ous
6. (R) prurit (S) us
7. (R) melan (CV) o (S) cyte
8. (R) pil (CV) o (R) erection
9. (R) fibr (CV) o (R) plas (S) ia
10. (P) circum (R) or (S) al
11. (P) inter (R) digit (S) al
12. (P) peri (R) an (S) al
13. (R) aller (R) gen
14. (R) carcin (S) oma

SECTION 16.3. SELF-TEST

1. pruritus
2. Alopecia
3. epidermis
4. subcutaneous
5. melanocyte
6. fibroplasia
7. intradermal
8. Circumoral
9. histamine
10. carcinoma
11. dermatitis
12. erythema
13. allergen
14. urticaria
15. Piloerection

Chapter 17 Answer Keys

SECTION 17.1. INTRODUCTION TO RELATED TERMS

1. (R) pharmac (CV) o (S) logy
2. (R) iatr (CV) o (R) gen (S) ic
3. (P) par (R) enter (S) al
4. (P) kilo (R) gram
5. (P) hecto (R) gram
6. (P) deca (R) gram
7. (P) deci (R) liter
8. (P) centi (R) meter
9. (P) milli (R) liter
10. (P) micro (R) gram
11. (P) per (R) cent
12. (P) ant (R) helmin (S) tic
13. (P) anti (R) pyr (CV) e (S) tic
14. (P) anti (R) bio (S) tic
15. (P) contra (R) indica (S) tion
16. (P) a (R) sep (S) sis

SECTION 17.5. SELF-TEST

1. iatrogenic
2. antipyretic
3. anthelmintic
4. kilogram
5. milliliter
6. subcutaneous
7. right eye
8. milligram
9. antibiotic
10. at bedtime
11. intravenous
12. contraindication
13. apothecary
14. two times daily
15. 2 drops
16. intramuscular
17. percent
18. Asepsis
19. three times daily before meals
20. right patient, right drug, right dosage, right route, right time

Glossary of Word Parts

-ad	suffix meaning toward
-al	suffix meaning pertaining to
-ar	suffix meaning pertaining to
-ary	suffix meaning pertaining to
-ase	suffix denoting a relationship to an enzyme
-asis	suffix meaning process or condition
-cal	suffix meaning pertaining to
-centesis	suffix meaning puncture of
-ectasis	suffix meaning expansion
-ectomy	suffix meaning to cut out, to excise
-elle	suffix meaning a small
-esis	suffix meaning process or condition
-gram	suffix meaning a recording or denoting a relationship to the metric basis of weight
-ia	suffix meaning a state, process, or condition
-iasis	suffix meaning process or condition
-ic	suffix meaning pertaining to
-ical	suffix meaning pertaining to
-ism	suffix meaning a state, process, or condition
-ist	suffix meaning one who specializes in
-itis	suffix meaning inflammation
-ive	suffix meaning pertaining to
-logy	suffix meaning the study of
-megaly	suffix meaning enlargement
-oid	suffix meaning resembling
-ole	suffix meaning a small
-olus	suffix meaning a small
-oma	suffix meaning tumor or swelling
-ory	suffix meaning pertaining to
-osis	suffix meaning process or condition
-ous	suffix meaning pertaining to
-paresis	suffix meaning weakness

-penia	suffix meaning deficiency
-physis	root meaning growth, to grow
-plegia	suffix meaning paralysis
-pnea	suffix meaning breathing
-poiesis	word termination meaning producing, production
-rrhage	suffix meaning to flow, escape
-sis	suffix meaning process or condition
-stasis	suffix meaning to stand still, to stop
-stomy	suffix meaning creation of a mouth or an opening
-tic	suffix meaning pertaining to
-tion	suffix meaning act, state of
-tomy	suffix meaning to cut, to incise
-trophy	suffix meaning growth, development
-ule	suffix meaning a small
-um	suffix creating a noun (i.e., indicating "the presence of")
-us	suffix creating a noun (i.e., indicating "the presence of")
a-	prefix meaning without, absence of
ab-	prefix meaning away
abdomin(o)-	combining form meaning abdomen
acoust(o)-	combining form meaning sound
ad-	prefix meaning toward
aden(o)-	combining form meaning gland
af-	prefix meaning toward
alg(o)-	combining form meaning pain
alges(o)-	combining form meaning pain
aliment(o)-	combining form meaning food, nutrients
alveol(o)-	combining form meaning alveolus
amyl(o)-	combining form meaning starch
an-	prefix meaning without, against
ana-	prefix meaning backward
ang(o)-	combining form meaning vessel
angi(o)-	combining form meaning vessel
anis(o)-	combining form meaning unequal, uneven
ante-	prefix meaning before
anter(o)-	combining form meaning before or front
anti-	prefix meaning without, against
arter(o)-	combining form meaning artery
arthr(o)-	combining form meaning joint
astr(o)-	combining form meaning star
atel(o)-	combining form meaning imperfect, incomplete
atri(o)-	combining form meaning atrium
atto-	metric prefix meaning one-quintillionth
audi(o)-	combining form meaning hearing
aur(o)-	combining form meaning ear
auto-	prefix meaning self

axi(o)-	combining form meaning axis
azot(o)-	combining form meaning nitrogen
baso-	prefix meaning blue, basic
bi-	prefix meaning two
bili(o)-	combining form meaning bile
bio-	root meaning life
blephar(o)-	combining form meaning eyelid
brachi(o)-	combining form meaning brachium (i.e., arm)
brady-	prefix meaning slow
bronch(o)-	combining form meaning bronchus
bucc(o)-	combining form meaning cheek
capn(o)-	combining form meaning carbon dioxide
carcin(o)-	combining form meaning cancer
cardi(o)-	combining form meaning heart
carp(o)-	combining form meaning carpus
caud(o)-	combining form meaning tail
cellul(o)-	combining form meaning cell
centi-	metric prefix meaning one-hundredth
centr(o)-	combining form meaning center, central
cerebell(o)-	combining form meaning cerebellum
cerebr(o)-	combining form meaning cerebrum (i.e., brain)
cervic(o)-	combining form meaning neck
chondr(o)-	combining form meaning cartilage
chrom(o)-	combining form meaning color
chromat(o)-	combining form meaning color
chyl(o)-	combining form meaning chyle
circum-	prefix meaning around
co-	prefix meaning together, jointly
coccyge(o)-	combining form meaning coccyx, tail
cochle(o)-	combining form meaning cochlea
conjunctiv(o)-	combining form meaning conjunctiva
contra-	prefix meaning opposed
corne(o)-	combining form meaning cornea
cost(o)-	combining form meaning rib
cox(o)-	combining form meaning hip
crani(o)-	combining form meaning head
crin(o)-	combining form meaning secrete
crypt(o)-	combining form meaning hidden
cyan(o)-	combining form meaning blue
cyst(o)-	combining form meaning bladder
cyt(o)-	combining form meaning cell
deca-	metric prefix meaning ten
deci-	metric prefix meaning one-tenth
deka-	metric prefix meaning ten
derm(o)-	combining form meaning dermis or skin

dermat(o)-	combining form meaning dermis or skin
dia-	prefix meaning through, between
dont(o)-	combining form meaning teeth
dors(o)-	combining form meaning back (i.e., dorsum)
duoden(o)-	combining form meaning duodenum
dys-	prefix meaning difficult
ec-	prefix meaning out, outward
ef-	prefix meaning out, outward
electr(o)-	combining form meaning electricity
en-	prefix meaning in, inward
encephal(o)-	combining form meaning brain
endo-	prefix meaning inside, within
endotheli(o)-	combining form meaning endothelium
enter(o)-	combining form meaning intestine
eosin(o)-	combining form meaning red
epi-	prefix meaning upon
epitheli(o)-	combining form meaning epithelium
erg(o)-	combining form meaning work
erythemat(o)-	combining form meaning red
erythr(o)-	combining form meaning red
esophag(o)-	combining form meaning esophagus
esthes(o)-	combining form meaning sensation
ethm(o)-	combining form meaning seive
ex-	prefix meaning out
extra-	prefix meaning outside
femor(o)-	combining form meaning femur
femto-	metric prefix meaning one-quadrillionth
fibul(o)-	combining form meaning fibula
gastr(o)-	combining form meaning stomach
gen(o)-	combining form meaning produce, production
giga-	metric prefix meaning billion
gingiv(o)-	combining form meaning gingiva (i.e., gums)
gloss(o)-	combining form meaning tongue
gluc(o)-	combining form meaning glucose (sugar)
glyc(o)-	combining form meaning glucose (sugar)
hecto-	metric prefix meaning hundred
hem(o)-	combining form meaning blood
hemat(o)-	combining form meaning blood
hemi-	prefix meaning half
hepat(o)-	combining form meaning liver
home(o)-	combining form meaning same, unchanging
humer(o)-	combining form meaning humerus
humor(o)-	combining form meaning liquid
hydr(o)-	combining form meaning water
hyper-	prefix meaning excessive, above normal

hypo-	prefix meaning deficient, below normal
hyster(o)-	combining form meaning uterus (womb)
iatr(o)-	combining form meaning physician
ile(o)-	combining form meaning ileum
inter-	prefix meaning between
intra-	prefix meaning inside, within
irid(o)-	combining form meaning iris
jejun(o)-	combining form meaning jejunum
kerat(o)-	combining form meaning cornea
kilo-	metric prefix meaning thousand
labi(o)-	combining form meaning lip
lacrim(o)-	combining form meaning tears
laryng(o)-	combining form meaning larynx
later(o)-	combining form meaning side
leuk(o)-	combining form meaning white
lingu(o)-	combining form meaning tongue
lip(o)-	combining form meaning fat
lith(o)-	combining form meaning stone
lumb(o)-	combining form meaning lumbus or loins
lymph(o)-	combining form meaning lymph
lys(o)-	combining form meaning dissolving, destruction, or dissolution
macro-	prefix meaning large
mast(o)-	combining form meaning breast
medi(o)-	combining form meaning middle
mega-	prefix meaning large or metric prefix meaning million
melan(o)-	combining form meaning black
mening(o)-	combining form meaning meninx or meninges (i.e., membrane)
mes(o)-	combining form meaning middle
meta-	prefix meaning after or beyond
metr(o)-	combining form meaning uterus
micro-	prefix meaning small or metric prefix meaning one-millionth
milli-	metric prefix meaning one-thousandth
mono-	prefix meaning one
morph(o)-	combining form meaning form, shape
multi-	prefix meaning many
muscul(o)-	combining form meaning muscle
my(o)-	combining form meaning muscle
myel(o)-	combining form meaning spinal cord or marrow
nano-	metric prefix meaning one-billionth
nas(o)-	combining form meaning nose
necr(o)-	combining form meaning dead, death
neo-	prefix meaning new

nephr(o)-	combining form meaning kidney
neur(o)-	combining form meaning nerve
neutr(o)-	combining form meaning neutral
nucle(o)-	combining form meaning nucleus
ocul(o)-	combining form meaning eye
olfact(o)-	combining form meaning smell
olig(o)-	combining form meaning small
ophthalm(o)-	combining form meaning eye
opt(o)-	combining form meaning sight
or(o)-	combining form meaning mouth
orch(o)-	combining form meaning testicle
orchi(o)-	combining form meaning testicle
orex(o)-	combining form meaning appetite
orth(o)-	combining form meaning straight
oste(o)-	combining form meaning bone
ot(o)-	combining form meaning ear
ovari(o)-	combining form meaning ovary
palm(o)-	combining form meaning palm (i.e., sole of forefeet of domestic animals)
palmar(o)-	combining form meaning palm (cf. palm(o)-)
palpebr(o)-	combining form meaning palpebra (i.e., eyelid)
pan-	prefix meaning all
pancreat(o)-	combining form meaning pancreas
para-	prefix meaning near, beyond
path(o)-	combining form meaning disease
peri-	prefix meaning around
peritone(o)-	combining form meaning peritoneum
phag(o)-	combining form meaning eat, eating
phalang(o)-	combining form meaning phalanx
pharmac(o)-	combining form meaning medicine
pharmaceut(o)-	combining form meaning pharmacist or pharmacy
pharyng(o)-	combining form meaning pharynx, throat
phil(o)-	combining form meaning affinity for
phleb(o)-	combining form meaning vein
phob(o)-	combining form meaning fear, aversion to
phot(o)-	combining form meaning light
physi(o)-	combining form meaning nature
pico-	metric prefix meaning one-trillionth
pil(o)-	combining form meaning hair
pin(o)-	combining form meaning drink, drinking
plant(o)-	combining form meaning sole (i.e., sole of hindfeet of domestic animals)
plantar(o)-	combining form meaning sole (cf. plant(o)-)
pleur(o)-	combining form meaning pleura
pneum(o)-	combining form meaning air or lung

pneumon(o)-	combining form meaning lung
poikil(o)-	combining form meaning varied, irregular
pollak(o)-	combining form meaning frequent
poly-	prefix meaning many, much
post-	prefix meaning after
poster(o)-	combining form meaning after or behind
pre-	prefix meaning before
pro-	prefix meaning before
prote(o)-	combining form meaning protein
pseud(o)-	combining form meaning false
pulmon(o)-	combining form meaning lung
py(o)-	combining form meaning pus
pyel(o)-	combining form meaning pelvis
pyr(o)-	combining form meaning fire, heat, fever
quadri-	prefix meaning four
radi(o)-	combining form meaning radius or ray
ren(o)-	combining form meaning kidney
reticul(o)-	combining form meaning net
retin(o)-	combining form meaning retina
retr(o)-	combining form meaning backward, behind
rhin(o)-	combining form meaning nose
rostr(o)-	combining form meaning nose
sacr(o)-	combining form meaning sacrum
scapul(o)-	combining form meaning scapula
scler(o)-	combining form meaning hard, sclera
scop(o)-	combining form meaning to view
semi-	prefix meaning partial
sial(o)-	combining form meaning saliva
skelet(o)-	suffix meaning skeleton
som(o)-	combining form meaning body
spermat(o)-	combining form meaning sperm
spher(o)-	combining form meaning ball, sphere
sphygm(o)-	combining form meaning pulse
splen(o)-	combining form meaning spleen
sten(o)-	combining form meaning narrow
stern(o)-	combining form meaning sternum
stomat(o)-	combining form meaning mouth or opening
sub-	prefix meaning below, under
sym-	prefix meaning with, together
syn-	prefix meaning with, together
tachy-	prefix meaning fast, rapid
tars(o)-	combining form meaning tarsus
tax(o)-	combining form meaning order
telo-	prefix meaning end
tera-	metric prefix meaning trillion

terat(o)-	combining form meaning monster
tetra-	prefix meaning four
thorac(o)-	combining form meaning thorax
thromb(o)-	combining form meaning clot
tibi(o)-	combining form meaning tibia
tox(o)-	combining form meaning poison
trache(o)-	combining form meaning trachea
trop(o)-	combining form meaning turn, turning, changing
tympan(o)-	combining form meaning tympanum (i.e., drum)
uln(o)-	combining form meaning ulna
uni-	prefix meaning one
ur(o)-	combining form meaning urine
urethr(o)-	combining form meaning urethra
urin(o)-	combining form meaning urine
uve(o)-	combining form meaning uvea
vas(o)-	combining form meaning vessel
vascul(o)-	combining form meaning vessel
ven(o)-	combining form meaning vein
ventr(o)-	combining form meaning belly
ventricul(o)-	combining form meaning ventricle
vertebr(o)-	combining form meaning vertebra
vestibul(o)-	combining form meaning vestibule (i.e., chamber)
viscer(o)-	combining form meaning organ
volvul(o)-	combining form meaning twist, twisting

Index